MUSCULOSKELETAL FATIGUE and

STRESS

FRACTURES

CRC Series in Exercise Physiology

Series Editor
Ira Wolinsky

Published Titles

CONCEPTS in FITNESS PROGRAMMING
Robert G. McMurray

EXERCISE and DISEASE MANAGEMENT
Brian C. Leutholtz and Ignacio Ripoll

PHYSIQUE, FITNESS, and PERFORMANCE
Thomas Battinelli

Forthcoming Titles

EXERCISE THROUGHOUT the LIFE CYCLE:
A Comprehensive Handbook
Richard R. Suminski and Jie Kang

PHYSICAL ACTIVITY and CANCER
Laurie Hoffman-Goetz

GROWTH, PHYSICAL ACTIVITY, and MOTOR
DEVELOPMENT in PREPUBERTAL CHILDREN
Toivo Jurimae and Jaak Jurimae

ENDURANCE EXERCISE and ADIPOSE TISSUE
Barbara Nicklas

EXERCISE and STRESS RESPONSE:
The Role of Stress Proteins
Marius Locke and Earl Noble

Preface

The famous American humorist Josh Billings once said, "The trouble with most folks ain't so much their ignorance as knowing so many things that ain't so." We all fall prey to "conventional wisdom," which is always plausible and therefore may not seem worth the effort to test. There are few areas in which this is as true as the field of exercise-related overuse injuries, and especially views about the causes and prevention of stress fractures. This edited volume summarizes the factual information about stress fractures and illustrates what is known and what is yet to be learned about these debilitating and costly fractures.

Much has been written about stress fractures, but the majority of information is found in widely dispersed journal articles that cover the disparate fields of sports medicine, radiology, veterinary medicine, orthopedics, anatomy, and military medicine. This information is brought together in one location, providing a holistic and well-rounded view of all aspects of the pathophysiology, clinical diagnosis, and treatment of stress fractures for easy reference by the physician, physical therapist, athletic trainer, veterinarian, or basic scientist. We believe that this volume provides the most comprehensive treatment of stress fracture etiology, prevention, and treatment since the classic book by Devas was published more than a quarter of a century ago. In the intervening years, there has been significant new information brought forth about stress fractures, based on epidemiologic and experimental studies. The book provides a complete picture of stress fracture pathophysiology, including the role that other tissues such as muscle may play in the prevention or acceleration of fracture. The first glimpse of the histological presentation of a stress fracture is provided, as well as new data describing *in vivo* measurements of strain in regions where stress fractures are prone to occur. The intent of *Musculoskeletal Fatigue and Stress Fractures* is to provide a badly needed update that summarizes current thought and integrates the most recent basic and clinical research and epidemiologic findings, related to stress fractures.

Musculoskeletal Fatigue and Stress Fractures is intended to be used as a reference for a wide spectrum of readers, including health care practitioners, research scientists, and others who work with animal or human populations subject to stress fractures. The chapters are written by highly respected experts in the fields of skeletal physiology, sports medicine, and orthopedics, and describe the epidemiology and pathophysiology of stress fractures, animal models used to study the injury, as well as new directions for prevention, diagnosis, and treatment. Chapters on prevention and treatment of stress fractures will be of particular interest to athletic trainers, physical therapists, and sports physicians. Researchers may find this book helpful in summarizing the state of current experimental studies, and will readily notice that our understanding of stress fractures is hampered by the absence of a good animal model. For clinicians, this volume provides the best and most complete review of clinical diagnostic and treatment protocols that can be found. Athletic trainers will find information to help them improve performance and redesign training protocols for maximum efficiency.

The authors and editors hope that you will find this volume useful, and that it will challenge your own preconceived notions in ways that will stimulate further research and modification of treatment to ultimately benefit individuals at risk for these injuries.

David B. Burr
Chuck Milgrom

The Editors

David Burr is Professor and Chair of Anatomy and Cell Biology, and Professor of Orthopedic Surgery at the Indiana University School of Medicine. He earned his Ph.D. in anthropology from the University of Colorado in 1977, and joined Indiana University following appointments at the University of Kansas Medical Center (1977 to 1980) and West Virginia University Health Sciences Center (1980 to 1990). He serves on editorial boards for *Bone, The Journal of Biomechanics,* and *The Journal of Bone and Mineral Metabolism.* He is a member of the American Association of Anatomists, the International Bone and Mineral Society, the Orthopedic Research Society, the American Society for Biomechanics, and Sigma Xi. His research activities include the study of biological and mechanical aspects of age-related bone and cartilage changes, and bone remodeling physiology using both animal models and cell culture. He has spent more than 10 years studying the pathophysiology of stress fractures using animal and human models. He is the author of more than 130 research articles, and is co-author of two books on the structure, function, and mechanics of bone.

Chuck Milgrom is Professor of Orthopedic Surgery at the Hadassah University Hospital and Hebrew University Medical School in Jerusalem, Israel. He earned his M.D. from the State University of New York in 1975 and completed his orthopedic training at the Maimonides Medical Center in Brooklyn. He has worked closely with the medical branch of the Israeli Defense Forces, where he serves as a reserve officer, on a series of epidemiological and intervention stress fracture and overuse studies that began in 1982. He has studied human *in vivo* tibial and metatarsal strains that occur during physical activities, and ways to modify them using orthotics and shoe gear. These and associated epidemiological studies have been the basis for developing bone-strengthening exercises. He is the author of more than 80 research articles related to stress fracture, overuse injuries, and bone microdamage.

Contributors

Thomas Beck
Johns Hopkins Outpatient Center
Baltimore, MD

Kim Bennell
School of Physiotherapy
University of Melbourne
Victoria, Australia

David B. Burr
Department of Anatomy
Indiana University School of Medicine
Indianapolis, IN

Dennis Carter
Department of Mechanical Engineering
Stanford University
Stanford, CA

Roland Chisin
Department of Nuclear Medicine
Hadassah University Hospital
Jerusalem, Israel

Seth Donahue
Musculoskeletal Research Lab
Department of Orthopedics
The Pennsylvania State University
Hershey, PA

Kenneth Egol
Department of Orthopedic Surgery
NYU Hospital for Joint Diseases
New York, NY

Ingrid Ekenman
Department of Orthopedic Surgery
Huddinge University Hospital
Huddinge, Sweden

Aharon Finestone
Hadassah Medical Organization
Jerusalem, Israel

Victor Frankel
Hospital for Joint Diseases
Orthopaedic Institute
New York, NY

Eitan Friedman
The Susanne Levy-Gertner Oncogenics
 Unit
Sackler School of Medicine
Tel-Hashomer, Israel

Susan K. Grimston
Program in Occupational Therapy
Washington University School of
 Medicine
St. Louis, MO

Antero Hulkko
Keski-Pohjanmaa Central Hospital
Kikkola, Finland

Yoji Kawaguchi
Department of Orthopedic Surgery
Kagawa Medical School
Kagawa, Japan

Jiliang Li
Department of Orthopedic Surgery
Kagawa Medical School
Kagawa, Japan

R. Bruce Martin
Orthopedic Research Lab
Sacramento, CA

Charles Milgrom
Department of Orthopaedics
Hadassah University Hospital
Jerusalem

Satoshi Mori
Department of Orthopedic Surgery
Kagawa Medical School
Kagawa, Japan

David Nunamaker
School of Veterinary Medicine
University of Pennsylvania
Kennett Square, PA

Sakari Orava
Tohtoritalo 41400 Hospital
Turku, Finland

Mitchell Schaffler
Department of Orthopedics
Mount Sinai School of Medicine
New York, NY

Richard Shaffer
Naval Health Research Center
San Diego, CA

Jushua Shemer
Ministry of Health
Jerusalem, Israel

Iris Vered
The Susanne Levy-Gertner Oncogenics
  Unit
Sackler School of Medicine
Tel-Hashomer, Israel

Scott A. Yerby
St. Francis Medical Technologies
Concord, CA

Contents

Chapter 1
Incidence and Prevalence of Stress Fractures in Military and Athletic
Populations..1
Richard A. Shaffer

Chapter 2
Risk Factors for Developing Stress Fractures.......................................15
Kim Bennell and Susan Grimston

Chapter 3
Factors Associated with the Development of Stress Fractures in Women.............35
Kim Bennell and Susan Grimston

Chapter 4
The Role of Age in the Development of Stress and Fatigue Fractures 55
Antero Hulkko and Sakari Orava

Chapter 5
The Prediction of Stress Fractures 73
Thomas J. Beck

Chapter 6
Bone Fatigue and Stress Fractures..85
Scott A. Yerby and Dennis R. Carter

Chapter 7
The Genetic Basis for Stress Fractures...105
Eitan Friedman, Iris Vered, and Jushua Shemer

Chapter 8
The Role of Strain and Strain Rates in Stress Fractures.......................119
Charles Milgrom

Chapter 9
The Role of Muscular Force and Fatigue in Stress Fractures.............131
Seth W. Donahue

Chapter 10
The Histological Appearance of Stress Fractures................................151
Satoshi Mori, Jiliang Li, and Yoji Kawaguchi

Chapter 11
Bone Fatigue and Remodeling in the Development of Stress Fractures 161
Mitchell B. Schaffler

Chapter 12
The Role of Bone Remodeling in Preventing or Promoting Stress Fractures 183
R. Bruce Martin

Chapter 13
Bucked Shins in Horses 203
David Nunamaker

Chapter 14
Rabbits As an Animal Model for Stress Fractures 221
David B. Burr

Chapter 15
Prevention of Stress Fractures by Modifying Shoe Wear 233
Aharon S. Finestone

Chapter 16
Exercise Programs That Prevent or Delay the Onset of Stress Fracture 247
Charles Milgrom and Richard Shaffer

Chapter 17
Pharmaceutical Treatments That May Prevent or Delay the Onset of Stress
Fractures 259
David B. Burr

Chapter 18
Physical Diagnosis of Stress Fractures 271
Ingrid Ekenman

Chapter 19
The Role of Various Imaging Modalities in Diagnosing Stress Fractures 279
Roland Chisin

Chapter 20
Early Diagnosis and Clinical Treatment of Stress Fractures 295
Charles Milgrom and Eitan Friedman

Chapter 21
Problematic Stress Fractures 305
Kenneth A. Egol and Victor H. Frankel

Index 321

Incidence and Prevalence of Stress Fractures in Military and Athletic Populations

Richard A. Shaffer

CONTENTS

Introduction 2
Problems in Estimating Incidence and Prevalence 2
    Case Definition 3
    Estimating the Population Base 3
    Active Versus Passive Surveillance 4
    Duration of Injury 5
    Individual Risk Variation 5
    Study Design 5
Incidence 6
    Military Populations 6
        Military Recruits 6
        Military Training (Non-Recruit) 8
        Military Populations (Non-Training) 8
    Athletic Populations 9
        Runners 9
        Team Sports 10
Summary 10
References 11

0-8493-0317-6/01/$0.00+$.50
© 2001 by CRC Press LLC

INTRODUCTION

It has become customary to begin any discussion about stress fractures by crediting Breithaupt with the first description of "the syndrome of painful swollen feet associated with marching" among Prussian soldiers in 1855.[1] For 125 years following his description, stress fractures were almost exclusively described in military populations. However, in the last 20 to 25 years, the condition often labeled "stress fracture" has become increasingly seen in non-military populations. This is primarily due to dramatic increases in sports and exercise participation. As a larger segment of the population adopts a lifestyle that includes vigorous, weight bearing activities such as running, soccer, or gymnastics, stress fractures become a growing concern for clinicians and athletic trainers. The epidemiology of stress fractures should begin with a discussion of the incidence and prevalence of these injuries in athletic and military populations.

Most reports from U.S. military recruit populations find the incidence of lower extremity stress fractures is 0.2 to 4.0% in men,[2-9] and 1 to 7% in women.[9-11] Other countries have reported incidence among military recruits as high as 49%.[12] In non-recruit military populations, the few reports providing incidence find approximately 1 to 2% of personnel per year developing stress fractures.[13-15] In non-military athletic populations, the highest incidence is reported in members of track and field teams, with rates from 10 to 31%.[16,17] Other activities with high rates of stress fractures are lacrosse, figure skating, crew, gymnastics, ballet, basketball, soccer, and aerobic dance.[16] The incidence of stress fractures in competitive runners is 2 to 8% in men and 13 to 37% in women.[18-24] A short review of stress fracture incidence such as provided above is potentially misleading because of problems in estimating incidence and prevalence. These rates should be used with caution, especially when performing comparisons between sports or cohorts of individuals. The methodology of establishing rates of stress fracture will be discussed in this chapter, followed by details of the incidence and prevalence in military and athletic populations.

PROBLEMS IN ESTIMATING INCIDENCE AND PREVALENCE

It is hard to imagine a discussion of incidence (new cases in a time frame) and prevalence (existing cases at a point in time) using an outcome more difficult than stress fractures. Many fundamentals of the study of distribution and determinants of a disease/injury in populations (epidemiology) are not easily applied to stress fractures. The first problem in stress fracture incidence and prevalence is case definition. The label of stress fracture is not uniformly accepted by clinicians to apply to the broad range of osseous reactions resulting from excessive weight bearing activity. Stress fracture, stress reaction, fatigue fracture, pathologic fracture, and periostitis are terms that are often used interchangeably. The case definition for stress fracture varies among authors. The use of different denominators, such as population base or amount of exercise exposure, result in rates of stress fractures that are difficult to compare, and vary widely in the literature. Active versus passive surveillance can yield different rates of stress fractures in the same population. Highly competitive athletes, or military trainees intent on finishing a program, can be recalcitrant in reporting stress fractures for fear of the activity restriction required for treatment. The duration of injury has a broad range, depending on the criteria of recovery, which causes confusion between reported incidence and prevalence. Stress fractures can occur in multiple sites in the same individual. Recurrence of the injury in the same individual can happen in a short time frame. The risk, and therefore the incidence, varies within an individual over time, according to physical condition and changes in activity. Finally, the rates of stress fracture in the literature are derived from reports that use a wide variety of case series and study design methodologies in selected populations which have limited generalization outside their study cohort.

Case Definition

Historically, there has been lack of consensus about the diagnostic criteria for stress fractures. Many authors have concerns about using the term stress fracture when often no fracture line can be seen in the radiographs of affected bone. During the last ten years, however, considerable progress has been made on a case definition of stress fracture.[25] The most commonly used case definition in recent reports is a history of localized pain of insidious onset, which worsens with progressive activity and is relieved by rest.[6,25-30] In addition, a recent change in activity, exercise, or training is included in the history. Radiographs are often performed as a matter of clinical habit, usually to rule out frank fracture, but radionuclide studies are used to confirm the clinical diagnosis of stress fracture.[5,25,31-33] Progression to stress fracture occurs in stages, however, and as with any insidious disease process, the question is at what stage of the physiologic reaction to physical stress should a patient be counted as having a stress fracture. Consequently, case definitions for stress fracture reports have become more consistent, but there is still a need to consider the stage of the physiologic response to activity in bone when presenting incidence in various military and athletic populations.

Another issue is whether to count the number of individuals with at least one stress fracture or to count the number of pathologic sites. Stress fractures often occur at more than one anatomical site in the same individual at the same time. Reports indicate that 11 to 50% of military and athletic populations will have more than one stress fracture at a time.[3,12,17,34,35] A rate which uses the number of individuals with at least one stress fracture is the most intuitively understandable and appropriate when determining risk factors for stress fracture, or how stress fractures affect a training program. However, the use of the number of pathologic sites of stress fracture is appropriate when stress fractures occur with long temporal separation in the same individual, or when anatomic site-specific rates are indicated. The most pragmatic solution to this situation is to report the number of individuals with at least one stress fracture as well as the total number of clinically distinct stress fractures within each individual.

Estimating the Population Base

Although the diagnosis of stress fracture according to standard criteria and the definition of stress fracture are important to establish incidence, the appropriate determination of the population base is critical to comparison of rates among military and athletic groups. Many reports provide only case numbers with no reference to the population at risk. The size of the population base is generally reported in one of three categories: (1) the number of individuals making up the cohort from which the stress fracture cases were acquired; (2) a combination of the number of individuals coupled with the accumulated time at risk to form a person-time measure (density); and (3) a measure of accumulated exposure to physical activity or training in the population. Arguably the latter category provides the best comparison of incidence between populations, but reference to exposure is very seldom seen in the literature. For populations with similar frequency, intensity, and duration of exercise, a density measure of the population base enables appropriate comparison of stress fracture incidence. However, most reports of stress fracture incidence with reference to a population base simply provide the number of individuals assessed for stress fracture. Although it is often hard to compare these rates, using a cohort denominator provides a general idea of the percentage of a population who will be forced to modify their training or exercise programs and/or seek medical attention due to stress fractures.

Active Versus Passive Surveillance

Case ascertainment of stress fracture in most reports relies on the patient's seeking medical care (passive surveillance). While this method of determining incidence is common for most outpatient problems, stress fractures by nature occur most often in highly motivated military or athletic populations, which may lead to underreporting. Athletic populations are usually aware of the length of time for rehabilitation required after stress fracture diagnosis and don't want to reduce their training. Typically, dedicated athletes are motivated to "run through" a wide variety of aches and pains. Military populations may have the same concern, but in addition, individuals in military training programs know that they may be set back or separated from training for a stress fracture. Within both military and athletic populations, symptom reporting also differs by attributes such as gender and age. In one population of military trainees, men tended to underreport injuries by more than 25%, while women reported all of their injuries in the same training program.[36]

Stress fracture incidence is higher when military trainees are actively assessed for stress fracture, and subjects demonstrating symptomatology are then scanned using scintigraphy.[12,33,37] There is no dispute that cases diagnosed using this method meet the definition of stress fracture, or at least stress reaction. The concern, however, is that these stress fracture cases include a proportion of trainees who might not voluntarily have brought their symptoms to the attention of clinicians, or are stress reactions that are identified earlier in the process of the injury, prior to development of a fracture.

Both active and passive methods of case ascertainment have important purposes, but consistency is critical when comparing rates. The active method of finding cases is most important on the individual level. Individuals identified by this method have at least begun the bone injury process for which intervention may be indicated. In addition, when investigating risk factors for stress fracture, active case ascertainment will minimize the misclassification bias that is a result of labeling subjects as stress fracture free, when in reality they are progressing through the injury process but are not reporting or are not aware of their symptoms. Passive methods, which are usually the easiest means of finding cases, are appropriate when determining the impact of stress fracture on a population. If an individual is able to continue an exercise program or military training even while symptomatic, the stress fracture does not impact the population or the program. Intervening with true stress fractures, even in reluctant individuals, is important to prevent further damage to the bone, but often individuals can complete a training program or season by "sticking it out" and then heal during breaks from the rigorous activity.

Duration of Injury

The differentiation between incidence and prevalence can be confusing for stress fractures in populations. Prevalence of an injury is a function of the incidence and duration of the injury.[38] Stress fractures are injuries with insidious onset and a long rehabilitation. Depending on the criteria for diagnosis and full recovery, the duration of injury can vary widely. Because stress fractures are long duration injuries, a small incidence rate can result in a substantially larger prevalence rate in the same population.[25] Even more concerning is the possibility that the same stress fracture could be counted twice over a period of time. As with the two methods of case ascertainment, both incidence and prevalence are useful as measures of the impact of stress fractures on a population, however, when comparing rates it is important to be sure which type of rates are presented.

Individual Risk Variation

A fundamental property of incidence is that it determines the risk of a problem in a population.[38] Conversely, in the absence of bias, as risk varies, so does incidence. Assuming that an individual's risk for stress fracture changes over time,[2,25,39] the incidence of stress fracture in a population can vary simply due to individual attributes. Further, as individuals adapt to their physical stressors or exercise programs, their risk declines. The time when incidence is calculated can determine the magnitude of the measure in a population. Published reports from military recruit populations show that even observation periods as short as two months can have a wide variation in incidence rates.[7,36,40] If the incidence rates were determined in a three-week time period at the beginning of U.S. Marine Corps recruit training, the incidence of stress fracture can be over twice as high as the next three-week period. In athletic populations, highly trained runners can experience increased risk corresponding to change in mileage, running frequency, or equipment.[41,42] The ramification of these changes in risk is that incidence rates should be compared among populations with risk factors that are comparable.

Study Design

The final consideration for making inferences about stress fracture incidence is the method of data collection used by the investigators. Stress fracture rates in the literature are derived from a variety of study designs. Many reports are comprised of a series of stress fracture cases seen in a clinical setting. These case series reports seldom include a population base and therefore cannot represent stress fracture incidence. A popular method for the determination of stress fracture incidence is to survey a group of athletes or military personnel and simply ask them about their history of stress fractures in a specified time period. The rates from this method are better labeled as prevalence. This method allows the calculation of rates, but due to sampling methods, the population base can be of questionable value in generalizing to other populations. Case ascertainment can be improved by confirming self-report stress fracture history with medical record review.

A more rigorous methodology, often considered the gold standard for determining incidence, is to prospectively follow a cohort of stress fracture-free individuals for a specified time period and document new stress fractures.[38] Inferences from this prospective cohort design can be limited due to sampling of the cohort or the method of case ascertainment. However, this design provides the most useful incidence rates when the cohort has good external validity, and bias is minimized in the ascertainment of stress fractures.

One final method has recently become available with computerized medical records. Databases of outpatient records can be searched for stress fracture diagnosis and the number of these cases adjusted to the appropriate population base. This method of surveillance is prone to a variety of biases in development of the case database, as well as concerns about determination of the applicable population base. Nevertheless, this method can provide useful large sample incidence rates.

INCIDENCE

Clearly the most studied population in the stress fracture literature is military recruits.[25,38,43] In contrast to military recruit populations, reports of stress fracture incidence in military training programs other than recruit training (i.e., officer training, special warfare, advanced infantry training), are not so common. Further, the incidence of stress fractures in military operational populations (trained units) has only recently been addressed. Reports about stress fractures in non-military populations have become more frequent. The majority of the literature is from running populations who are recreational runners or are part of a track and field team.

Military Populations

Military Recruits

The incidence of stress fractures in recruit populations varies for a number of reasons. The attributes of the training program (length, physical rigor, and exercise schedule) have the most direct effect on the magnitude of the incidence rate.[2,7,11,25,43,44] Differences in case ascertainment policies also lead to a variation in stress fracture rates.[25] However, even with these expected variations, the stress fracture incidence in recruit populations is acceptably established. Each year the U.S. military trains approximately 200,000 recruits (89% male). The percentage of male U.S. recruits suffering at least one stress fracture ranges from 0.2 to 4.0%, with Navy and Air Force programs on the low end of that range, and Army and Marine Corps programs on the high end.[2,3,8-11,25,40,44,45] The rates for female recruits are higher than their male counterparts and also have a wider variation. Earlier reports were that 8 to 13% of women will develop at least one stress fracture during recruit training in the U.S military.[46,47] More recent reports, however, report a range of 1 to 7% among women.[10,11,25,44,48,49] As with the men, the Navy and Air Force are on the low end of that range, with the Army and Marine Corps on the high end.

Studies from Israeli recruit populations demonstrate markedly higher stress fracture rates than U.S. populations.[12,33,37,50,51] This contrast has been the source of considerable investigation and discussion. In several studies, about a third of Israeli recruits were diagnosed with at least one stress fracture during their 14 week program.[37,51] Other studies report a stress fracture rate as high as 50% in some Israeli recruit cohorts.[12] Much of the difference between these rates and the incidence in U.S. recruits is due to methods of case identification. Studies reporting the highest incidence from Israeli recruits have employed active case identification methods, whereas rates in U.S. populations have come from passive surveillance methods. Some authors have suggested that case definitions differ in the Israeli and U.S reports.[25] These methodological differences notwithstanding, the Israeli recruit training programs do tend to result in higher stress fracture incidence than U.S. recruit populations.

Recruit studies often use prospective cohort designs to determine stress fracture incidence rates. These studies start with injury-free populations who are monitored for stress fractures throughout training. When all recruits, or a statistically valid sample, are used, these rates are the best estimates of stress fracture incidence. These studies also allow the best comparison, since measures of person-time or exposure time can be used. For example, in one cohort, 4.0% of U.S. Marine Corps recruits had at least one stress fracture.[2] In another cohort, 3.0% of U.S. Army recruits had a least one stress fracture.[7] However, Marine Corps recruit training is 12 weeks, while Army recruit training is 8 weeks. Using person-time measures as denominators, the incidence density of stress fractures becomes 1.3 per 100 recruit-months for the Marine Corps and 1.4 per 100 recruit-months for the Army. With additional information from the training schedule of a program, it is possible to calculate rate per exposure, such as 33 stress fractures per 100 hours of vigorous (≥6 metabolic equivalents [METs]) activity in U.S. Marine Corps recruit training.

When passive surveillance methods are used for case identification in recruit populations, the tendency of individuals to report symptoms of stress fracture should be expected to vary. The most common reasons for variations in symptom reporting are stage in training and gender differences.[2,7,11,25,36] Recruits in the early stages of training tend to report their symptoms more readily than recruits near graduation. In 1996, the U.S. Marine Corps added an extremely rigorous three-day event at the end of training called The Crucible. Prior to The Crucible, very few stress fractures were reported during the last two weeks of training.[2,9] Once The Crucible was implemented, there was a significant increase in stress fracture symptom reporting during the last week of training.[45] These stress fractures were injuries which recruits likely would have hesitated to report, knowing that reporting the injuries could result in delay of graduation. However, the physical intensity of The Crucible was too much to endure with the pain of a stress fracture.

In addition to stage of training, gender has also been shown to affect symptom reporting.[36] In one study which passively monitored a group of male and female recruits during training and then examined them at the end of training, women reported symptoms significantly more often than men. When differences in symptom reporting were removed, men and women had similar injury rates.

Over the years, there has a been a change in the distribution of stress fractures by anatomical location. Historically, the foot was the most common site,[5,47] but more recently the tibia has become the most common, and accounts for 40 to 50% of all stress fractures in men[2,3,9,25] and 25 to 35% in women.[44,49] The most interesting gender difference is that men present with very few stress fractures (5 to 15%) above the knee,[9] whereas women may have as many as 50% in the femur and pelvis.[10]

Military Training (Non-Recruit)

Very few studies have focused on stress fractures in training populations other than recruits. These other training programs can vary from a few weeks to a year in duration. In the six month program which trains U.S. Navy SEALS, 9.0% of male trainees were diagnosed with at least one stress fracture.[52] In the 10 week U.S. Marine Corps officer candidate program, a stress fracture incidence of 7.0% was seen in men and 11% in women.[53] In a two month study of U.S Army officer cadets, 1.0% of men and 10.0% of women had at least one stress fracture.[54]

Military Populations (Non-Training)

Operational populations have a wide variety of physical activity requirements. For example, infantry units with high field training requirements can be expected to have a higher stress fracture incidence than personnel assigned to a large medical facility (which does not have day-to-day field training requirements). The data that exists from studies of operational populations indicates that 1.0 to 2.0% of these populations will suffer a stress fracture in a 12 month period.[13-15] Another study surveyed 2,312 active duty U.S. Army women and found that 16.1% reported ever having a stress fracture diagnosis.[55]

Another indication of stress fracture incidence in "trained" populations comes from the recent establishment of a database of outpatient encounters in the U.S. military. The rates of pathologic fracture among men and women in the four military services are presented in Table 1.[56] The inferences from these rates must be limited. The number of cases is defined as all outpatient encounters captured by the surveillance system with an assigned ICD-9 code of pathologic fracture. Exercise-induced stress fracture does not have a specific code in the ICD-9 system. Pathologic fractures other than stress fractures are included in these rates, however, this young military population is not prone to bone diseases of older populations. The population base

Table 1   Outpatient Rate of Pathologic Fractures (ICD-9 #73310) Among the U.S. Military in 1998

Service	Men		Women		Total	
	Rate*	Person Years	Rate*	Person Years	Rate*	Person Years
Army	1.83	407,903	8.73	70,762	2.85	478,665
Navy	0.71	359,484	6.78	51,903	1.48	411,387
Air Force	0.07	299,684	0.12	65,266	0.08	364,950
Marine Corps	2.82	162,146	4.45	9,567	2.91	171,713
Total	1.21	1,229,217	5.17	197,498	1.75	1,426,715

* Rate per 100 person years
Source: DMSS, 1999

for these rates is all personnel on active duty for the specified time period, stratified by gender.

Athletic Populations

Runners

In 1998, there were 10.7 million runners in the U.S. according to the American Sports Data survey. The definition of a runner for this survey was a person who runs at least 100 times a year. In addition, the Road Runners Club of America reported that 1.18 million runners completed the 100 largest races in 1998. While a reasonable amount of running clearly has physical and mental health benefits, one of the risks of running is injury.[57] Surveys of road race participants have shown that approximately 50% of runners have had injuries in the past 12 months.[23,41,58] Prospective studies of runners have shown that 35 to 50% of runners are injured within a 12 month period.[57] Reports from clinical case series of running injuries have shown that lower extremity stress fractures account for 6 to 15% of these injuries.[59,60] Approximately 462,000 stress fractures can be expected in a 12 month time period from running, assuming injuries to 42% of runners, of which 11% are stress fractures. This extrapolated 12 month incidence rate of 4.6% is consistent with the rates reported from studies of stress fractures in runners.[61,62]

In one survey of recreational runners, 8.3% of men and 13.2% of women self-report a stress fracture during their running careers.[62] The history of stress fractures in a survey of collegiate female distance runners is much higher (37%).[18] The most common site of stress fractures in male and female recreational runners was the tibia and fibula (males 45%, females 42%), followed by the forefoot (males 35%, females 34%).[62] The remaining sites in men were heel (9.6%), pelvis (7.4%), and femur (3.2%). The remaining sites in women were the pelvis (12.0%), heel (6.0%), and femur (6.0%). In one of the larger case series of runner's stress fractures, the most common site was the tibia (34%), followed by the fibula (24%), metatarsals (20%), femur (14%), and pelvis (6%).[63]

Team Sports

Stress fracture incidence and prevalence in team sports is difficult to determine for two reasons: (1) the heterogeneous types of activity, seasons, and teams; and (2) lack of population-based rates reported in the literature. The literature on stress fractures does support that clinicians dealing with exercise-induced pain in athletes should always consider stress fracture when making the diagnosis. Further, the suspicion of stress fracture should increase when the sport includes running as part of the training regimen and there has been a recent change in the training schedule.

Stress fractures are a common injury in sports where running is part of the training program. In two prospective studies of track and field athletes, 10% and 20% of men, as well as 31 and 22% of women developed a stress fracture in a 12 month period.[16,17,64] The event with the most stress fractures was distance running. Stress fractures were a higher percentage than expected (20%) of all injuries in these athletes.[17] Other sports with reported incidence of stress fractures in collegiate athletes during the 12 month period were lacrosse, crew, basketball, football, and soccer. The most common site of stress fracture was the tibia. A noteworthy finding in one study was that 20.6% of stress fractures were in the shaft of the femur.[16]

Three other sports have reported rates of stress fractures. These reports do have a population base, but identify stress fractures from the past. Ballet dancers have a high prevalence of stress fractures, with 22.2 and 31.5% of dancers reporting at least one stress fracture.[65,66] The most common site of fracture in these dancers was the metatarsals (63%). Ballet dancers also have a high rate of multiple fractures, with 27 fractures in 17 individuals. Another group of athletes with a high reported rate of stress fractures is figure skaters. In a group of 42 world class skaters, 21.5% reported ever having a stress fracture during their careers.[67] In male and female skaters, the lumbosacral spine accounted for the majority of stress fractures (males 33%, females 45%). Finally, the stress fracture history of 42 male and 74 female elite gymnasts was assessed by medical record review.[68] During the typical observation period of three years for men and two years for women, 16% of men and 24% of women were diagnosed with stress fractures.

In reports of case series of stress fractures, running is by far the most common sport engaged in at the time of the injury (61 to 72% of stress fractures).[35,69,70] The second most frequent sport that stress fracture patients participate in is ball sports (8 to 16%), followed by racket sports, figure skating, ballet, and gymnastics.

SUMMARY

Stress fractures are common in military training populations and athletes, and make up a large component of injuries seen in sports medicine clinics. When assessing the incidence of stress fractures in a specified population, it is important to consider the methods used to establish the rates. Military recruit populations have well established rates of stress fractures. In athletic populations, stress fracture rates are highest in those sports which include running as part of the training regimen.

REFERENCES

1. Breithaupt, J., Zur pathologic des menschlichen fusses, *Med. Ztg.,* Berlin, 36, 169, 1855.
2. Almeida, S.A., Williams, K.M., Shaffer, R.A., and Brodine, S.K., Epidemiological patterns of musculoskeletal injuries and physical training, *Med. Sci. Sports Exerc.,* 31,1176, 1999.
3. Beck, T.J., Ruff, C.B., Mourtada, F.A., Shaffer, R.A., Williams, K.M., Kao, G.L., Sartoris, D.J., and Brodine, S.K., Dual-energy X-ray absorptiometry derived structural geometry for stress fracture prediction in male U.S. Marine Corps recruits, *J. Bone Miner. Res.,* 11, 645, 1996.
4. Garcia, J.E., Grabhorn, L.L., and Franklin, K.J., Factors associated with stress fractures in military recruits, *Mil. Med.,* 152, 45, 1987.
5. Gilbert, R.S. and Johnson, H.A., Stress fractures in military recruits – a review of twelve years' experience, *Mil. Med.,* 131, 716, 1966.
6. Greaney, R.B., Gerber, F.H., Laughlin, R.L., Kmet, J.P., Metz, C.D., Kilcheski, T.S., Rao, B.R., and Silverman, E.D., Distribution and natural history of stress fractures in U.S. Marine recruits, *Radiology,* 146, 339,1983.
7. Jones, B.H., Cowan, D.N., Tomlinson, J.P., Robinson, J.R., Polly, D.W., and Frykman, P.N., Epidemiology of injuries associated with physical training among young men in the army, *Med. Sci. Sports Exerc.,* 25, 197, 1993.
8. Scully, T.J. and Besterman, G., Stress fracture — a preventable training injury, *Mil. Med.,* 147, 285, 1982.
9. Shaffer, R.A., Brodine, S.K., Almeida, S.A., Williams, K.M., and Ronaghy, S., Use of simple measures of physical activity to predict stress fractures in young men undergoing a rigorous physical training program, *Am. J. Epidemiol.,* 149, 236, 1999.
10. Kelly, E.W., Jonson, S.R., Cohen, M.E., and Shaffer, R.A., Stress fractures of the pelvis in female navy recruits: an analysis of possible mechanisms of injury, *Mil. Med.,* 165, 142, 2000.
11. Knapik, J., Cuthie, J., Canham, M., Hewitson, W., Laurin, M., Nee, M., Hoedebecke, E., Hauret, K., Carroll, D., and Jones, B., Epidemiology Consultation No. 29-HE-7513-98, Injury Incidence, Injury Risk Factors, and Physical Fitness of U.S. Army Basic Trainees at Ft Jackson, South Carolina, U.S. Army Center for Health Promotion and Preventive Medicine, Aberdeen, MD, 1997.
12. Giladi, M., Milgrom, C., Simkin, A., and Danon, Y., Stress fractures. Identifiable risk factors, *Am. J. Sports Med.,* 19, 647, 1991.
13. Fleming, J.L., One-year prevalence of lower extremity injuries among active duty military soldiers, *Mil. Med.,* 153, 476, 1988.
14. Milgrom, C., Giladi, M., Chisin, R., and Dizian, R., The long-term followup of soldiers with stress fractures, *Am. J. Sports Med.,* 13, 398, 1985.
15. Shaffer, R., Final Report: Musculoskeletal injury among select operational U.S. Navy and Marine Corps populations, Naval Health Research Center, San Diego, CA, 1999.
16. Johnson, A.W., Weiss, C.B., Jr., and Wheeler, D.L., Stress fractures of the femoral shaft in athletes — more common than expected. A new clinical test, *Am. J. Sports Med.,* 22, 248, 1994.
17. Bennell, K.L., Malcolm, S.A., Thomas, S.A., Wark, J.D., and Brukner, P.D., The incidence and distribution of stress fractures in competitive track and field athletes. A twelve-month prospective study, *Am. J. Sports Med.,* 24, 21, 1996.
18. Barrow, G.W. and Saha, S., Menstrual irregularity and stress fractures in collegiate female distance runners, *Am. J. Sports Med.,* 16, 209, 1988.

19. Belkin, S.C., Stress fractures in athletes, *Orthop. Clin. N. Am.,* 11, 735, 1980.
20. Blair, S.N., Kohl, H.W., and Goodyear, N.N., Rates and risks for running and exercise injuries: studies in three populations, *Res. Q. Exerc. Sport.,* 58, 221, 1987.
21. Brill, P.A. and Macera, C.A., The influence of running patterns on running injuries, *Sports Med.,* 20, 365, 1995.
22. Clement, D.B., Taunton, J.E., Smart, G.W., and McNicol, K.L., A survey of overuse running injuries, *Physician Sportsmed.,* 9, 47, 1981.
23. Jacobs, S.J. and Berson, B.L., Injuries to runners: a study of entrants to a 10,000 meter race, *Am. J. Sports Med.,* 14, 151, 1986.
24. Powell, K.E., Kohl, H.W., Caspersen, C.J., and Blair, S.N., An epidemiological perspective on the causes of running injuries, *Physician Sportsmed.,* 14, 100, 1986.
25. Jones, B.H., Harris, J.M., Vinh, T.N., and Rubin, C., Exercise-induced stress fractures and stress reactions of bone: epidemiology, etiology, and classification, *Exerc. Sport Sci. Rev.,* 17, 379, 1989.
26. Worthen, B.M. and Yanklowitz, B.A., The pathophysiology and treatment of stress fractures in military personnel, *J. Am. Podiatry Assoc.,* 68, 317, 1978.
27. Hershman, E.B. and Mailly, T., Stress fractures, *Clin. Sports Med.,* 9, 183, 1990.
28. Jackson, D.W. and Strizak, A.M., Stress fractures in runners, excluding the foot, in *Symposium on the Foot and Leg in Running Sports, Coronado, California, September 1980,* Mack, R.P., Ed., C. V. Mosby, St. Louis, 1982, 109.
29. Knapp, T.P. and Garrett, W.E., Jr. Stress fractures: general concepts, *Clin. Sports Med.,* 16, 339, 1997.
30. Markey, K.L., Stress fractures, *Clin. Sports Med.,* 6, 405, 1987.
31. Arendt, E.A. and Griffiths, H.J., The use of MR imaging in the assessment and clinical management of stress reactions of bone in high-performance athletes, *Clin. Sports Med.,* 16, 291, 1997.
32. Deutsch, A.L., Coel, M.N., and Mink, J.H., Imaging of stress injuries to bone. Radiography, scintigraphy, and MR imaging, *Clin. Sports Med.,* 16, 275, 1997.
33. Giladi, M., Nili, E., Ziv, Y., Danon, Y.L., and Aharonson, Z., Comparison between radiography, bone scan, and ultrasound in the diagnosis of stress fractures, *Mil. Med.,* 149, 459, 1984.
34. Bennell, K.L., Malcolm, S.A., Thomas, S.A., Ebeling, P.R., McCrory, P.R., Wark, J.D., and Brukner, P.D., Risk factors for stress fractures in female track-and-field athletes: a retrospective analysis, *Clin. J. Sport Med.,* 5, 229, 1995.
35. Matheson, G.O., Clement, D.B., McKenzie, D.C., Taunton, J.E., Lloyd-Smith, D.R., and MacIntyre, J.G., Stress fractures in athletes. A study of 320 cases, *Am. J. Sports Med.,* 15, 46 1987.
36. Almeida, S.A., Trone, D.W., Leone, D.M., Shaffer, R.A., Patheal, S.L., and Long, K., Gender differences in musculoskeletal injury rates: a function of symptom reporting? *Med. Sci. Sports Exerc.,* 31, 1807, 1999.
37. Milgrom, C., Giladi, M., Stein, M., Kashtan, H., Margulies, J.K., Chisin, R., Steinberg, R., and Aharonson, Z., Stress fractures in military recruits. A prospective study showing an unusually high incidence, *J. Bone Jt. Surg.,* 67, 732, 1985.
38. Gordis, L., *Epidemiology,* W.B. Saunders, Philadelphia, 1996.
39. Bennell, K., Matheson, G., Meeuwisse, W., and Brukner, P., Risk factors for stress fractures, *Sports Med.,* 28, 91, 1999.
40. Jones, B.H. and Knapik, J.J., Physical training and exercise-related injuries. Surveillance, research and injury prevention in military populations, *Sports Med.,* 27, 111, 1999.

41. Macera, C.A., Pate, R.R., Powell, K.E., Jackson, K.L., Kendrick, J.S., and Craven, T.E., Predicting lower-extremity injuries among habitual runners, *Arch. Int. Med.,* 149, 2565, 1989.
42. Macera, C.A., Lower extremity injuries in runners. Advances in prediction, *Sports Med.,* 13, 50, 1992.
43. Bennell, K.L. and Brukner, P.D., Epidemiology and site specificity of stress fractures, *Clin. Sports Med.,* 16, 179, 1997.
44. Jones, B.H., Amoroso, P.J., and Canham, M.L., Atlas of injuries in the U.S. Armed Forces, *Mil. Med.,* S, 164, 1999.
45. Shaffer, RA., Unpublished data, 2000.
46. Reinker, K.A. and Ozburne, S., A comparison of male and female orthopaedic pathology in basic training, *Mil. Med.,* 144, 532, 1979.
47. Brudvig, T.J., Gudger, T.D., and Obermeyer, L., Stress fractures in 295 trainees: a one-year study of incidence as related to age, sex, and race, *Mil. Med.,* 148, 666, 1983.
48. Shaffer, R.A., Brodine, S.K., Ito, S.I., and Le, A.H., Epidemiology of illness and injury among U.S. Navy and Marine Corps female training populations, *Mil. Med.,* 164, 17, 1999.
49. Institute of Medicine, Reducing stress fracture in physically active military women, in *Committee on Military Nutrition Research,* Food and Nutrition Board, Ed., National Academy Press, Washington, D.C., 1998, 117.
50. Volpin, G., Petronius, G., Hoerer, D., and Stein, H., Lower limb pain and disability following strenuous activity, *Mil. Med.,* 154, 294, 1989.
51. Milgrom, C., Finestone, A., Shlamkovitch, N., Rand, N., Lev, B., Simkin, A., and Wiener, M., Youth is a risk for stress fracture: a study of 783 infantry recruits, *J. Bone Jt. Surg.,* 76(B), 20, 1994.
52. Kaufman, K.R., Brodine, S.K., Shaffer, R.A., Johnson, C.W., and Cullison, T.R., The effect of foot structure and range of motion on musculoskeletal overuse injuries, *Am. J. Sports Med.,* 27, 585, 1999.
53. Winfield, A.C., Moore, J., Bracker, M., and Johnson, C.W., Risk factors associated with stress reactions in female Marines, *Mil. Med.,* 162, 698, 1997.
54. Protzman, R.R., Physiologic performance of women compared to men. Observations of cadets at the United States Military Academy, *Am. J. Sports Med.,* 7, 191, 1979.
55. Friedl, K.E., Nuovo, J.A., Patience, T.H., and Dettori, J.R., Factors associated with stress fracture in young army women: indications for further research, *Mil. Med.,* 157, 334, 1992.
56. DMSS, Defense Medical Surveillance System, Aberdeen, MD, 1999.
57. Koplan, J.P., Powell, K.E., Sikes, R.K., Shirley, R.W., and Campbell, C.C., An epidemiologic study of the benefits and risks of running, *JAMA,* 248, 3118, 1982.
58. Marti, B., Vader, J.P., Minder, C.E., and Abelin, T., On the epidemiology of running injuries. The 1984 Bern Grand-Prix study, *Am. J. Sports Med.,* 16, 285,1988.
59. James, S.L., Bates, B.T., and Osternig, L.R., Injuries to runners, *Am. J. Sports Med.,* 6, 40, 1978.
60. Brubaker, C.E. and James, S.L., Inuries to runners, *J. Sports Med.,* 2, 189, 1974.
61. Bovens, A.M., Janssen, G.M., Vermeer, H.G., Hoeberigs, J.H., Janssen, M.P., and Verstappen, F.T., Occurrence of running injuries in adults following a supervised training program, *Int. J. Sports Med.,* 10(S), 186, 1989.
62. Brunet, M.E., Cook, S.D., Brinker, M.R., and Dickinson, J.A., A survey of running injuries in 1505 competitive and recreational runners, *J. Sports Med. Phys. Fitness,* 30, 307, 1990.

63. McBryde, A.M., Jr., Stress fractures in runners, *Clin. Sports Med.,* 4, 737, 1985.
64. Bennell, K.L., Malcolm, S.A., Thomas, S.A., Ebeling, P.R., McCrory, P.R., Wark, J.D., and Brukner, P.D., Risk factors for stress fractures in track and field athletes. A twelve-month prospective study, *Am. J. Sports Med.,* 24, 810, 1996.
65. Frusztajer, N.T., Dhuper, S., Warren, M.P., Brooks-Gunn, J., and Fox, R.P., Nutrition and the incidence of stress fractures in ballet dancers, *Am. J. Clin. Nutr.,* 51, 779, 1990.
66. Kadel, N.J., Teitz, C.C., and Kronmal, R.A., Stress fractures in ballet dancers, *Am. J. Sports Med.,* 20, 445, 1992.
67. Peacina, M., Bojaniac, I., and Dubravaciac, S., Stress fractures in figure skaters, *Am. J. Sports Med.,* 18, 277, 1990.
68. Dixon, M. and Fricker, P., Injuries to elite gymnasts over 10 yr, *Med. Sci. Sports Exerc.,* 25, 1322, 1993.
69. Hulkko, A. and Orava, S., Stress fractures in athletes, *Int. J. Sports Med.,* 8, 221, 1987.
70. Rupani, H.D., Holder, L.E., Espinola, D.A., and Engin, S.I., Three-phase radionuclide bone imaging in sports medicine, *Radiology,* 156, 187, 1985.

CHAPTER 2

Risk Factors for Developing Stress Fractures

Kim Bennell and Susan Grimston

CONTENTS

Introduction 16
Level 2 — Measureable Bone Components 17
    Bone Density 17
    Bone Geometry 17
Level 3 — Controller 19
Level 4 — Functional Stimuli 20
    Mechanical 20
    Training — Mechanical Loading 20
        Physical Fitness — Loading History 21
        Training Regimen — Mechanical Loading Regimen 22
    Gait Mechanics 22
        Lower Extremity Alignment and Foot Type 22
        Muscle Flexibility and Joint Range of Motion 25
    Impact Attenuation 26
        Training Surface 26
        Muscular Strength and Fatigue 26
        Body Size and Composition 26
    Physiological 27
Level 5 — Constraints 27
    Nutrition 28
    Psychological Traits 28
Summary 29
References 29

INTRODUCTION

Prevention of stress fractures is a major goal of sports medicine practitioners. To prevent injury there must be a clear understanding of the causative factors and the mechanisms by which they interact. With this knowledge, preventive measures can be evaluated. This chapter reviews the role of risk factors in the pathogenesis of stress fractures. Risk factors specifically related to women are discussed in further detail in Chapter 3.

Because stress fractures represent failure of bone to adapt to mechanical load, it is useful to consider risk factors in the context of how they influence the adaptation process. This will be conceptualized using a five-level research model (Figure 1) described by Grimston, and based on the mechanostat theory proposed by Frost.[2] In this model, development of a stress fracture indicates that loading has exceeded the mechanical competence of the skeleton (Level 1). Mechanical competence depends on several properties of bone tissue (Level 2) including bone density, geometry, and microarchitecture. All bone properties are governed by bone cellular dynamics. These cellular activities are controlled by the mechanostat (Level 3), which is the mechanosensory system of bone responsible for sensing strain, comparing it with threshold or 'set point' strain and then activating an appropriate adaptive biological response. Functional stimuli (Level 4) fall into three broad categories of mechanical, physiological, and pharmacological, and are factors that affect bone and stimulate a response by the mechanostat. Finally, there are overriding constraints on bone health (Level 5); those that are predetermined, and those that are a function of environmental influences.

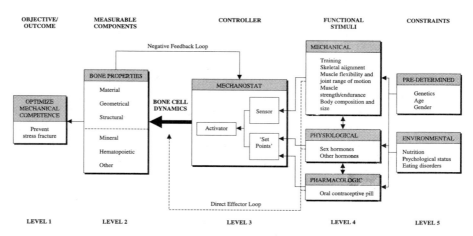

Figure 1   Research model based on mechanostat theory, showing the five distinct levels influencing bone adaptation to mechanical load. Relevant risk factors for stress fractures are highlighted in the model. Adapted from Grimston, S.K., *Med. Sci. Sports Exerc.*, 25, 1993. With permission.

LEVEL 2 — MEASURABLE BONE COMPONENTS

Bone mineral density and bone geometry are factors influencing bone's mechanical competence that have been measured in relation to stress fractures in athletes and military personnel.

Bone Density

The association between fragility fractures and low bone density has been well established in persons with osteoporosis. Clinically, bone density measurements are used to predict the likelihood of fracture.[3-4] However, unlike the elderly population, most active young people have bone density within the normal range, and in many cases it is well above that of their age-matched, less active counterparts.[5,6] Nevertheless, it is feasible that the level of bone density required by physically active individuals to resist repetitive strains without developing fatigue fractures may be greater than that of the less active population who subject their bones to much lower forces. It is usually only during special circumstances, such as endocrine disorders in the female athlete, that bone density is clinically decreased and bone strength lowered (see Chapter 3).

Results of studies investigating the relationship between bone density and stress fracture in male athletes and military recruits are shown in Table 1,[7-11] while those for females are discussed in Chapter 3. All studies included measures of bone density at lower limb sites, where the stress fractures generally occurred.

Very little prospective evidence exists to support a clear causal relationship between bone density and risk of stress fractures in men. Giladi et al.[7] found no significant difference in tibial bone density in 91 recruits who developed stress fractures compared with 198 controls. Similar findings were reported in a prospective cohort study of track and field athletes[9] and in a cross-sectional study of runners with and without history of tibial stress fracture.[11] Although Beck et al.[8] found significantly lower tibial and femoral bone density in 23 male recruits who developed stress fractures compared with 587 controls, this result may be explained by differences in body weight, as the stress fracture recruits were 11% lighter. An older cross-sectional study using dual photon absorptiometry to measure bone density at proximal hip sites in military recruits also reported lower bone density in those with a history of stress fracture.[10] It is important to ensure that groups are matched in body weight, a major predictor of bone density. Alternatively, body weight should be controlled statistically in order to determine the independent relationship between bone density and stress fractures.

Conflicting results could indicate that populations of active individuals with stress fractures are heterogenous in terms of bone density. In addition, it is likely that other independent factors contribute to the risk of fracture in physically active males.

Bone Geometry

Bone strength is also related to bone geometry. The structural properties of long bones vary with age and gender and are largely dependent on body size,[12] although

Table 1   Summary of studies investigating the relationship between bone density and stress fractures in men. Studies are ordered according to the strength of their study design and then chronologically.

Reference	Study Design	Subjects	Sample Size	Tech[n]	Sites	Results % Diff †
Giladi et al. 1991[7]	PC	Military	91 — SF 198 — NSF	SPA	Tibial shaft	−6.0%
Beck et al. 1996[8]	PC	Military	23 — SF 587 — NSF	DXA	Femur Tibia Fibula	−3.9%* −5.6%* −5.2%
Bennell et al. 1996[9]	PC	Track & field aths	10 — SF 39 — NSF	DXA	Upper limb Thoracic spine Lumbar spine Femur Tibia/fibula Foot	−4.9% −4.1% −0.8% −2.9% −4.0% −0.3%
Pouilles et al. 1989[10]	XS	Military	41 — SF 48 — NSF	DPA	Femoral neck Wards triangle Trochanter	−5.7%* −7.1%* −7.4%*
Crossley et al. 1999[11]	XS	Athletes	23 — SF 23 — NSF	DXA	Tibial shaft	8.1%

PC = observational analytic prospective cohort; XS = observational descriptive cross-sectional; DPA = dual photon absorptiometry; DXA = dual energy x-ray absorptiometry; SPA = single photon absorptiometry; Tech[n] = technique.
* $p < 0.05$
† Results are given as the % difference comparing stress fracture subjects (SF) with non-stress fracture subjects (NSF).
Adapted from Brukner, P.D. and Bennell, K.L., *Crit. Rev. Phys. Rehab. Med.*, 9, 163, 1997.

even among individuals of similar age and build there is great variation in bone geometry. In addition, within any long bone, the geometry is complex and changes continuously along its length. There is much greater variation in structural geometry than in bone material properties, including bone mineral density.[13] Thus, differences in bone geometry might partly explain differences in stress fracture predisposition.

A prospective observational cohort study of 295 male Israeli military recruits showed that those who developed stress fractures had narrower tibias in the mediolateral plane (measured radiographically) than those without stress fractures.[14] The cross-sectional moment of inertia about the anteroposterior axis ($CSMI_{AP}$), an estimate of the ability of bone to resist mediolateral bending, was shown to be an even better indicator of stress fracture risk than tibial width.[15,16] Calculations of $CSMI_{AP}$ were made based on the assumption that the tibia is an elliptical ring with an eccentric hole, which does not truly describe the cross-sectional shape of the tibia.

The above results were supported by a prospective study of more than 600 military recruits undergoing basic training. Bone mineral data acquired from a dual energy x-ray absorptiometer (DXA) were used to derive cross-sectional geometric properties of the tibia, fibula, and femur.[8] This method is likely to be more accurate than radiographs, as it does not entail assumptions of cross-sectional shape or manual measurements of cortical thickness. The results showed that even after adjusting for differences in body weight, the stress fracture recruits had smaller tibial width, cross-sectional area, moment of inertia, and modulus than the non-stress fracture group. The average difference in tibial bone size of the stress fracture group compared to those who did not fracture was 10.6%, which is greater than the 4.4% found by Milgrom et al.[15]

There is also evidence to suggest that smaller bones are risk factors for stress fracture in athletes. In a cross-sectional study of 46 male runners, computed tomography scanning was used to evaluate tibial geometry at the level of the middle and distal third.[11] Runners with a history of tibial stress fracture had significantly smaller tibial cross-sectional areas than the non-stress fracture group after adjusting for body mass and height. This difference was about 8.4%. The significance of bone geometry has not been investigated in physically active females.

Even if bone geometry plays a role in stress fracture development, large scale screening of tibial geometry using plain radiographs or DXA techniques is impractical and costly. With further research, it may be possible to develop surrogate indicators of tibial geometry via simple anthropometric measurements.

LEVEL 3 — CONTROLLER

It is generally acknowledged that some mechanosensory systems[17] respond to changes in bone's mechanical environment and orchestrate bone cell dynamics such that some form of adaptation takes place. At this stage the presence of a controller of bone cell dynamics has not been experimentally verified, and remains a conceptual model.

Changes in bone cell dynamics may influence the risk of stress fracture (see Chapters 11 and 12). Stress fractures develop if microdamage cannot be successfully repaired by the remodeling process and accumulates to form symptomatic "macrocracks" in bone.[18] Depressed bone remodeling may not allow normal skeletal repair of naturally occurring microdamage. Accelerated remodeling resulting from excessive bone strain or from the influence of systemic factors may also weaken bone, because bone resorption occurs before new bone is formed. This could promote the initiation of microdamage at remodeling sites.[19]

Because direct assessment of bone remodeling in humans is invasive and impractical, measurement of biochemical markers of bone turnover may prove useful in a clinical setting to aid in identification of individuals most at risk for stress fracture. A prospective cohort study of 104 male military recruits showed that a single measurement of plasma hydroxyproline (a nonspecific indicator of bone resorption) was significantly higher in five recruits who subsequently sustained stress fractures than in those who remained uninjured.[20] While this supports the concept that elevated bone turnover may be a stimulus for stress fracture development, hydroxyproline is not specific to bone and thus the elevated levels may reflect non-skeletal sources.

A limited number of cross-sectional studies have measured biochemical markers of bone turnover in small samples of female athletes with and without a history of stress fracture.[21-23] These studies showed no difference in bone turnover levels between groups, however, they were based on single measurements of relatively insensitive markers. Furthermore, measurements were taken at variable times after the stress fracture occurred and may not reflect bone turnover prior to the injury.

A 12-month prospective study in track and field athletes measured monthly bone turnover levels using osteocalcin, pyridinium cross-links, and N-telopeptides of type 1 collagen.[24] Athletes who developed stress fractures had similar baseline and monthly levels of bone turnover compared with their non-stress fracture counterparts, suggesting that neither single nor multiple measurements of bone turnover are clinically useful predictors of the likelihood of athletic stress fractures. However, this does not negate a possible pathogenetic role of local changes in bone remodeling at stress fracture sites, as turnover markers exhibit high biological variability and reflect the integration of all bone remodeling throughout the skeleton. If trabecular bone, with its greater metabolic activity, contributes more to bone turnover levels than cortical bone, this may explain the relative insensitivity of bone turnover markers to predict stress fractures which are primarily cortical lesions.

LEVEL 4 — FUNCTIONAL STIMULI

Functional stimuli are divided into three categories: mechanical, physiological, and pharmacological. Only the first two will be discussed in relation to stress fractures in this chapter. Discussion of the role of oral contraceptives will be reserved for Chapter 3.

Mechanical

Mechanical stimuli are strains induced through mechanical usage that are sensed and compared to existing thresholds to determine cellular response. Training influences bone strain and is affected by four factors. The volume of training is a function of the total number of strain cycles received by the bone, whereas the intensity of training (load per unit time — pace, speed) is a function of the frequency of strain cycles applied to the bone. The magnitude of each strain and duration of each strain cycle are functions of body weight, muscular shock absorption capability, and lower extremity biomechanical alignment. Impact attenuation is both intrinsic (muscular factors) and extrinsic (equipment and training surfaces). Eccentric muscular strength is important, but more important is the muscle's ability to resist fatigue. Muscular fatigue is a function of metabolic adaptations that occur with training. Foot type and lower extremity biomechanical alignment may affect gait mechanics, but altered gait may also occur from fatigue, disease, and injury (Figure 2). The relationship between these factors and stress fractures will be discussed in the following sections.

Training — Mechanical Loading

Repetitive, subthreshold mechanical loading arising from physical activity contributes to stress fracture development. However, the contribution of each training component (type, volume, intensity, frequency, and rate of change) has not been elucidated. Training may also influence bone indirectly through changes in levels of circulating hormones, particularly sex hormones,[25-27] and through effects on soft tissue composition where increase in muscle mass may be protective of stress fractures.

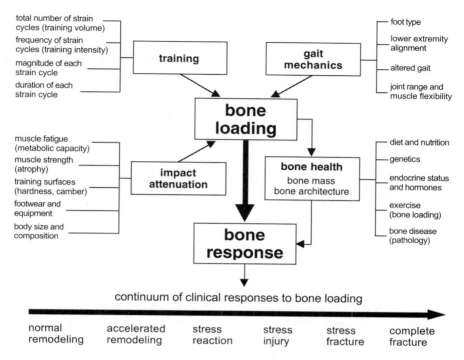

Figure 2 Contribution of risk factors to stress fracture pathogenesis. From Brukner, P., Bennell, K., and Matheson, G., *Stress Fractures.*, Blackwell Science, Melbourne, 1999. With permission.

Physical Fitness — Loading History

Military studies on the role of mechanical loading history, as reflected in measures of physical fitness, have been conflicting. The majority of data support the hypothesis that dramatic changes in bone's mechanical environment can precipitate changes in cellular dynamics that could potentiate development of a stress fracture. For example, a recent study by Shaffer[28] demonstrated that high risk recruits with poor physical fitness and low levels of prior physical activity suffered more than three times as many stress fractures as low risk recruits. Similar findings have been reported by others using self-reporting to assess previous physical activity levels,[57] and these appear to be independent of gender.[30,31] However, a relationship between physical fitness and stress fracture risk is less apparent when standardized fitness tests such as timed run and predicted VO_2 max are employed.[7,32,33]

Poor physical conditioning does seem to increase the risk of stress fractures in military recruits, probably because the mechanical loading experienced by unfit individuals during intensive training represents a dramatic change in skeletal load. However, this may not necessarily apply to athletes, where stress fractures often occur in well-conditioned individuals who have been training for years.

Training Regimen — Mechanical Loading Regimen

Controlled external loading studies in animals clearly demonstrate a differential skeletal response to various parameters of the loading regimen.[34,35] Load magnitude and rate are the most powerful determinants of bone cellular dynamics. It is therefore apparent that different aspects of the mechanical loading regimen influence stress fracture development.

Measurement of ground reaction force can provide an indirect measure of the magnitude and rate of external load on the lower extremity during physical activity.[36] In two cross-sectional studies, Grimston and colleagues[37,38] found significant differences in ground reaction force during running between stress fracture and non stress fracture groups. However, in their initial study the forces were higher in the stress fracture group, while in the subsequent study they were lower. Sample characteristics and testing procedures differed between the two studies, which may have contributed to the inconsistent findings. A more recent cross-sectional study in 46 male runners failed to support a role for external loading kinetics in stress fracture development.[11]

Military studies have shown that various training modifications can decrease the incidence of stress fractures in recruits. These interventions include rest periods,[39,40] elimination of running and marching on concrete,[41,42] use of running shoes rather than combat boots,[42,43] and reduction of high impact activity.[40,44,45] These measures may reduce stress fracture risk by allowing time for bone microdamage to be repaired and by decreasing the magnitude and rate of the load applied to bone.

In contrast, there is little controlled research in athletes. Most are anecdotal observations or case series where training parameters are examined only in athletes with stress fractures. For example, surveys reporting that up to 86% of athletes can identify some change in their training prior to the onset of the stress fracture[46,47] do not provide a similar comparison with uninjured athletes. Other researchers have blamed training "errors" in a varying proportion of cases but do not adequately define these errors.[48-51] A greater volume of training has been linked to an increased incidence of stress fractures in runners[52] and ballet dancers.[53]

Gait Mechanics

Lower Extremity Alignment and Foot Type

Lower limb and foot alignment influence the distribution, magnitude, and rate of mechanical loading as well as muscle activity. Footwear and orthotics can affect skeletal alignment (see Chapter 15). While associations between stress fractures and various factors influencing skeletal alignment have been studied in military populations, there are few data pertaining to athletes. Furthermore, the way in which the factors were defined and assessed was inconsistent, and reliability and validity issues were often not addressed. Studies evaluating a link between skeletal alignment and stress fractures are summarized in Table 2.

The structure of the foot will partly determine the amount of force absorbed by the bones in the foot and how much force is transferred to proximal bones such as the tibia during ground contact. The high arched (pes cavus) foot is more rigid and

Table 2 Studies investigating the association between skeletal alignment and stress fractures. Studies are ranked first according to the strength of their study design and then chronologically.

Reference	Study Design	Subjects	Sample Size	Factors Analysed	Method of Measurement	Results
Friberg 1982[59]	XS&PC	Army-Finland	371-M	Leg length difference	X-ray-WB	Increased incidence with increased difference
Giladi et al. 1985[54]	PC	Army-Israel	295-M	Foot type	Observation-NWB	SF risk greater in high arch than low arch
Giladi et al. 1987[62]	PC	Army-Israel	295-M	Genu valgum/varum	Observation	No relationship with SF
				Tibial torsion	NS	No relationship with SF
				Gait intoe/outtoe	Observation	No relationship with SF
Montgomery et al. 1989[57]	PC	SEAL-U.S.	505-M	Genu recurvatum	Distance heels to bed-supine	No relationship with SF
				Genu valgum/varum	Distance b/n condyles-WB	No relationship with SF
				Q angle	Goniometer-supine	No relationship with SF
				Foot type	Observation-WB	No relationship with SF
Simkin et al. 1989[55]	PC	Army-Israel	295-M	Foot type	X-ray-WB	High arch-higher risk of fem and tibial SF
						Low arch-higher risk of MT SF
Milgrom et al. 1994[63]	PC	Army-Israel	783-M	Genu valgum/varum	Distance b/n condyles	No relationship with SF
Bennell et al. 1996[9]	PC	Athletes	53-F/58-M	Leg length difference	Tape measure-NWB	Leg length diff-higher incidence of SF
Cowan et al. 1996[60]	PC	Army-U.S.	294-M	Genu valgum/varum	Observation-NWB	No relationship with SF
				Foot type	Observation-WB	No relationship with SF
				Genu valgum/varum	Computer digitization of photographs showing highlighted anatomic	Increased SF risk with increased valgus
				Genu recurvatum		No relationship with SF
				Q angle		Q angle >15° = increased risk for SF
Winfield et al. 1997[30]	PC	Marines-U.S.	101-F	Leg length difference	landmarks-WB	No relationship with SF
				Q angle	NS	No relationship with SF
Hughes 1985[61]	XS	Army-U.S.	47-M	Forefoot varus	Goniometer-NWB	Greater FFV 8.3 times at risk of MT SF

Table 2 (continued) Studies investigating the association between skeletal alignment and stress fractures. Studies are ranked first according to the strength of their study design and then chronologically.

Reference	Study Design	Subjects	Sample Size	Factors Analysed	Method of Measurement	Results
Brunet et al. 1990[52]	XS	Athletes	375-F/1130-M	Rearfoot valgus	Goniometer-WB	No relationship with SF
				Leg length difference	Self-report questionnaire	Leg length diff — higher SF risk
Brosh and Arcan 1994[56]	XS	NS	42-M	Foot type	Self-report questionnaire	No relationship with SF
				Foot type	Contact pressure display	Higher arches = increased SF risk
Ekenman et al. 1996[64]	XS	Athletes	29-SF M&F 30-NSF M&F	Foot type	Contact pressure during gait	No relationship with SF
				Rearfoot valgus	NS	
				Forefoot varus	NS	
Matheson et al. 1987[58]	CS	Athletes	320	Subtalar varus	>3°	Not related to site of SF
				Foot type	NS	Pron-tib & tarsal SF; cavus-MT & fem SF
				Forefoot varus	>2°	Not related to site of SF
				Genu valgum/varum	Distance b/n condyles	Not related to site of SF
				Tibial varum	>10°	Not related to site of SF

CS = case series; PC = prospective cohort; XS = cross-sectional; M = male; F = female; NS = not stated; NWB = non-weight bearing; WB = weight bearing; b/n = between; MT = metatarsal; SF = stress fracture; FFV = forefoot varus

Adapted From Brukner, P., Bennell, K., and Matheson, G., *Stress Fractures*, Blackwell Science, Melbourne, 1999. With permission.

less able to absorb shock, resulting in more force passing to the tibia and femur. The low arched (pes planus) foot is more flexible, allowing stress to be absorbed by the musculoskeletal structures of the foot. Pes planus is also often associated with prolonged pronation or hyperpronation. This can induce a great amount of torsion on the tibia, and may exacerbate muscle fatigue as the muscles have to work harder to control the excessive motion, especially at toe-off. Theoretically, either foot type could predispose to stress fracture. Several studies have indicated that the risk of stress fracture is greater for male recruits with high foot arches than with low arches,[54-56] although not all have corroborated these findings.[57] Most of the athlete studies are case series, which do not allow comparison of injured and uninjured athletes. While pes planus may be the most common foot type in athletes presenting to sports clinics with stress fractures,[46,48] it may be equally as common a foot type in athletes who remain uninjured. The relationship between foot type and stress fracture may vary depending on the site of stress fracture.[55,58] Therefore, studies may fail to find an association between certain foot types and stress fractures because the data have not been analyzed separately by stress fracture site.

There is evidence that leg length discrepancy increases the likelihood of stress fractures in both military[59] and athletic[9,52] populations, but the injury does not seem to occur on either the shorter or longer leg preferentially. Other alignment features include the presence of genu varum, valgum, or recurvatum, Q angle, and tibial torsion. Of these, only increased Q angle has been found in association with stress fractures,[60] although this is not a universal finding.[30,57]

The literature suggests that foot type may play a role in stress fracture development, but the exact relationship probably depends upon the anatomical location of the injured region and the activities undertaken by the individual. However, leg length discrepancy does appear to be a risk factor in both military and civilian populations. The failure to find an association between other biomechanical features and stress fractures in cohort studies does not necessarily rule out their importance. A thorough biomechanical assessment is an essential part of treatment and prevention of stress fractures. Until the contribution of biomechanical abnormalities to stress fracture risk is clarified through scientific research, correction of such abnormalities should be attempted.

Muscle Flexibility and Joint Range of Motion

The role of flexibility is difficult to evaluate, as flexibility encompasses a number of characteristics including active joint mobility, ligamentous laxity, and muscle length. Numerous variables have been assessed, including range of rearfoot inversion/eversion, ankle dorsiflexion/plantarflexion, knee flexion/extension, and hip rotation/extension, together with length of calf, hamstring, quadriceps, hip adductors, and hip flexor muscles.[9,30,57,61-64] Of these, only increased range of hip external rotation[7,62,63] and decreased range of ankle dorsiflexion[61] have been associated with stress fracture development, and even these findings have been inconsistent.

The difficulty in assessing the role of muscle and joint flexibility in stress fractures may relate to a number of factors, including the relatively imprecise methods of measurement, the heterogeneity of these variables, and the fact that both increased and decreased flexibility may be contributory.

Impact Attenuation

Training Surface

Training surface has long been considered a contributor to stress fracture development.[65] Anatomical and biomechanical problems can be accentuated by cambered or uneven surfaces, while ground reaction forces are increased by less compliant surfaces.[66,67] Alternatively, running on softer surfaces may hasten muscle fatigue. There are no data that assess the relationship of training surface with stress fractures. This may be due to difficulty in accurately quantifying running surface parameters, and to sampling bias. However, it may still be prudent to advise athletes to minimize time spent training on hard, uneven surfaces.

Muscular Strength and Fatigue

Muscle strength and endurance are critical in stress fracture development (see Chapter 9). Some investigators consider that muscles act dynamically to cause stress fractures by increasing bone strain at sites of muscle attachment.[68,69] However, under normal circumstances muscles exert a protective effect by contracting to reduce bending strains on cortical bone surfaces.[70] Following fatiguing exercise, bone strain, and particularly strain rate, is increased,[71,72] more in younger versus older persons.[72]

Studies measuring muscle strength or endurance[7,33,63,64] have generally failed to find an association with stress fracture occurrence. Some indirect evidence for muscle fatigue as a risk factor comes from a study by Grimston and colleagues.[38] They found that during the latter stages of a 45 minute run, women with a past history of stress fracture recorded increased ground reaction forces, whereas in the control group ground reaction forces did not vary during the run.

Measurements of muscle size may indicate the ability of a muscle to generate force. Male recruits with larger calf circumference developed significantly fewer femoral and tibial stress fractures.[73] This finding was also evident in female athletes, but not male athletes.[9] In order to establish a causal relationship, the effectiveness of a calf strengthening program in reducing incidence of stress fractures should be evaluated in a randomized, controlled trial.

Body Size and Composition

Body size and soft tissue composition could directly affect stress fracture risk by influencing the forces applied to bones. For example, heavier individuals generate higher forces during physical activity.[74] These factors could also have indirect effects on stress fracture risk via bone density or menstrual function.

A number of potential risk factors related to body size and composition have been reported in the stress fracture literature including height, weight, body mass index, skinfold thickness, total and regional lean mass and fat mass, limb and segment lengths, and body girth and width.[9,23,53,75,76] No study has found an association between these factors and stress fracture incidence. This lack of association may be because athletes of a particular sport tend to be relatively homogenous in terms of somatotype and body composition, or because a potential relationship may be non-linear. Furthermore, these parameters are unlikely to be stable and their measurement in cross-sectional studies may not reflect their status prior to injury.

Body size may be a risk factor in military recruits, where size variations are likely to be greater than in athletes. In a recent study, the incidence of stress fracture was greater in smaller individuals.[8] The authors surmised that this may be because of common training requirements where similar weight packs and other equipment are carried regardless of recruit body weight. On the other hand, overweight individuals may be at increased risk for stress fracture as these populations tend to be less physically active. Nevertheless, most military studies have failed to find an association between stress fractures and various parameters of body size and composition in either gender.[7,30,31,45]

Physiological

Endogenous hormones, particularly sex hormones, are essential for skeletal health. (The relationship between menstrual disturbances and stress fractures in females is discussed in Chapter 3). The role of sex hormones in men has not been well investigated, but the results of a limited number of studies have failed to establish a relationship between lowered circulating testosterone levels and osteopenia[77-79] or stress fractures.[80] From a clinical perspective, it is important to clarify that although some male athletes do present with reduced testosterone levels, these concentrations are generally still within the normal range for adult men. Therefore, stress fracture risk may not be increased and detrimental effects on bone density may not be as dramatic as those described for females with athletic amenorrhoea where estradiol levels are well below normal.

Although alterations in calcium metabolism could affect bone remodeling and bone density and thus predispose to stress fracture, there is no evidence to support such a relationship. Single measurements of serum calcium, parathyroid hormone, 25 OH-vitamin D and 1,25-dihydroxy vitamin D did not differ between stress fracture and non-stress fracture groups in military recruits[81] or athletes.[21-23] These findings may reflect the sampling procedures, as single measurements were taken at some time point following stress fracture. Conversely, since many of these biochemical parameters are tightly regulated, alterations in calcium metabolism may not be a factor in stress fracture development in healthy individuals. Other endocrine factors that have the potential to influence bone health and hence stress fracture risk include glucocorticoids, growth hormone, and thyroxin but these have not been assessed.

LEVEL 5 — CONSTRAINTS

The fifth level of the model reflects the overriding constraints on bone health which influence the impact of the respective functional stimuli and therefore indirectly influence risk of stress fracture. These comprise predetermined factors such as gender, genetics, and age (see Chapters 3, 4 and 7), and factors that are a function of environmental influences such as nutrition and psychological traits, although these may also be partly genetically pre-determined.

Nutrition

Dietary deficiencies, in particular dietary calcium, may contribute to the development of stress fractures by influencing bone density and bone remodeling.[82-85] However, it is difficult to clarify the role of diet as (1) accurate assessment of habitual dietary intake is problematic; (2) nutrients may exert their effects on bone over a number of years and hence measurement of current intake may not represent lifetime status; (3) calcium balance is negatively influenced by other dietary factors, and (4) calcium operates as a threshold nutrient, whereby intake above a certain level produces no additional effects on bone.[86]

The only randomized intervention study assessing the relationship of calcium intake to stress fracture development was conducted in military recruits. Schwellnus and Jordaan[87] found a similar incidence of stress fractures during a nine-week training program in 247 male recruits taking 500 mg supplementation of calcium daily, and 1151 controls. This result does not appear to support a role for calcium in stress fracture prevention. However, nine weeks is probably not long enough for any calcium effects to become apparent, particularly at cortical lower limb sites where the bone turnover rate is slower. Furthermore, both groups already had a baseline dietary calcium intake greater than 800 mg/day. This intake may have been sufficient to protect against stress fracture, with additional calcium offering no added benefit. No studies have evaluated the effect of calcium supplementation on stress fracture incidence in individuals whose usual dietary calcium intake is low.

A recent cross-sectional study in female military recruits did not find a difference in dietary calcium intake between the stress fracture and non-stress fracture groups,[31] confirming the results of the intervention study in male recruits. There is also scant evidence to show that lower calcium intake is associated with an increased risk for stress fracture in athletes. While one study found that current calcium intake was significantly lower in the stress fracture group,[22] other studies in athletes have failed to confirm this.[9,21,37,53,88,89] Negative influences on calcium balance can include high intake of salt, protein, phosphorus, caffeine, and alcohol. At present, there are no reports of any association between these and the incidence of stress fractures in athletes.[9,21,22,88,89]

Psychological Traits

There is little information about a link between psychological traits and stress fractures, particularly in athletes. Of the three prospective studies conducted in the military, two failed to find an association between psychological factors and incidence of stress fractures.[7,45] The other found that low achievement and high obedience personality traits were related to increased incidence of stress fractures.[90] A mechanism for this relationship is not clear, but high achievement and motivation could be related to greater training volume and intensity or perhaps disordered eating patterns (see Chapter 3). Whether the results may be extrapolated directly to athletes involved in voluntary exercise is unknown.

SUMMARY

It is apparent that there are a number of proposed factors which may directly or indirectly influence the risk of stress fracture. Many of these factors have not been proven by studies to date, but this may relate to the complex inter-relationships between these factors and the difficulty in conducting clinical research. Although most study designs in this area do not permit the assignment of causality, general factors which have been shown to be associated with stress fractures in physically active individuals include smaller bones, leg length discrepancy, muscle fatigue, and training factors.

REFERENCES

1. Grimston, S.K., An application of mechanostat theory to research design: a theoretical model, *Med. Sci. Sports Exerc.*, 25, 1293, 1993.
2. Frost, H.M., Structural adaptations to mechanical usage (SATMU): redefining Wolff's Law, *Anat. Rec.*, 226, 403, 1990.
3. Cummings, S.R., et al., Bone density at various sites for prediction of hip fractures, *Lancet*, 341, 72, 1993.
4. Melton, L.J., et al., Long-term fracture prediction by bone mineral assessed at different skeletal sites, *J. Bone Miner. Res.*, 8, 1227, 1993.
5. Bennell, K.L., et al., Bone mass and bone turnover in power athletes, endurance athletes and controls: a 12-month longitudinal study, *Bone*, 20, 477, 1997.
6. Bass, S., et al., Exercise before puberty may confer residual benefits in bone density in adulthood: studies in active prepubertal and retired female gymnasts, *J. Bone Miner. Res.*, 13, 500, 1998.
7. Giladi, M., et al., Stress fractures: identifiable risk factors, *Am. J. Sports Med.*, 19, 647, 1991.
8. Beck, T.J., et al., Dual-energy x-ray absorptiometry derived structural geometry for stress fracture prediction in male U.S. Marine Corps recruits, *J. Bone Miner. Res.*, 11, 645, 1996.
9. Bennell, K.L., et al., Risk factors for stress fractures in track and field athletes: a 12 month prospective study, *Am. J. Sports Med.*, 24, 810, 1996.
10. Pouilles, J.M., et al., Femoral bone density in young male adults with stress fractures, *Bone*, 10, 105, 1989.
11. Crossley, K., et al., Ground reaction forces, bone characteristics and tibial stress fracture in male runners, *Med. Sci. Sports Exerc.*, 31, 1088, 1999.
12. Miller, G.J. and Purkey, W.W., The geometric properties of paired human tibiae, *J. Biomech.*, 13, 1, 1980.
13. Martens, M., et al., The geometrical properties of human femur and tibia and their importance for the mechanical behaviour of these bone structures, *Acta Orthop. Traum. Surg.*, 98, 113, 1981.
14. Giladi, M., et al., Stress fractures and tibial bone width. A risk factor, *J. Bone Jt. Surg.*, 69(B), 326, 1987.
15. Milgrom, C., et al., An analysis of the biomechanical mechanism of tibial stress fractures among Israeli infantry recruits, *Clin. Orthop. Rel. Res.*, 231, 216, 1988.

16. Milgrom, C., et al., The area moment of inertia of the tibia: a risk factor for stress fractures, *J. Biomech.*, 22, 1243, 1989.

17. Cowin, S.C., Moss-Salentijn, L., and Moss, M.L., Candidates for the mechanosensory system in bone, *J. Biomech. Eng.*, 113, 191, 1991.

18. Li, G., et al., Radiographic and histologic analyses of stress fracture in rabbit tibias, *Am. J. Sports Med.*, 13, 285, 1985.

19. Johnson, L.C., et al., Histogenesis of stress fractures, *J. Bone Jt. Surg.*, 45(A), 1542, 1963.

20. Murguia, M.J., et al., Elevated plasma hydroxyproline. A possible risk factor associated with connective tissue injuries during overuse, *Am. J. Sports Med.*, 16, 660, 1988.

21. Carbon, R., et al., Bone density of elite female athletes with stress fractures, *Med. J. Aust.*, 153, 373, 1990.

22. Myburgh, K.H., et al., Low bone density is an etiologic factor for stress fractures in athletes, *Ann. Intern. Med.*, 113, 754, 1990.

23. Warren, M.P., et al., Scoliosis and fractures in young ballet dancers, *N. Engl. J. Med.*, 314, 1348, 1986.

24. Bennell, K.L., et al., A 12-month prospective study of the relationship between stress fractures and bone turnover in athletes, *Calcif. Tissue Int.*, 63, 80, 1998.

25. Wheeler, G.D., et al., Endurance training decreases serum testosterone levels in men without changes in luteinizing hormone pulsatile release, *J. Clin. Endocrinol. Metab.*, 72, 422, 1991.

26. De Souza, M.J., et al., High frequency of luteal phase deficiency and anovulation in recreational women runners: blunted elevation in follicle-stimulating hormone observed during luteal-follicular transition, *J. Clin. Endocrinol. Metab.*, 83, 4220, 1998.

27. Morris, F.L., Payne, W.R., and Wark, J.D., The impact of intense training on endogenous estrogen and progesterone concentrations and bone mineral acquisition in adolescent rowers, *Osteoporosis Int.*, 10, 361, 1999.

28. Shaffer, R.A., et al., Use of simple measures of physical activity to predict stress fractures in young men undergoing a rigorous physical training program, *Am. J. Epidemiol.*, 149, 236, 1999.

29. Gardner, L.I., et al., Prevention of lower extremity stress fractures: a controlled trial of a shock absorbent insole, *Am. J. Public Health*, 78, 1563, 1988.

30. Winfield, A.C., et al., Risk factors associated with stress reactions in female marines, *Mil. Med.*, 162, 698, 1997.

31. Cline, A.D., Jansen, G.R., and Melby, C.L., Stress fractures in female army recruits — implications of bone density, calcium intake, and exercise, *J. Am. Coll. Nutr.*, 17, 128, 1998.

32. Swissa, A., et al., The effect of pretraining sports activity on the incidence of stress fractures among military recruits, *Clin. Orthop. Rel. Res.*, 245, 256, 1989.

33. Hoffman, J.R., et al., The effect of leg strength on the incidence of lower extremity overuse injuries during military training, *Mil. Med.*, 164, 153, 1999.

34. Rubin, C.T. and Lanyon, L.E., Regulation of bone formation by applied dynamic loads, *J. Bone Jt. Surg.*, 66-A, 397, 1984.

35. Rubin, C.T. and Lanyon, L.E., Regulation of bone mass by mechanical strain magnitude, *Calcif. Tissue Int.*, 37, 411, 1985.

36. Nigg, B.M., Biomechanics, load analysis and sports injuries in the lower extremities, *Sports Med.*, 2, 367, 1985.

37. Grimston, S.K., et al., Bone mass, external loads, and stress fractures in female runners, *Int. J. Sport Biomech.*, 7, 293, 1991.

38. Grimston, S.K., et al., External loads throughout a 45 minute run in stress fracture and non-stress fracture runners, *J. Biomech.*, 27, 668, 1994.
39. Worthen, B.M. and Yanklowitz, B.A.D., The pathophysiology and treatment of stress fractures in military personnel, *J. Am. Podiatric Med. Assoc.*, 68, 317, 1978.
40. Scully, T.J. and Besterman, G., Stress fracture — a preventable training injury, *Mil. Med.*, 147, 285, 1982.
41. Reinker, K.A. and Ozburne, S., A comparison of male and female orthopaedic pathology in basic training, *Mil. Med.*, Aug, 532, 1979.
42. Greaney, R.B., et al., Distribution and natural history of stress fractures in U.S. marine recruits, *Radiology*, 146, 339, 1983.
43. Proztman, R.R., Physiologic performance of women compared to men, *Am. J. Sports Med.*, 7, 191, 1979.
44. Pester, S. and Smith, P.C., Stress fractures in the lower extremities of soldiers in basic training, *Orthop. Rev.*, 21, 297, 1992.
45. Taimela, S., et al., Risk factors for stress fractures during physical training programs, *Clin. J. Sports Med.*, 2, 105, 1992.
46. Sullivan, D., et al., Stress fractures in 51 runners, *Clin. Orthop. Rel. Res.*, 187, 188, 1984.
47. Goldberg, B. and Pecora, C., Stress fractures. A risk of increased training in freshman, *Physician Sportsmed.*, 22, 68, 1994.
48. Taunton, J.E., Clement, D.B., and Webber, D., Lower extremity stress fractures in athletes, *Physician Sportsmed.*, 9, 77, 1981.
49. McBryde, A.M., Stress fractures in runners, *Clin. Sports Med.*, 4, 737, 1985.
50. Courtenay, B.G. and Bowers, D.M., Stress fractures: clinical features and investigation, *Med. J. Aust.*, 153, 155, 1990.
51. Pecina, M., Bojanic, I., and Dubravcic, S., Stress fractures in figure skaters, *Am. J. Sports Med.*, 18, 277, 1990.
52. Brunet, M.E., et al., A survey of running injuries in 1505 competitive and recreational runners, *J. Sports Med. Phys. Fitness*, 30, 307, 1990.
53. Kadel, N.J., Teitz, C.C., and Kronmal, R.A., Stress fractures in ballet dancers, *Am. J. Sports Med.*, 20, 445, 1992.
54. Giladi, M., et al., The low arch, a protective factor in stress fractures. A prospective study of 295 military recruits, *Orthop. Rev.*, 14, 709, 1985.
55. Simkin, A., et al., Combined effect of foot arch structure and an orthotic device on stress fractures, *Foot Ankle*, 10, 25, 1989.
56. Brosh, T. and Arcan, M., Toward early detection of the tendency to stress fractures, *Clin. Biomech.*, 9, 111, 1994.
57. Montgomery, L.C., et al., Orthopedic history and examination in the etiology of overuse injuries, *Med. Sci. Sports Exerc.*, 21, 237, 1989.
58. Matheson, G.O., et al., Stress fractures in athletes. A study of 320 cases, *Am. J. Sports Med.*, 15, 46, 1987.
59. Friberg, O., Leg length asymmetry in stress fractures. A clinical and radiological study, *J. Sports Med.*, 22, 485, 1982.
60. Cowan, D.N., et al., Lower limb morphology and risk of overuse injury among male infantry trainees, *Med. Sci. Sports Exerc.*, 28, 945, 1996.
61. Hughes, L.Y., Biomechanical analysis of the foot and ankle for predisposition to developing stress fractures, *J. Orthop. Sports Phys. Therapy*, 7, 96, 1985.
62. Giladi, M., et al., External rotation of the hip. A predictor of risk for stress fractures, *Clin. Orthop. Related Res.*, 216, 131, 1987.

63. Milgrom, C., et al., Youth as a risk factor for stress fracture. A study of 783 infantry recruits, *J. Bone Jt. Surg.*, 76-B, 20, 1994.

64. Ekenman, I., et al., A study of intrinsic factors in patients with stress fractures of the tibia, *Foot Ankle Int.*, 17, 477, 1996.

65. Devas, M.B. and Sweetnam, R., Stress fractures of the fibula. A review of fifty cases in athletes, *J. Bone Jt. Surg.*, 38B, 818, 1956.

66. McMahon, T.A. and Greene, P.R., The influence of track compliance on running, *J. Biomech.*, 12, 893, 1979.

67. Steele, J.R. and Milburn, P.D., Effect of different synthetic sport surfaces on ground reactions forces at landing in netball, *Int. J. Sport Biomech.*, 4, 130, 1988.

68. Stanitski, C.L., McMaster, J.H., and Scranton, P.E., On the nature of stress fractures, *Am. J. Sports Med.*, 6, 391, 1978.

69. Meyer, S.A., Saltzman, C.L. and Albright, J.P., Stress fractures of the foot and leg, *Clin. Sports Med.*, 12, 395, 1993.

70. Scott, S.H. and Winter, D.A., Internal forces at chronic running injury sites, *Med. Sci. Sports Exerc.*, 22, 357, 1990.

71. Yoshikawa, T., et al., The effects of muscle fatigue on bone strain, *J. Exp. Biol.*, 188, 217, 1994.

72. Fyhrie, D.P., et al., Effect of fatiguing exercise on longitudinal bone strain as related to stress fracture in humans, *Ann. Biomed. Eng.*, 26, 660, 1998.

73. Milgrom, C., The Israeli elite infantry recruit: a model for understanding the biomechanics of stress fractures, *J. R. Coll. Surg. Edinburgh*, 34, S18, 1989.

74. Frederick, E.C. and Hagy, J.L., Factors affecting peak vertical ground reaction forces in running, *Int. J. Sport Biomech.*, 2, 41, 1986.

75. Lloyd, T., et al., Women athletes with menstrual irregularity have increased musculoskeletal injuries, *Med. Sci. Sports Exerc.*, 18, 374, 1986.

76. Barrow, G.W. and Saha, S., Menstrual irregularity and stress fractures in collegiate female distance runners, *Am. J. Sports Med.*, 16, 209, 1988.

77. MacDougall, J.D., et al., Relationship among running mileage, bone density, and serum testosterone in male runners, *J. Appl. Physiol.*, 73, 1165, 1992.

78. Hetland, M.L., Haarbo, J., and Christiansen, C., Low bone mass and high bone turnover in male long distance runners, *J. Clin. Endocrinol. Metab.*, 77, 770, 1993.

79. Smith, R. and Rutherford, O.M., Spine and total body bone mineral density and serum testosterone levels in male athletes, *Eur. J. Appl. Physiol.*, 67, 330, 1993.

80. Skarda, S.T. and Burge, M.R., Prospective evaluation of risk factors for exercise-induced hypogonadism in male runners, *West. J. Med.*, 169, 9, 1998.

81. Mustajoki, P., Laapio, H., and Meurman, K., Calcium metabolism, physical activity, and stress fractures, *Lancet*, 2, 797, 1983.

82. Lanyon, L.E., Rubin, C.T., and Baust, G., Modulation of bone loss during calcium insufficiency by controlled dynamic loading, *Calcif. Tissue Int.*, 38, 209, 1986.

83. Specker, B.L., Evidence for an interaction between calcium intake and physical activity on changes in bone mineral density, *J. Bone Miner. Res.*, 11, 1539, 1996.

84. Johnston, C.C., et al., Calcium supplementation and increases in bone mineral density in children, *N. Engl. J. Med.*, 327, 82, 1992.

85. Lee, W.T.K., et al., Double-blind, controlled calcium supplementation and bone mineral accretion in children accustomed to a low-calcium diet, *Am. J. Clin. Nutr.*, 60, 744, 1994.

86. Matkovic, V. and Heaney, R.P., Calcium balance during human growth: evidence for threshold behaviour, *Am. J. Clin. Nutr.*, 55, 992, 1992.

87. Schwellnus, M.P. and Jordaan, G., Does calcium supplementation prevent bone stress injuries? A clinical trial, *Int. J. Sport Nutr.,* 2, 165, 1992.
88. Frusztajer, N.T., et al., Nutrition and the incidence of stress fractures in ballet dancers, *Am. J. Clin. Nutr.,* 51, 779, 1990.
89. Warren, M.P., et al., Lack of bone accretion and amenorrhea: evidence for a relative osteopenia in weight bearing bones, *J. Clin. Endocrinol. Metab.,* 72, 847, 1991.
90. Taimela, S., Kujala, U.M. and Osterman, K., Intrinsic risk factors and athletic injuries, *Sports Med.,* 9, 205, 1990.

CHAPTER 3

Factors Associated with the Development of Stress Fractures in Women

Kim Bennell and Susan Grimston

CONTENTS

Introduction 36
Level 5 — Constraints 36
    Predetermined 36
    Environmental Constraints 36
        Calcium Intake 36
        Disordered Patterns of Eating 38
Level 4 — Functional Stimuli 39
    Mechanical 39
    Physiological Stimuli 39
        Effects of Amenorrhea on Bone Mass 40
        Mechanisms of Low Bone Mass in Amenorrhea 40
        Relationship Between Amenorrhea and Stress Fractures 41
        Shortened Luteal Phase 43
        Age of Menarche 43
    Pharmacology 44
        Effects of Oral Contraceptive Pill Use on Bone Density 44
        Effects of the Oral Contraceptive Pill on Stress Fracture Risk 44
Level 3 — Controller 45
Level 2 — Bone Properties 45
Summary 48
References 48

INTRODUCTION

The number of physically active women has increased over the last several decades and much research has focused on their unique medical concerns, particularly in the area of skeletal health. Although general risk factors for stress fractures (see Chapter 2) apply equally to both genders, other factors specific to women impact upon the ability of bone to successfully adapt to mechanical load. These factors may explain the higher incidence of stress fracture in females compared with their male counterparts.[1-9] Based on the five level research model described in Chapter 2 (Figure 1), predetermined genetic and environmental factors determine a number of functional stimuli and bone properties specific to women. These will be outlined in relation to their influence on bone density and ultimately stress fracture risk.

LEVEL 5 — CONSTRAINTS

Predetermined

The overriding constraint determining risk of stress fracture in women is genetics. Female chromosomes determine a number of factors that ultimately influence bone strength. Genetic factors affect bone geometry, skeletal alignment, hormonal milieu (in particular estrogen), and the response of bone to pharmacological stimuli such as the oral contraceptive pill (OCP). Genes can also influence psychological traits and behaviors which may impact on training habits and susceptibility to eating disorders and menstrual disturbances.

Environmental Constraints

Women appear to be more susceptible to environmental influences than men, resulting in the preoccupation of many women, especially physically active women, with body weight and shape.[10] Restricted dietary intake combined with excessive exercise may be strategies used by women to achieve the "ideal" body. Peers and popular culture influence weight control beliefs and behaviors in women.[11] The increasing difference in body size and shape of the average young woman from the ideal promoted by the media[12] may be partly responsible for the phenomenon of body dissatisfaction. Furthermore, certain sports place weight restrictions on their participants, while others emphasize leanness for success.

Calcium Intake

Dietary surveys of various sporting groups often reveal inadequate intakes of macro- and micro-nutrients, especially in women.[13,14] The skeleton serves as a calcium reservoir, and when it is called upon to meet dietary insufficiencies bone strength may be compromised. However, in children and adolescents, higher calcium retention efficiency means that only in severe cases of dietary restriction will bone mineral accrual be affected. These situations are seldom observed in Western culture.[15,16] In amenorrheic and postmenopausal women, greater calcium intake is needed to retain calcium balance because of increased urinary calcium losses associated with low estrogen levels.[17] Other nutritional factors such as increased sodium and protein intake can also increase urinary calcium losses and thus affect calcium balance.

Despite the importance of calcium for bone health, the evidence for a relationship between estimated dietary calcium intake and bone density is inconclusive and probably varies depending on life stage. Large longitudinal studies[18,19] and calcium intervention studies[20] have failed to find an effect of high or low levels of calcium intake on bone density or rates of bone loss in premenopausal women. This suggests that during the premenopausal years, the effect of genetics and other environmental factors on bone mass may be greater than that of dietary calcium.[21] However, calcium may be more important in amenorrheic physically active women where the effects of calcium deficiency and hypogonadism may be additive.[22] This is supported by the findings of Wolman,[23] who reported a linear relationship between calcium intake and lumbar spine trabecular bone density in both amenorrheic and eumenorrheic athletes, although at all levels of calcium intake, bone density was lower in the amenorrheic group.

Given the imprecision of methods for assessing current and lifetime calcium intake and the confounding effect of other nutrients, it is not surprising that most studies have failed to establish a definite link between low calcium intake and stress fracture development in either athletic[24-29] or military[30] populations. Ballet dancers have been found to consume less than the recommended daily allowance for calcium regardless of their stress fracture status.[25,28] These results suggest that other factors may be more important as risk factors in dancers. In female track and field athletes, calcium intake, assessed using four day food records as well as food frequency questionnaires, was similar in those with and without stress fractures.[29] This does not necessarily exclude calcium deficiency as a risk factor for stress fracture, as the majority of athletes in this study were consuming more than their recommended daily allowance of 800 mg/day and hence would not be regarded as calcium deficient. While historical calcium intake may be more relevant for current skeletal health, the only study to assess this found that a calcium index, based on variability in calcium intake during the ages of 12 to 23 years, was similar in female runners with and without stress fractures.[26]

The results of studies from one research group do support a role for calcium in preventing stress fracture development. In a cross-sectional design, Myburgh et al.[31] found a significantly lower intake of calcium in athletes with shin soreness compared with a matched control group. However, since exact diagnoses were not made, stress fracture may not have been the only pathology included in the shin soreness group. A follow-up study in athletes with scintigraphically-confirmed stress fractures showed similar results.[32] Current calcium intake was significantly lower in the stress fracture group, at 87% of recommended daily intake for that population. It is possible that while calcium intake may be considered adequate based on recommended daily intake levels, it may be inadequate in terms of stress fracture risk.

Disordered Patterns of Eating

Female athletes report a greater frequency of disordered eating patterns than male athletes,[33] especially in sports emphasizing leanness and/or those competing at higher levels.[34] A recent study also highlighted the problem in military populations, where an 8% prevalence of eating disorders was found in women on active duty in the Army.[35] Many female athletes are undernourished, reporting seemingly insufficient energy intakes to meet the demands of exercise training. Low caloric intake has been hypothesized as one of the mechanisms for menstrual disturbances in sportswomen, as amenorrheic athletes often have lower energy intakes than eumenorrheic athletes.[36,37] Lower fat intake[38] and vegetarianism[39,40] are also more likely in amenorrheic athletes. Undernutrition manifests as low body weight and low body fat, and while these factors have been linked with menstrual dysfunction, the exact relationship has not been clarified.[41-43]

The independent effects of disordered eating on bone mass are often hard to elucidate, given the difficulty in controlling for confounding factors such as body weight and menstrual disturbances.[44,45] Certainly the effects of extreme eating disorders such as anorexia nervosa on bone are profound, with marked osteopenia and insufficiency fractures common.[46-48] The severity of osteopenia in anorexia is greater than in patients with hypothalamic amenorrhea and is critically dependent upon nutritional factors in addition to the degree or duration of estrogen deficiency. Lean body mass is also an important predictor of bone loss in women with anorexia.[48] Less extreme forms of disordered eating may also have detrimental effects on bone mass, as undernutrition appears to be a common feature in physically active individuals with osteopenia.

Disordered eating patterns appear to be associated with increased risk of stress fracture. Ballet dancers with stress fractures were more likely to restrict caloric intake, avoid high-fat dairy foods, consume low-calorie products, have a self-reported history of an eating disorder, and have lower percentages of ideal body weight than those without stress fractures.[25] Similarly, in a cross-sectional study of young adult female track and field athletes, those with a history of stress fracture scored higher on the EAT-40 test (a validated test relating to dieting, bulimia, food preoccupation, and oral control) and were more likely to engage in restrictive eating patterns and dieting than those without stress fractures.[49] In this group followed prospectively, four-day food records revealed a lower fat diet in females who went on to develop stress fractures during the year of the study.[29] More recently, a large multi-center survey of 2298 U.S. collegiate athletes revealed that pathogenic weight-control behavior is associated with a twofold increased risk of stress fracture.[50]

In summary, there is currently little evidence to support low calcium intake as a risk factor for stress fractures in otherwise healthy recreational and elite athletes or military recruits. Conversely, abnormal and restrictive eating behaviors do seem to increase the likelihood of fracture. Disordered eating, amenorrhea, and osteopenia often occur simultaneously in athletic females, a syndrome that has been referred to as the 'female athlete triad.'[51] Conversely, the female athlete triad has not been shown to be a clinically significant problem in military women.[52] Undernutrition may have a direct influence on bone properties (Level 2), or an indirect influence via effects on hormonal status and body composition. Healthy eating habits should be promoted in all individuals. If one is concerned about dietary intake in physically active females, food records as well as biochemical and anthropometric indices should be used to assess dietary adequacy and nutritional status, and appropriate nutritional counselling provided.

LEVEL 4 — FUNCTIONAL STIMULI

Mechanical

Most of the mechanical factors that influence stress fracture development are common to both genders. However, there are genetically determined differences between the genders, particularly with regard to skeletal alignment and body composition, that could play a role in increasing the risk of stress fracture in women.

In general, females are shorter than males and thus have to take relatively longer strides when marching in formation with men in military drills. This has been blamed partly for a higher incidence of pelvic stress fractures in women. Measures to reduce mechanical loading in female recruits, including self-selected step length, have been successful in reducing stress fracture incidence.[53] Women also have a wider pelvis with an increased Q angle at the knee compared with men. The Q angle refers to the angle formed by the intersection of the line of pull of the quadriceps muscles and the patellar tendon, measured through the center of the patella. Generally, an increased Q angle has been thought to increase biomechanical stresses in the lower limb. However, in female Marine trainees, a narrow pelvis ($\leq$26 cm) was associated with a 3.6 times greater risk of stress fracture.[54] An explanation for this finding is not clear, but it is possible that a narrow pelvis in this group of female Marines was a marker for some other risk factor for stress fractures.

Body composition differs between genders, women having a greater percentage of body fat mass and less muscle mass in relation to body size. Men are stronger than women because of this greater muscle mass but, per unit of muscle mass, the female is equally strong. Given the importance of muscle activity to stress fracture development, this difference in absolute muscle mass may confer a difference in stress fracture risk between genders, but this hypothesis has not been formally tested. Furthermore, if bone mass is adjusted to muscle mass, gender differences may not be apparent.

Physiological Stimuli

One of the key differences between the genders influencing stress fracture risk is the role of sex hormones in skeletal health. Physically active females have a higher prevalence of menstrual disturbances including delayed menarche, anovulation, abnormal luteal phase, oligomenorrhea, and amenorrhea compared with the general female population.[37,50,55,56] Amenorrhea is generally defined as less than three menstrual cycles per year or no cycles for the past six months, while oligomenorrhea is defined as 3 to 6 cycles per year.[57] Younger, nulliparous women of excessive leanness who train intensely, particularly in sports such as ballet, gymnastics, light weight rowing, and distance running appear to be at greater risk for developing menstrual disturbances.[56,58] Athletic amenorrhea is the term used to describe menstrual disturbances which occur in conjunction with physical activity in women.

Effects of Amenorrhea on Bone Mass

The detrimental effects of athletic amenorrhea on bone mass were first identified in the 1980s by several authors.[59-62] Since then, numerous others have shown lower axial bone density in athletes with amenorrhea or oligomenorrhea compared with their eumenorrheic counterparts.[60,63-65] Appendicular bone density may also be affected,[64-66] but this has been a less consistent finding. Thus in athletes, exercise-induced osteogenic benefits are lessened when training is associated with menstrual dysfunction.[67]

The reversibility of bone loss observed with amenorrhea has been a concern due to the long–term consequences on bone mass. Drinkwater et al.[68] followed up athletes with amenorrhea 15.5 months after they regained menses, and showed a 6% increase in vertebral bone density, although this still remained below normal levels of cyclic athletes and non-athletes. The resumption of menses was also associated with an increase in body weight and reduction in exercise level. However, it was later reported[69] that bone gain in these athletes slowed to 3% the following year and ceased after two years, still well below the average for their age group, suggesting that bone mass may never fully recover. Micklesfield et al.[70] also showed that despite resumption of menses, previously irregularly menstruating runners still had reduced vertebral bone mass compared with regularly menstruating runners. History of menstrual irregularity is therefore detrimental to the maintenance of peak bone mass.

Mechanisms of Low Bone Mass in Amenorrhea

There are probably multiple mechanisms responsible for the deleterious effects of menstrual disturbances on bone density. However, the main cause is thought to be low-circulating estrogens, since these have important indirect[71-74] and possibly direct[75-77] skeletal effects. Compared with their eumenorrheic counterparts, amenorrheic athletes have significantly lower plasma estradiol levels, resembling those of postmenopausal women.[60,78,79]

Recently, however, this primary mechanism for bone loss has been questioned.[80] Evidence for this is related to findings of bone turnover studies[80,81] and to the fact that amenorrheic athletes appear to be less responsive to estrogen therapy[82,83] than women with ovarian failure. The postmenopausal state is characterised by increased bone turnover with an excess of bone resorption.[84] Conversely, recent data show that the pattern of bone remodeling in amenorrheic athletes is atypical of an estrogen deficient state with either no change[79,85] or an apparent reduction in bone turnover and reduced bone formation.[86] Other work suggests that undernutrition and its metabolic consequences may underlie the bone remodeling imbalance and bone loss in active amenorrheic women.[81,87,88] Bone formation markers were shown to be lowest in amenorrheic runners with the lowest body mass index,[81] demonstrating a relationship with undernutrition. However, these findings do not preclude estrogen deficiency playing a role, as undernutrition may also cause ovarian suppression.[89]

Relationship Between Amenorrhea and Stress Fractures

The relationship between amenorrhea or oligomenorrhea and stress fracture risk has been the subject of numerous studies, mainly retrospective cross-sectional surveys of runners and ballet dancers.[28,90-95] Many of these studies are characterized by small samples and low questionnaire response rates. In other studies, subjects are specifically recruited according to certain criteria; either stress fracture history or menstrual status.[24-27,32,62,63,96,97] Categorization of menstrual status is based on number of menses per year, rather than on analysis of hormonal levels, and definitions of menstrual status vary between studies. Where hormonal assessment is included, most are single measurements, often non-standardized with respect to menstrual cycle phase. The length of exposure to amenorrhea also differs within and between studies, and this may influence stress fracture risk.

Despite the methodology limitations, the findings generally show that stress fractures are more common in athletes with menstrual disturbances[24-26,28,29,32,49,54,62,90-93,95,96] (Figure 1). Athletes with menstrual disturbances have a relative risk for stress fracture that is between two to four times greater than that of their eumenorrheic counterparts. However, in ballet dancers, logistic regression analysis showed that amenorrhea for longer than six months' duration was an independent contributor to the risk of stress fracture and that the estimated risk was 93 times that of a dancer with regular menses.[28] While this risk seems extraordinarily high, there were only six dancers with regular menses in this sample of 54 dancers, and this may have affected the statistical analyses.

The risk of multiple stress fractures also seems to be increased in women with menstrual disturbances.[93,94] Clark et al. [94] found that while amenorrheic and eumenorrheic groups reported a similar prevalence of single stress fractures, 50% of the

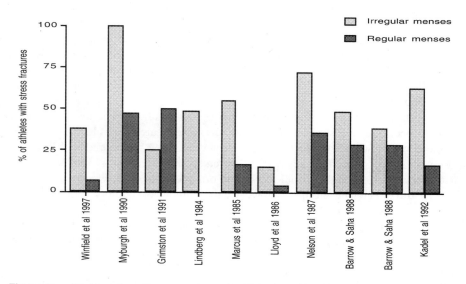

Figure 1a Studies where the percentage of athletes/recruits with stress fractures could be compared in groups with and without menstrual irregularity

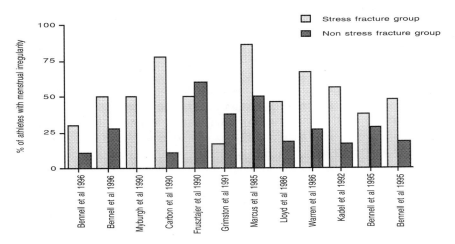

Figure 1b   Studies where the percentage of athletes/recruits with menstrual irregularity could be compared in groups with and without stress fractures. Adapted from Brukner, P.D., and Bennell, K.L., *Crit. Rev. Phys. Rehab. Med.*, 9, 161, 1997. With permission.

amenorrheic runners reported multiple stress fractures compared with only 9% of those regularly menstruating. In female distance runners, the amenorrheic group was the only one to have a runner who had sustained six stress fractures whereas in the 120 eumenorrheic runners, none had more than three stress fractures.[93]

Grimston and colleagues[98] developed a menstrual index that summarized previous and present menstrual status. The index quantified the average number of menses per year since menarche. They found no relationship between this menstrual index and the incidence of stress fractures in 16 female runners. Conversely, track and field athletes with a lower menstrual index, indicating fewer menses per year since menarche, were at greater risk of stress fracture than those with a higher index.[29] Barrow and Saha[93] also found that lifetime menstrual history affected the risk of stress fracture. They showed the incidence of stress fracture to be 29% in the regular group and 49% in the very irregular group.

Menstrual disturbances may also predispose to stress fracture in female recruits. In a prospective cohort study of 101 female Marines, the incidence of stress fractures in those with fewer than 10 periods per year was 37.5%, compared with 6.7% in those with 10 to 13 periods per year.[54] Conversely, in a study of 49 female soldiers with stress fractures and 78 soldiers with no orthopedic injuries, menstrual patterns did not differ between groups.[30] However, the number of soldiers with menstrual disturbances was relatively low.

The mechanism by which menstrual disturbances increases stress fracture risk is not known, as menstrual disturbances often co-exist with other factors such as low calcium intake,[37] greater training load,[99] and lower body fat or body mass index.[43,58,88] Since these were not always controlled for in the studies discussed, it is difficult to ascertain which are the most important contributory factors.

Given the association between menstrual irregularity and risk of stress fracture, it is important to question physically active females about their current and past menstrual status and then seek appropriate medical opinion if necessary. Since menstrual disturbances are often found together with eating disorders and osteopenia, the "female athlete triad", the presence of one of these factors should alert the practitioner to the possibility of the others.

Shortened Luteal Phase

Although amenorrhea is the most obvious sign of reproductive hormone disturbance, exercise may cause subtle changes in reproductive hormone levels that are too small to produce amenorrhea.[88,100] A decrease in progesterone production associated with short luteal phases and anovulation can be present in women despite normal menstrual cycle duration and normal flow characteristics.[101,102] These menstrual disturbances may be induced by relatively low volumes of exercise, and following abrupt onset of training.[100]

The role of progesterone in maintenance of skeletal health is still contentious. While there is *in vitro* evidence to show promotion of bone formation with progesterone particularly in cortical bone,[103-105] results from clinical studies are contradictory. In a prospective study involving eumenorrheic women, two thirds of whom were runners, Prior et al.[106] found that recurrent short luteal phase cycles and anovulation were associated with spinal bone loss of approximately 2 to 4% per year. These results were supported more recently by another 12 month prospective study[107] in premenopausal runners. Serum progesterone levels and the proportion of the total menstrual cycle spent in luteal phase also have been found to be significant predictors of lumbar spine bone density,[108] as well as rate of change of bone mass at this site.[106] However, a cross-sectional study failed to find a significant difference in spinal bone density between groups with short and long luteal phase lengths.[109] Despite the possible detrimental effects of luteal phase deficiency on bone, a link between this and stress fracture risk has not yet been formally sought.

Age of Menarche

Menarche is attained later in athletes compared with non-athletes, especially in sports such as ballet, gymnastics, and running.[110-112] The relationship between age of menarche and risk of stress fracture is unclear. Some authors have found that athletes with stress fractures have a later age of menarche[24,27,29,91] while others have found no difference.[25,28,32] In a prospective cohort study, age of menarche was an independent risk factor for stress fracture in female track and field athletes, with the risk increasing by a factor of 4.1 for every additional year of age at menarche.[29]

An association between delayed menarche and stress fractures may be due to a lower rate of bone mineral accretion during adolescence and therefore decreased peak bone mass.[113-115] In large cohorts of healthy adolescents and pre– and post–menopausal women, the most common finding is that a later age of menarche is related to lower bone density.[113,115-119] However, this does not imply a causal relationship, since other factors such as genetic background may be major determinants of both variables.

A later age of menarche has also been found in association with amenorrhea, lowered energy intake, decreased body fat or weight, and excessive premenarcheal training.[95,120,121] All of these could feasibly influence stress fracture risk. Whatever the reason for an association, athletes should be questioned about when they commenced their periods. A later age of menarche could then be used as a marker to identify a possible predisposition for fracture.

Pharmacology

Effects of Oral Contraceptive Pill Use on Bone Density

The main pharmacological agent impacting on skeletal health in physically active women is the oral contraceptive pill (OCP). Most of the studies addressing the relationship between OCP use and bone density involve cross-sectional or longitudinal designs in healthy non-athletic cohorts. Confounding variables are often not well controlled and include smoking, alcohol intake, past menstrual status, body composition, dietary intake, and physical activity levels.

Some studies in healthy women have shown greater bone mass in current or past users of the OCP compared with non-users.[122-124] Conversely, a number of others have failed to find an association between the OCP and bone mass in both normally active women[19,125-128] and in sportswomen.[23,129-131] More unexpectedly, there have been several recent reports of detrimental effects of the OCP on bone mass[132-135] and fracture risk.[136] However, the clinical implications of these negative findings should be kept in perspective until further more scientifically rigorous studies are conducted. These studies will help to establish whether reported detrimental effects are due to actual prevention of bone accretion or to methodological issues such as lifestyle factors and history of menstrual disturbances in OCP users, which are also associated with low bone density (Prior, J., personal communication).

Despite the fact that the OCP is commonly prescribed as a treatment, the ability of the OCP to improve bone mass in amenorrheic athletes has not been well investigated. Randomized, controlled trials in this area are extremely difficult to conduct and require large sample sizes.[137] Improvements in bone density do not seem to be as great[83,138] as those demonstrated with hormone replacement therapies in postmenopausal women.[139]

Effects of the Oral Contraceptive Pill on Stress Fracture Risk

Some authors have claimed that regular use of the OCP may protect against stress fracture development by providing an exogenous source of estrogen to improve bone quality and/or density. There have been no randomized intervention trials to show that use of the OCP reduces the stress fracture rate in athletes, particularly in those with prior or current menstrual disturbances.

Two prospective cohort studies, one in athletes[29] and one in female Marines,[54] have failed to support a protective effect of OCP use on stress fracture development although numbers in the stress fracture groups were relatively small (n = 10 and 12, respectively).

The results of cross-sectional studies are contradictory. Barrow and Saha[93] found that runners using the OCP for at least one year had significantly fewer stress fractures (12%) than non-users (29%). This was supported by the findings of Myburgh et al.[32] Conversely, no difference in OCP use was reported in ballet dancers with and without stress fractures.[28] However, few dancers were taking the OCP. Since these studies are retrospective in nature, it is not known whether the athletes were taking the OCP prior to or following the stress fracture episode. In addition, athletes may or may not take the OCP for reasons that could influence stress fracture risk. It is not known whether the risk of stress fracture is decreased in athletes with menstrual disturbances who subsequently take the OCP.

LEVEL 3 — CONTROLLER

The mechanosensory system is responsible for changes in bone cell dynamics via a feedback system driven by mechanical strains whose values fall outside physiological set points. The set points determine the sensitivity of bone cells to mechanical stimuli. It is generally thought that the set points are genetically defined, and vary depending upon the skeletal region.[140] However, hormonal and other influences can alter these set points, thereby modulating the effect of mechanical loading. It is felt that low estrogen levels increase the set points for mechanical strain such that higher mechanical loads are required to maintain or increase bone mass in the presence of estrogen deficiency.[22,141] While some forms of exercise (such as gymnastics or rowing) may produce strains sufficient to reach these increased set points in amenorrheic physically active women, other forms (such as running) may be of insufficient magnitude, and hence bone loss results.[142] Thus, predisposition to stress fracture can be influenced by the interaction of functional stimuli (Level 4) with the controlling mechanism for bone adaptation (Level 3).

LEVEL 2 — BONE PROPERTIES

In males, bone geometry has been related to stress fracture development, with smaller bones associated with greater risk (see Chapter 2). Women have smaller bones than males,[143] and if both engage in exactly the same training (mechanical loading) regimen, one could predict a higher risk for fracture in females. No study has correlated bone geometry with stress fracture incidence in active female populations.

Women on average have a smaller peak bone mass than men because their skeletons are physically smaller. However, a gender difference in bone density is not nearly as clear-cut and probably varies from site to site.[144] Given the prevalence of menstrual disturbances in active women and the effects of these on bone cellular dynamics, low bone density could feasibly be associated with a greater likelihood of stress fractures in women than in men. There are eight studies to date investigating

Table 1 Summary of studies investigating the relationship between bone density and stress fractures in females. Studies are ordered according to the strength of study design and then chronologically.

Reference	Study Design	Subjects	Sample Size	Tech[n]	Sites	Results % Diff [†]
Bennell et al. 1996[29]	PC	Track & field athletes	10 — SF 36 — NSF	DXA	Upper limb Thoracic spine Lumbar spine Femur Tibia/fibula Foot	-3.3% -6.7% -11.9%* -2.2% -4.2% -6.6%*
Carbon et al. 1990[24]	XS	Various athletes	9 — SF 9 — NSF	DPA SPA	Lumbar spine Femoral neck Distal radius Ultradistal radius	-4.0%* -7.0% -7.7% 0.0%
Frusztajer et al. 1990[25]	XS	Ballet dancers	10 — SF 10 — NSF	DPA SPA	Lumbar spine 1st metatarsal Radial shaft	-4.1% 0.0% 0.0%
Myburgh et al. 1990[32]	XS	Various athletes	25 — SF 25 — NSF (19 F,6 M)	DXA	Lumbar spine Femoral neck Wards triangle Trochanter Intertrochanter Proximal femur	-8.5%* -6.7%* -9.0%* -8.6%* -5.5% -6.5%*
Grimston et al. 1991[26]	XS	Runners	6 — SF 8 — NSF	DPA	Lumbar spine Femoral neck Tibial shaft	8.2%* 7.6%* 9.7%
Bennell et al. 1995[49]	XS	Track & field athletes	22 — SF 31 — NSF	DXA	Lumbar spine Lower limb Tibia/fibula	-3.5% -0.9% -2.0%
Cline et al. 1998[30]	XS	Military	49 — SF 78 — NSF		Lumbar spine Femoral neck Wards triangle Trochanter Radial shaft	-2.4% 0% -2.2% 0% 1.5%
Lauder et al. 2000[145]	XS	Military	27 — SF 158 — NSF	DXA	Lumbar spine Femoral neck	1.3% -1.6%

PC = observational analytic prospective cohort; XS = observational descriptive cross-sectional; DPA = dual photon absorptiometry; DXA = dual energy x-ray absorptiometry; SPA = single photon absorptiometry; Tech[n] = technique.

* Statistically significant
† Results are given as the % difference comparing stress fracture subjects (SF) with non-stress fracture subjects (NSF).

Adapted from Brukner, P.D. and Bennell, K.L., *Crit. Rev. Phys. Rehab. Med.,* 9, 163, 1997 and Bennell et al., *Scand. J. Sci. Med. Sport.,* 7, 269, 1997. With permission.

this relationship,[24-26,29,30,32,49,145] but only one has been prospective in design.[29] The results are contradictory which may reflect differences in populations (military versus athletic), type of sport (running, dancing, track and field), measurement techniques (single or dual photon absorptiometry, dual energy x-ray absorptiometry), and bone regions studied (Table 1). A problem with cross-sectional studies is that the stress fracture and non-stress fracture groups were often inadequately matched and differed on other factors thought to influence bone density and stress fracture risk, such as menstrual status, body composition, and training levels. Multivariate statistical analyses were not performed to take into account the influence of these confounding factors. It was also unclear how long after injury the bone density measurements were taken. It is possible that enforced immobilization or reduced activity levels following stress fracture may have led to a decrease in bone density.

For osteoporotic fractures, bone density measurements of the bone at risk for fracture are generally the best predictor of eventual fracture, although bone density at other sites is also predictive. To best provide evidence for a causal relationship between low bone density and stress fracture, measurements ideally should be taken at bone sites where stress fractures occur. Four studies included bone density measurements at lower limb sites while the others measured the lumbar spine, radius, and/or proximal femur only. These latter sites may not necessarily reflect the bone status at stress fracture sites.

Unlike studies in males, there is greater evidence to suggest that lower bone density may play a role in stress fracture development in women. In the only prospective cohort study, female track and field athletes who sustained stress fractures had significantly lower total body bone mineral content and lower bone density at the lumbar spine and foot than those without a fracture.[29] The subgroup of women who developed tibial stress fractures had 8.1% lower bone density at the tibia/fibula. This deficit located at the site of fracture supports a possible cause–and–effect relationship, although the number in this subgroup was small. An important point to note is that while bone density was lower in the athletes with stress fractures, it nevertheless remained, as a group, higher than or similar to bone density of less active non-athletes. This implies that the level of bone density required by physically active individuals for short-term bone health may be greater than that required by the general population. It also implies that the stress fracture individuals in this study would not have been identified as being at risk based on normative DXA values. At present there are no normative data bases specific to athletes of different sports to enable legitimate comparisons of bone density.

Findings of the cross-sectional studies are contradictory. One study of 14 female runners actually found significantly higher lumbar spine and femoral neck bone density in the stress fracture group.[26] The authors speculated that greater external loading forces measured in the stress fracture subjects during running may have been responsible for their higher bone density. Others have either reported no difference or significantly lower bone density in the stress fracture group. In a recent study, multivariate analyses revealed a strong negative association between femoral neck bone density and probability of stress fracture in 27 military recruits compared with 158 controls.[145]

The relationship between bone density and stress fracture development is still not clearly established, although there is evidence that low bone density as a risk factor may be more common in women. In general, it would seem that bone densitometry does not have a place as a general screening tool to predict risk of stress fracture in otherwise healthy individuals. However, bone densitometry may be warranted in women with multiple stress fracture episodes or with menstrual disturbances.

SUMMARY

Being a female imparts an additional set of risk factors for stress fracture, over and above those shared by both genders, which may explain the seemingly greater incidence of this bony injury in women. Differences in bone density, bone geometry, skeletal alignment, and hormonal milieu may jeopardize the ability of bone to adapt to identical mechanical loads in women. Furthermore, environmental influences to which women may be more prone may manifest themselves as eating disorders or inappropriate training habits. The interrelationship of disordered eating, menstrual dysfunction, and osteopenia, commonly known as the "female athlete triad" may have direct or indirect effects on the mechanical competence of bone and result in symptomatic stress fracture.

REFERENCES

1. Protzman, R.R. and Griffis, C.C., Comparative stress fracture incidence in males and females in an equal training environment, *Athletic Training,* 12, 126, 1977.
2. Brudvig, T.J.S., Gudger, T.D., and Obermeyer, L., Stress fractures in 295 trainees: a one-year study of incidence as related to age, sex, and race, *Mil. Med.,* 148, 666, 1983.
3. Jones, H., et al., Exercise-induced stress fractures and stress reactions of bone: epidemiology, etiology, and classification, *Exerc. Sports Sci. Rev.,* 17, 379, 1989.
4. Pester, S. and Smith, P.C., Stress fractures in the lower extremities of soldiers in basic training, *Orthop. Rev.,* 21, 297, 1992.
5. Jones, B.H., et al., Intrinsic risk factors for exercise-related injuries among male and female army trainees, *Am. J. Sports Med.,* 21, 705, 1993.
6. Brunet, M.E., et al., A survey of running injuries in 1505 competitive and recreational runners, *J. Sports Med. Phys. Fitness,* 30, 307, 1990.
7. Dixon, M. and Fricker, P., Injuries to elite gymnasts over 10 yr, *Med. Sci. Sports Exerc.,* 25, 1322, 1993.
8. Goldberg, B. and Pecora, C., Stress fractures. A risk of increased training in freshman, *Phys. Sportsmed.,* 22, 68, 1994.
9. Johnson, A.W., Weiss, C.B., and Wheeler, D.L., Stress fractures of the femoral shaft in athletes-more common than expected. A new clinical test, *Am. J. Sports Med.,* 22, 248, 1994.
10. Hausenblas, H.A. and Carron, A.V., Eating disorder indices and athletes: an integration, *J. Sport Exerc. Psychol.,* 21, 230, 1999.
11. Field, A.E., et al., Relation of peer and media influences to the development of purging behaviors among preadolescent and adolescent girls, *Arch. Ped. Adolescent Med.,* 153, 1184, 1999.
12. Spitzer, B.L., Henderson, K.A., and Zivian, M.T., Gender differences in population versus media body sizes: a comparison over four decades, *Sex Roles,* 40, 545, 1999.
13. Ronsen, O., Sundgot-Borgen, J., and Maehlum, S., Supplement use and nutritional habits in Norwegian elite athletes, *Scand. J. Med. Sci. Sports.,* 9, 28, 1999.
14. Ziegler, P.J., Nelson, J.A., and Jonnalagadda, S.S., Nutritional and physiological status of US national figure skaters, *Int. J. Sport Nutr.,* 9, 345, 1999.
15. Abrams, S.A., et al., Calcium and magnesium balance in 9- to 14-year-old children, *Am. J. Clin. Nutr.,* 66, 1172, 1997.

16. Martin, A.D., et al., Bone mineral and calcium accretion during puberty, *Am. J. Clin. Nutr.,* 66, 611, 1997.

17. Heaney, R.P., Recker, R.R., and Saville, P.D., Menopausal changes in calcium balance performance, *J. Lab. Clin. Med.,* 92, 953, 1978.

18. Riggs, B.L., et al., Dietary calcium intake and rates of bone loss in women, *J. Clin. Inv.,* 80, 979, 1987.

19. Mazess, R.B. and Barden, H.S., Bone density in premenopausal women: effects of age, dietary intake, physical activity, smoking, and birth-control pills, *Am. J. Clin. Nutr.,* 53, 132, 1991.

20. Smith, E.L., et al., Calcium supplementation and bone loss in middle-aged women, *Am. J. Clin. Nutr.,* 50, 833, 1989.

21. Kanis, J.A., Calcium nutrition and its implications for osteoporosis. 1. Children and healthy adults, *Eur. J. Clin. Nutr.,* 48, 757, 1994.

22. Dalsky, G.P., Effect of exercise on bone: permissive influence of estrogen and calcium, *Med. Sci. Sports Exerc.,* 22, 281, 1990.

23. Wolman, R.L., et al., Dietary calcium as a statistical determinant of spinal trabecular bone density in amenorrhoeic and estrogen-replete athletes, *Bone Miner.,* 12, 415, 1992.

24. Carbon, R., et al., Bone density of elite female athletes with stress fractures, *Med. J. Aust.,* 153, 373, 1990.

25. Frusztajer, N.T., et al., Nutrition and the incidence of stress fractures in ballet dancers, *Am. J. Clin. Nutr.,* 51, 779, 1990.

26. Grimston, S.K., et al., Bone mass, external loads, and stress fractures in female runners, *Int. J. Sport Biomech.,* 7, 293, 1991.

27. Warren, M.P., et al., Lack of bone accretion and amenorrhea: evidence for a relative osteopenia in weight bearing bones, *J. Clin. Endocrinol. Metab.,* 72, 847, 1991.

28. Kadel, N.J., Teitz, C.C., and Kronmal, R.A., Stress fractures in ballet dancers, *Am. J. Sports Med.,* 20, 445, 1992.

29. Bennell, K.L., et al., Risk factors for stress fractures in track and field athletes: a 12 month prospective study, *Am. J. Sports Med.,* 24, 810, 1996.

30. Cline, A.D., Jansen, G.R. and Melby, C.L., Stress fractures in female army recruits — implications of bone density, calcium intake, and exercise, *J. Am. Coll. Nutr.,* 17, 128, 1998.

31. Myburgh, K.H., Grobler, N., and Noakes, T.D., Factors associated with shin soreness in athletes, *Phys. Sportsmed.,* 16, 129, 1988.

32. Myburgh, K.H., et al., Low bone density is an etiologic factor for stress fractures in athletes, *Ann. Intern. Med.,* 113, 754, 1990.

33. Johnson, C., Powers, P.S., and Dick, R., Athletes and eating disorders: the National Collegiate Athletic Association study, *Int. J. Eating Disorders,* 26, 179, 1999.

34. Picard, C.L., The level of competition as a factor for the development of eating disorders in female collegiate athletes, *J. Youth Adolescence,* 28, 583, 1999.

35. Lauder, T.D., et al., Abnormal eating behaviors in military women, *Med. Sci. Sports Exerc.,* 31, 1265, 1999.

36. Nelson, M.E., et al., Diet and bone status in amenorrheic runners, *Am. J. Clin. Nutr.,* 43, 910, 1986.

37. Kaiserauer, S., et al., Nutritional, physiological, and menstrual status of distance runners, *Med. Sci. Sports Exerc.,* 21, 120, 1989.

38. Deuster, P.A., et al., Nutritional intakes and status of highly trained amenorrheic and eumenorrheic women runners, *Fertil. Sterility,* 46, 636, 1986.

39. Brooks, S.M., et al., Diet in athletic amenorrhoea, *Lancet,* 1, 559, 1984.
40. Barr, S.I., Vegetarianism and menstrual cycle disturbances: is there an association?, *Am. J. Clin. Nutr.,* 70, 549S, 1999.
41. Carlberg, K.A., et al., Body composition of oligo/amenorrheic athletes, *Med. Sci. Sports Exerc.,* 15, 215, 1983.
42. Sanborn, C.F., Albrecht, B.H., and Wagner, W.W., Athletic amenorrhea: lack of association with body fat, *Med. Sci. Sports Exerc.,* 19, 207, 1987.
43. Rosetta, L., Harrison, G.A., and Read, G.F., Ovarian impairments of female recreational distance runners during a season of training, *Ann. Hum. Biol.,* 25, 345, 1998.
44. Brooks-Gunn, J., Warren, M.P., and Hamilton, L., The relation of eating problems and amenorrhea in ballet dancers, *Med. Sci. Sports Exerc.,* 19, 41, 1987.
45. Gadpaille, W.J., Sanborn, C.F., and Wagner, W.W., Athletic amenorrhea, major affective disorders, and eating disorders, *Am. J. Psych.,* 144, 939, 1987.
46. Rigotti, N.A., et al., The clinical course of osteoporosis in anorexia nervosa. A longitudinal study of cortical bone mass, *JAMA,* 265, 1133, 1991.
47. Grinspoon, S., et al., Severity of osteopenia in estrogen-deficient women with anorexia nervosa and hypothalamic amenorrhea, *J. Clin. Endocrinol. Metab.,* 84, 2049, 1999.
48. Soyka, L.A., et al., The effects of anorexia nervosa on bone metabolism in female adolescents, *J. Clin. Endocrinol. Metab.,* 84, 4489, 1999.
49. Bennell, K.L., et al., Risk factors for stress fractures in female track-and-field athletes: a retrospective analysis, *Clin. J. Sports Med.,* 5, 229, 1995.
50. Nattiv, A., Puffer, J.C., and Green, G.A., Lifestyles and health risks of collegiate athletes — a multi-center study, *Clin. J. Sports Med.,* 7, 262, 1997.
51. Otis, C.L., et al., American College of Sports Medicine position stand. The female athlete triad, *Med. Sci. Sports Exerc.,* 29, I-x, 1997.
52. Lauder, T.D., et al., The female athlete triad: prevalence in military women, *Mil. Med.,* 164, 630, 1999.
53. Pope, R.P., Prevention of pelvic stress fractures in female army recruits, *Mil. Med.,* 164, 370, 1999.
54. Winfield, A.C., et al., Risk factors associated with stress reactions in female marines, *Mil. Med.,* 162, 698, 1997.
55. Malina, R.M., et al., Age at menarche and selected menstrual characteristics in athletes at different competitive levels and in different sports, *Med. Sci. Sports Exerc.,* 10, 218, 1978.
56. Skierska, E., Age at menarche and prevalance of oligo/amenorrhea in top Polish athletes, *Am. J. Hum. Biol.,* 10, 511, 1998.
57. Keen, A.D. and Drinkwater, B.L., Irreversible bone loss in former amenorrheic athletes, *Osteoporosis Int.,* 7, 311, 1997.
58. Wolman, R.L. and Harries, M.G., Menstrual abnormalities in elite athletes, *Clin. Sports Med.,* 1, 95, 1989.
59. Cann, C.E., et al., Decreased spinal mineral content in amenorrheic women, *JAMA,* 251, 626, 1984.
60. Drinkwater, B.L., et al., Bone mineral content of amenorrheic and eumenorrheic athletes, *N. Engl. J. Med.,* 311, 5, 277, 1984.
61. Linnell, S.L., et al., Bone mineral content and menstrual regularity in female runners, *Med. Sci. Sports Exerc.,* 16, 343, 1984.
62. Marcus, R., et al., Menstrual function and bone mass in elite women distance runners, *Ann. Intern. Med.,* 102, 158, 1985.
63. Rutherford, O.M., Spine and total body bone mineral density in amenorrheic endurance athletes, *J. Appl. Physiol.,* 74, 2904, 1993.

64. Micklesfield, L.K., et al., Bone mineral density in mature, premenopausal ultramarathon runners, *Med. Sci. Sports Exerc.*, 27, 688, 1995.
65. Tomten, S.E., et al., Bone mineral density and menstrual irregularities — a comparative study on cortical and trabecular bone structures in runners with alleged normal eating behavior, *Int. J. Sports Med.*, 19, 92, 1998.
66. Pettersson, U., et al., Low bone mass density at multiple skeletal sites, including the appendicular skeleton in amenorrheic runners, *Calcif. Tissue Int.*, 64, 117, 1999.
67. Morris, F.L., Payne, W.R., and Wark, J.D., The impact of intense training on endogenous estrogen and progesterone concentrations and bone mineral acquisition in adolescent rowers, *Osteoporosis Int.*, 10, 361, 1999.
68. Drinkwater, B.L., et al., Bone mineral density after resumption of menses in amenorrheic athletes, *JAMA*, 256, 380, 1986.
69. Drinkwater, B.L., Bruemner, B., and Chesnut lll, C.H., Menstrual history as a determinant of current bone density in young athletes, *JAMA*, 263, 545, 1990.
70. Micklesfield, L.K., et al., Long-term restoration of deficits in bone mineral density is inadequate in premenopausal women with prior menstrual irregularity, *Clin. J. Sports Med.*, 8, 155, 1998.
71. Feyen, J.H.M. and Raisz, L.G., Prostaglandin production by calvariae from sham operated and oophorectomized rats: effect of 17β-estradiol in vivo, *Endocrinology*, 121, 819, 1987.
72. Heaney, R.P., et al., Calcium absorption in women: relationships to calcium intake, estrogen status, and age, *J. Bone Miner. Res.*, 4, 469, 1989.
73. Girasole, G., et al., 17β-estradiol inhibits interleukin-6 production by bone marrow-derived stromal cells and osteoblasts in vitro, *J. Clin. Invest.*, 89, 883, 1992.
74. Jilka, R.L., et al., Increased osteoclast development after estrogen loss: mediation by interleukin-6, *Science*, 257, 88, 1992.
75. Eriksen, E., et al., Evidence of estrogen receptors in normal human osteoblast-like cells, *Science*, 241, 84, 1988.
76. Komm, B.S., et al., Estrogen binding, receptor mRNA, and biologic response in osteoblast-like osteosarcoma cells, *Science*, 241, 81, 1988.
77. Pensler, J.M., et al., Osteoclasts isolated from membranous bone in children exhibit nuclear estrogen and progesterone receptors, *J. Bone Miner. Res.*, 5, 797, 1990.
78. Myerson, M., et al., Total body bone density in amenorrheic runners, *Obstet. Gynecol.*, 79, 973, 1992.
79. Hetland, M.L., et al., Running induces menstrual disturbances but bone mass is unaffected, except in amenorrheic women, *Am. J. Med.*, 95, 53, 1993.
80. Zanker, C.L., Bone metabolism in exercise associated amenorrhea: the importance of nutrition, *Br. J. Sports Med.*, 33, 228, 1999.
81. Zanker, C.L. and Swaine, I.L., Relation between bone turnover, oestradiol, and energy balance in women distance runners, *Br. J. Sports Med.*, 32, 167, 1998.
82. Hergenroeder, A.C., Bone mineralisation, hypothalamic amenorrhea and sex steroid therapy in female adolescents and young adults, *J. Pediatr.*, 126, 683, 1995.
83. Hergenroeder, A.C., et al., Bone mineral changes in young women with hypothalamic amenorrhea treated with oral contraceptives, medroxyprogesterone, or placebo over 12 months, *Am. J. Obstet. Gynecol.*, 176, 1017, 1997.
84. Prince, R.L., et al., The effects of menopause and age on calciotropic hormones: a cross-sectional study of 655 healthy women aged 35 to 90, *J. Bone Miner. Res.*, 10, 835, 1995.
85. Stacey, E., et al., Decreased nitric oxide levels and bone turnover in amenorrheic athletes with spinal osteopenia, *J. Clin. Endocrinol. Metab.*, 83, 3056, 1998.

86. Zanker, C.L. and Swaine, I.L., Bone turnover in amenorrheic and eumenorrheic women distance runners, *Scand. J. Med. Sci. Sport,* 8, 20, 1998.

87. Thissen, J.P., Ketelslegers, J.M., and Underwood, L.E., Nutritional regulation of the insulin-like growth factors, *Endocrin. Rev.,* 15, 80, 1994.

88. De Souza, M.J., et al., High frequency of luteal phase deficiency and anovulation in recreational women runners: blunted elevation in follicle-stimulating hormone observed during luteal-follicular transition, *J. Clin. Endocrinol. Metab.,* 83, 4220, 1998.

89. Bonen, A., Exercise-induced menstrual cycle changes: a functional, temporary adaptation to metabolic stress, *Sports Med.,* 17, 373, 1994.

90. Lloyd, T., et al., Women athletes with menstrual irregularity have increased musculoskeletal injuries, *Med. Sci. Sports Exerc.,* 18, 374, 1986.

91. Warren, M.P., et al., Scoliosis and fractures in young ballet dancers, *N. Engl. J. Med.,* 314, 1348, 1986.

92. Nelson, M.E., et al., Elite women runners: association between menstrual status, weight history and stress fractures, *Med. Sci. Sports Exerc.,* 19, S13, 1987.

93. Barrow, G.W. and Saha, S., Menstrual irregularity and stress fractures in collegiate female distance runners, *Am. J. Sports Med.,* 16(3), 209, 1988.

94. Clark, N., Nelson, M., and Evans, W., Nutrition education for elite female runners, *Physician Sports Med.,* 16, 124, 1988.

95. Tomten, S.E., Prevalance of menstrual dysfunction in Norwegian long-distance runners participating in the Oslo marathon games, *Scand. J. Med. Sci. Sport,* 6, 164, 1996.

96. Lindberg, J.S., et al., Exercise-induced amenorrhea and bone density, *Ann. Intern. Med.,* 101, 647, 1984.

97. Cook, S.D., et al., Trabecular bone density and menstrual function in women runners, *Am. J. Sports Med.,* 15, 503, 1987.

98. Grimston, S.K., et al., Menstrual, calcium, and training history: relationship to bone health in female runners, *Clin. Sports Med.,* 2, 119, 1990.

99. Guler, F. and Hascelik, Z., Menstrual dysfunction rate and delayed menarche in top athletes of team games, *Sports Med. Training Rehabil.,* 4, 99, 1993.

100. Williams, N.I., et al., Effects of short-term strenuous endurance exercise upon corpus luteum function, *Med. Sci. Sports Exerc.,* 31, 949, 1999.

101. Beitins, I.Z., et al., Exercise induces two types of human luteal dysfunction: confirmation by urinary free progesterone, *J. Clin. Endocrinol. Metab.,* 72, 1350, 1991.

102. Prior, J.C. and Vigna, Y.M., Ovulation disturbances and exercise training, *Clin. Obstet. Gynecol.,* 34, 180, 1991.

103. Snow, G.R. and Anderson, C., The effects of continuous progestogen treatment on cortical bone remodeling activity in beagles, *Calcif. Tissue Int.,* 37, 282, 1985.

104. Karambolova, K.K., Snow, G.R., and Anderson, C., Surface activity on the periosteal and corticoendosteal envelopes following continuous progestogen supplementation in spayed beagles, *Calcif. Tissue Int.,* 38, 239, 1986.

105. Snow, G.R. and Anderson, C., The effects of 17β-estradiol and progestogen on trabecular bone remodeling in oophorectomized dogs, *Calcif. Tissue Int.,* 39, 198, 1986.

106. Prior, J.C., et al., Spinal bone loss and ovulatory disturbances, *N. Engl. J. Med.,* 323, 1221, 1990.

107. Petit, M.A., Prior, J.C., and Barr, S.I., Running and ovulation positively change cancellous bone in premenopausal women, *Med. Sci. Sports Exerc.,* 31, 780, 1999.

108. Snead, D.B., et al., Reproductive hormones and bone mineral density in women runners, *J. Appl. Physiol.,* 72, 2149, 1992.

109. Barr, S.I., Prior, J.C., and Vigna, Y.M., Restrained eating and ovulatory disturbances: possible implications for bone health, *Am. J. Clin. Nutr.,* 59, 92, 1994.
110. Malina, R.M., Menarche in athletes: a synthesis and hypothesis, *Ann. Hum. Biol.,* 10, 1, 1983.
111. Stager, J.M. and Hatler, L.K., Menarche in athletes: the influence of genetics and prepubertal training, *Med. Sci. Sport Exerc.,* 20, 369, 1988.
112. Bennell, K.L., et al., Bone mass and bone turnover in power athletes, endurance athletes and controls: a 12-month longitudinal study, *Bone,* 20, 477, 1997.
113. Lu, P.W., et al., Bone mineral density of total body, spine, and femoral neck in children and young adults: a cross-sectional and longitudinal study, *J. Bone Miner. Res.,* 9, 1451, 1994.
114. Young, D., et al., Determinants of bone mass in 10- to 26-year-old females: a twin study, *J. Bone Miner. Res.,* 10, 558, 1995.
115. McKay, H.A., et al., Peak bone mineral accrual and age at menarche in adolescent girls — a 6-year longitudinal study, *J. Pediatr.,* 133, 682, 1998.
116. Katzman, D.K., et al., Clinical and anthropometric correlates of bone mineral acquisition in healthy adolescent girls, *J. Clin. Endocrinol. Metab.,* 73, 1332, 1991.
117. Armamento-Villareal, R., et al., Estrogen status and heredity are major determinants of premenopausal bone loss, *J. Clin. Inv.,* 90, 2464, 1992.
118. Elliot, J.R., et al., Historical assessment of risk factors in screening for osteopenia in a normal Caucasian population, *Aust. N.Z. J. Med.,* 23, 458, 1993.
119. Fox, K.M., et al., Reproductive correlates of bone mass in elderly women, *J. Bone Miner. Res.,* 8, 901, 1993.
120. Frisch, R.E., et al., Delayed menarche and amenorrhea of college athletes in relation to age of onset of training, *JAMA,* 246, 1559, 1981.
121. Moisan, J., Meyer, F., and Gingras, S., A nested case-control study of the correlates of early menarche, *Am. J. Epidemiol.,* 132, 953, 1990.
122. Sowers, M.F., Wallace, R.B., and Lemke, J.H., Correlates of forearm bone mass among women during maximal bone mineralization, *Preventative Med.,* 14, 585, 1985.
123. Lindsay, J.R., Tohme, J., and Kanders, B., The effect of oral contraceptive use on vertebral bone mass in pre- and post-menopausal women, *Contraception,* 34, 333, 1986.
124. Recker, R.R., et al., Bone gain in young adult women, *JAMA,* 268, 2403, 1992.
125. Hreshchyshyn, M.M., et al., Associations of parity, breast-feeding, and birth control pills with lumbar spine and femoral neck bone densities, *Am. J. Obstet. Gynecol.,* 159, 318, 1988.
126. Rodin, A., Chapman, M., and Fogelman, I., Bone density in users of combined oral contraception. Preliminary reports of a pilot study, *Br. J. Fam. Plann.,* 16, 125, 1991.
127. Hansen, M.A., Assessment of age and risk factors on bone density and bone turnover in healthy premenopausal women, *Osteoporosis Int.,* 4, 123, 1994.
128. Garnero, P., Sornayrendu, E., and Delmas, P.D., Decreased bone turnover in oral contraceptive users, *Bone,* 16, 499, 1995.
129. Davee, A.M., Rosen, C.J., and Adler, R.A., Exercise patterns and trabecular bone density in college women, *J. Bone Miner. Res.,* 5, 245, 1990.
130. Taaffe, D.R., et al., Differential effects of swimming versus weight-bearing activity on bone mineral status of eumenorrheic athletes, *J. Bone Miner. Res.,* 10, 586, 1995.
131. Keay, N., Fogelman, I., and Blake, G., Bone mineral density in professional female dancers, *Br. J. Sports Med.,* 31, 143, 1997.
132. Polatti, F., et al., Bone mass and long-term monophasic oral contraceptive treatment in young women, *Contraception,* 51, 221, 1995.

133. Hartard, M., et al., Effects on bone mineral density of low-dosed oral contraceptives compared to and combined with physical activity, *Contraception,* 55, 87, 1997.

134. Register, T.C., Jayo, M.J., and Jerome, C.P., Oral contraceptive treatment inhibits the normal acquisition of bone mineral in skeletally immature young adult female monkeys, *Osteoporosis Int.,* 7, 348, 1997.

135. Prior, J., personal communication, 1998.

136. Cooper, C., et al., Oral contraceptive pill use and fractures in women: a prospective study, *Bone,* 14, 41, 1993.

137. Gibson, J.H., et al., Treatment of reduced bone mineral density in athletic amenorrhea: a pilot study, *Osteoporosis Int.,* 10, 284, 1999.

138. Cann, C.E., et al., Menstrual history is the primary determinant of trabecular bone density in women runners, *Med. Sci. Sports Exerc.,* 20, 59, 1988.

139. Prince, R.L., et al., Prevention of postmenopausal osteoporosis. A comparative study of exercise, calcium supplementation, and hormone-replacement therapy, *N. Engl. J. Med.,* 325, 1189, 1991.

140. Rubin, C.T. and Lanyon, L.E., Osteoregulatory nature of mechanical stimuli: Function as a determinant for adaptive remodeling in bone, *J. Orthop. Res.,* 5, 300, 1987.

141. Cheng, M.Z., Zaman, G., and Lanyon, L.E., Estrogen enhances the stimulation of bone collagen synthesis by loading and exogenous prostacyclin, but not prostaglandin E2 in organ cultures of rat ulnae, *J. Bone Miner. Res.,* 9, 805, 1994.

142. Robinson, T.L., et al., Gymnasts exhibit higher bone mass than runners despite similar prevalence of amenorrhea and oligomenorrhea, *J. Bone Miner. Res.,* 10, 26, 1995.

143. Miller, G.J. and Purkey, W.W., The geometric properties of paired human tibiae, *J. Biomech.,* 13, 1, 1980.

144. Bonjour, J.P., et al., Critical years and stages of puberty for spinal and femoral bone mass accumulation during adolescence, *J. Clin. Endocrinol. Metab.,* 73, 555, 1991.

145. Lauder, T.D., et al., The relation between stress fractures and bone mineral density: Evidence from active-duty army women, *Arch. Phys. Med. Rehab.,* 81, 73, 2000.

CHAPTER 4

The Role of Age in the Development of Stress and Fatigue Fractures

Antero Hulkko and Sakari Orava

CONTENTS

Introduction...55
Stress Fractures in Specific Age Categories 56
    Children, Age 0 to 6 Years 56
    Stress Fractures in Older Children and Early Adolescents, Age 7 to
        15 Years...56
    Stress Fractures in Late Adolescence, Age 16 to 19 Years 59
    Adults, (≥20 Years)..60
        Military Recruits and Career Soldiers..60
        Athletes 62
                Age in Large Series Including All Events 62
                Age and Location of the Stress Fracture 63
Age As a Risk Factor for Stress Fractures in Sports and Ballet..........................63
    Track and Field...63
    Running...64
    Ballet...65
Conclusions..65
References...66

INTRODUCTION

Most stress fractures have been shown to occur in adolescents or young adults engaged in competitive or recreational sports, ballet and other dancing, or basic military training.[9,11,15,40,54,59,72] However, there is a lack of valid epidemiological data pertaining to stress fracture incidence and prevalence in the general community.[9] Most athletic data originate from case or case series reports collected from populations with widely differing participation in various events. In those reports, often only the mean age of the whole group or the mean age of each gender is reported. The division into age groups has been variable, making comparison of the studies difficult.

An increasing number of prospective military and athletic cohort studies now evaluate the effect of age with multivariate analysis.[4,6,10,35,48,79,96,106,108]. These studies have provided us with more reliable information about stress fractures than the case series did. Conclusive evidence that age is important in stress fracture risk has not been given, however. Two recent reviews on the epidemiology of stress fractures and risk factors associated with them concluded only that age may be a risk factor for stress fractures.[9,11]

The role of age will be analyzed here in two ways. Stress fractures will be described according to specific age categories, then age as a risk factor for stress fractures in sports and ballet will be examined.

STRESS FRACTURES IN SPECIFIC AGE CATEGORIES

Children, Age 0 to 6 Years

Stress fractures are rare in healthy children under 7 years of age except for stress fractures of the tibia and fibula.[26,104] Recently increased physical activity, pathological hyperactivity, or a hyperkinetic neurological syndrome is usually the cause of stress fractures, but there are cases in which no etiological explanation can be found.[26,81,82] The most common stress fracture is stress fracture of the tibia. It is always located in the proximal third. A typical radiological finding is early and abundant callus, resembling in some cases osteosarcoma or chronic osteomyelitis.[26,28,32,104,110,124] In the fibula, the proximal third is nearly always affected.[26] The fibula may sustain a stress fracture at a younger age than any other bone. It has been described in 1 to 2 year-old infants after violent kicking or walker use.[26,65,107] Stress fractures of the metatarsals, tarsal bones, femur, or pelvis are uncommon in this age cohort.[18,26,103,109,114].

Stress Fractures in Older Children and Early Adolescents, Age 7 to 15 Years

The peak incidence of stress fractures in 7 to 15 year-old children occurs between 10 and 15 years, a time when the children become increasingly involved with organized sports.[2,23,25,52,76,86] In the U.S. more than half of boys and one quarter of girls in the 8 to 16 year-old range are engaged in some type of competitive sport.[86] Overuse injuries of all types are increasingly reported in this age group mainly because of increased training and competition levels.[97] There are also patients in this age group who sustain stress fractures without a history of competitive sports.[104] Stress fractures are not as common in this age group as in later adolescence and adulthood. The amount and intensity of training is significantly less in running and other track and

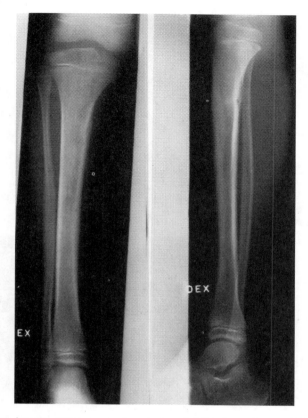

Figure 1 Stress fracture of the proximal posteromedial tibia in an 8 year old boy.

field events for these children,[52] and ground reaction forces are less during running and jumping due to lighter body weight. The bones are more compliant, and their capacity for remodeling and healing is greater than in adults.[63,73,110,111]

In a review of 23 published reports of stress fractures in children under 14 years old the most common sites were the tibia (51%), fibula (20%), pars interarticularis (15%), femur (3%), metatarsals (2%) and tarsal navicular (2%).[123] Stress fractures of the femur have been reported to comprise about 10% of all fractures.[76,118] The main difference when compared with adults is the greater number of pars interarticularis stress fractures, and the much smaller number of metatarsal and tarsal stress fractures. The posterior upper or lower thirds of the tibia are usually affected in prepubescent children (Figure 1).[26,89]

Isthmic spondylolysis (Figure 2) is present in 5 to 6% of the population. This is a fatigue fracture of the pars interarticularis of the lumbar vertebrae. Its incidence increases from less than 1% in children 5 years of age to 4.5% in children 7 years of age. The remaining 0.8 to 1% occurs between ages 11 and 16 years, presumably caused by athletic activity.[122] The highest incidence, 11%, has been found in young female gymnasts, in whom stress fractures of the lumbosacral spine accounted for 45% of all stress fractures.[27]

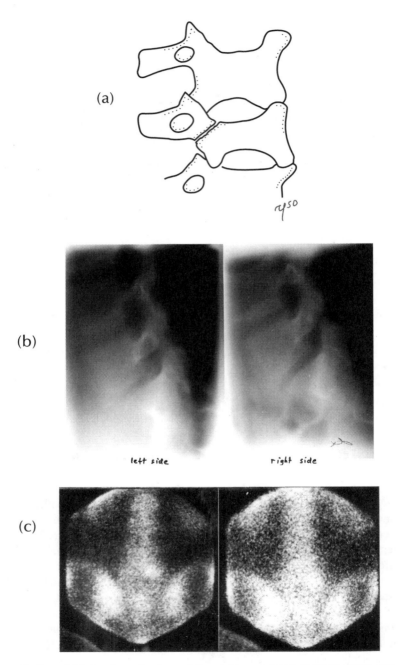

Figure 2 Spondylolytic stress fracture of the right pars interarticularis of the fifth lumbar vertebra. a. In a schematic drawing the stress fracture is shown in an oblique view as a collar on scotty dog's neck. b. In tomography the defect is seen on the right side (right picture). Left pars is intact (left picture). c. Isotope scan shows increased uptake on the right side.

Epiphyseal stress fractures are rare, but do occur.[74] They have been described in the proximal humerus,[13,21] medial epicondyle,[43] olecranon,[3,115] distal radius,[98,101] femoral head,[105] distal femur,[39] and proximal tibia.[22] They are rare compared with apophyseal overuse injuries.[1,105] In a series of 60 young gymnasts, only five showed stress-related changes in the distal radial growth plate.[19] The evidence in female gymnasts supports the plausibility of stress-related distal radial physeal arrest with secondary ulna radial length difference.[20]

Stress Fractures in Late Adolescence, Age 16 to 19 Years

The first athletic stress fracture was reported by Pirker in 1934.[95] The patient was an adolescent 18-year-old skier, swimmer, and handball player who suffered a transverse stress fracture of the femoral shaft during a training session. Adolescent athletes usually suffer less frequently than adults from overuse injuries,[88] but it has been claimed that the relative frequency of stress fractures in this age group is higher than in children and adults.[52,111] This is reflected in the remarkably low mean age (19 to 21 years) of athletes in several large athletic series. In a Finnish series of 368 athletic stress fractures,[54] there were 117 (31.8%) stress fractures in 16 to 19-year-old adolescents. The adolescent middle and long distance runners ran distances which did not differ significantly from those of adult runners. The adolescents ran 98.4 ± 31.5 km/week, and the adults ran 111.6 ± 49.7 km/week. It is likely that the training programs were not adequately tailored to the needs of this age group. In a Canadian study, the peak age for injured middle distance runners was in the 10 to 19-year-old group, with declining numbers in the older categories (20 to 29, 30 to 39 and ≥40 years).[69] In epidemiological studies of basketball, soccer, and Australian football, adolescents sustained an equal or greater amount of stress fractures as adults in the highest competitive level.[47,84,94] The incidence of stress fractures in young female basketball players seems to be increasing.[47]

The highest incidence of spondylolysis stress fracture of the pars interarticularis has been found in adolescents.[41] Low back pain in young athletes (mean age 15.8 years) was ascribed to this in about 50% of the cases.[77] Frequency is highest in athletes who perform movements involving repeated flexion and extension of the spine. Sports associated with pars interarticularis stress fracture are gymnastics, hockey, handball, soccer, weight lifting, and running.[27,41,45,66,120] Other stress fractures frequently seen in this age group are stress fractures of the toes (Figure 3),[91] patella,[93] and diaphyseal stress fractures of the humerus, radius, and ulna.[16,99,112]

The structural properties of the long bones vary with age and gender and are largely dependent on body size. In late adolescence the development of bones, ligaments, and muscles is still incomplete. Peak bone mass and strength are not reached until the early 20's.[83] The bones have not yet attained their peak mass or maximal length, size, width, cross-sectional area, and cross-sectional moment of inertia, which seem to be important in determining the risk of stress fractures.[24,78,83] It has been shown in human experimental studies that strain rates in the tibia, which may be causal for stress fracture, increase after fatigue with a greater increase in young as opposed to older persons.[34]

The muscles have not yet achieved their maximal strength, and there may be ligamentous laxity and muscle tightness predisposing to stress injuries.[48,67] Other

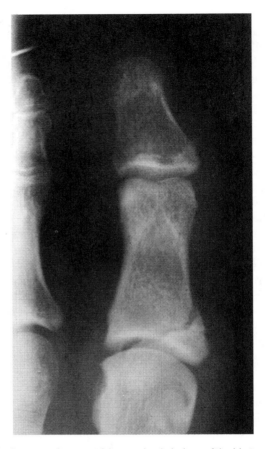

Figure 3   Intra-articular stress fracture of the proximal phalanx of the big toe in a 15 year-old girl.

factors, such as nutritional factors and hormonal status, may also explain a possible relationship between age and stress fracture risk.[11,83,119] The occurrence of stress fractures in females during late adolescence has a positive correlation with late menarche and menstrual disturbances (see Chapter 3). [5]

Adults, (≥20 Years)

Military Recruits and Career Soldiers

One population at very high risk for stress fractures is military recruits, who during their 1 to 4 month-long basic training period become exposed to vigorous physical activity, to which they often are not accustomed in civilian life. This training period has been used as a human laboratory in which it is possible to control external training factors and nutritional factors.

The mean age of the populations in some of the major cohort studies in which stress fracture incidence of the recruits has been studied varies from 18.4 to

20.2 years.[14,35,37,38,59] (Military recruits are often 17-19-years-old and belong to the late adolescent group, but for the sake of clarity the whole military population is discussed here.) Service in the armed forces is voluntary in the U.S., while it is compulsory in Israel. This is reflected by a greater age variation in the U.S. studies.

The influence of age on the occurrence of stress fractures in military populations has remained a controversial issue. There are three major studies which indicate that the risk for stress fractures increases with age.[14,35,59] Gardner et al.[35] carried out a prospective controlled study to determine the usefulness of an insole to prevent stress fractures. The median age for men was 19 years, and for women 20 years. The relative risk for stress fractures in the age group 18 to 20 years old (n = 2074) was 1.01, while it was 1.82 in the group 21 years and older (n = 934). When adjusted for previous physical activity, the relative risk for older recruits was 1.71.

Brudvig et al.[14] collected retrospective data on 339 stress fractures occurring in 295 army trainees in a training population of 20,422 trainees. The average age of male trainees developing stress fractures was 20.58 ± 4.53 years, and the average age of female trainees developing stress fractures was 22.46 ± 3.46 years. The rate of incidence was 1.27 in the age group 17 to 22 years, 2.32 in the age group 23 to 28 years, and 5.01 in the age group 29 to 34 years. The authors concluded that age is a factor in the development of stress fractures.

Jones et al.[59] followed 303 infantry recruits with a mean age of 20.2 ± 3.1 years and a median age of 19 years (17 to 35 years) for the 12-week basic training period. The relative risks for various factors related to stress fractures were evaluated with a logistic regression model. The relative risk for recruits under 24 years was 1.0, while it was 4.3 for those 24 years old and older. The trend of increasing risk with increasing age was significant ($p < 0.05$).

In contrast, there are military studies that argue against the hypothesis that stress fracture incidence increases with age. Winfield et al.[121] studied female officer candidates (ages 20 to 27 years). Younger individuals (<23 years) had a higher rate of bone stress reactions ($p < 0.01$). In a prospective cohort study by Milgrom and colleagues,[79] in the Israeli army the age of the recruits ranged from 17 to 26 years. For each year of increase in age from 17 to 26 years, the risk for stress fracture at all sites decreased by 28%. The authors suggested that the decreasing risk with age may be related to increased structural maturity, increased bone density, larger cross-sectional moment of inertia, or changes in bone quality in the older recruits. The number of recruits over the age of 19 was very small in this study.

There appear to be at least four explanations for the conflicting results:

1. The populations studied were different in age and pre-training physical condition. The results in studies carried out by Brudvig et al.[14] and Gardner et al.[35] may simply reflect lower fitness levels and higher body fat in older military trainees.[80]
2. The training methods and length of basic training periods were not similar.
3. The diagnostic methods varied. In U.S. studies the diagnosis was usually confirmed with radiographs, while in Israel bone scan was used.
4. The statistical methods varied from classical t– and Chi square tests in older studies to advanced multivariate analysis in the more recent studies. Brudvig's study[14] was retrospective, while the other studies were prospective.

In several recent prospective studies of stress fracture risk in military recruits using multivariate analysis, there was no association with age and stress fracture incidence. Evidence was found of other significant risk factors, i.e., small body dimension, small diaphyseal dimension of the tibia and femur relative to body weight, malalignment and length differences of the lower extremity, poor strength of the lower leg muscles, poor fitness, poor training procedures, and training in specific subunits.[4,33,38,48,96,106,108]

Jones states[61] that stress fracture incidence is lower with increasing age in career soldiers. The conclusion is based upon data of U.S. infantry soldiers and mixed groups of soldiers showing a declining trend for injuries with increasing age. Professional soldiers usually are in very good physical condition and in this respect they resemble well-conditioned runners. On the other hand, career soldiers are not exposed to sudden stress increases as are recruits.

Athletes

Age in Large Series Including All Events

Stress fractures in runners became a common stress injury in the 1970s.[55,87,74] By the 1980s up to 10% of injuries in sports medicine practices were stress fractures.[58] More recent reports of the distribution of stress fractures in various sports events indicate that the greatest percentage of stress fractures among civilians still occurs in young track and field athletes, especially runners, hurdlers, and jumpers.[6,36,40,54,72] The only exception among some representative series (Table 1) is the series from Seoul, South Korea, in which volleyball was the most common event.[44]

In a Finnish series representing all events and age categories, 59.5% of the stress fractures occurred in adults (≥20 years).[52] The mean patient age varies in some large case series from 19 to 30 years depending on the athletic population from which the case series has been collected.[6,15,29,31,36,42,44,54,64,72,74,88,102,116] The most important factor determining the mean age is the distribution between competitive and recreational athletes in the series.[52,56,57,72] The mean age of the competitive track and field athletes is usually a little over 20 years, while the mean age of recreational runners is over 30 years. Table 1 also shows that the mean age of the male athletes is higher than the mean age of the females. Women have a greater proportion of injuries presenting at a younger age[52,69] This is partly due to demographic factors, but there are also biologic factors explaining the phenomenon. Bennell et al.[5] found that female athletes

Table 1   Large Athletic Series Including All Events: Age and Sex

Reference	Sample Size	Males/ Females	Average Age (yrs)	Average Age, Male	Average Age, Female
Matheson et al., Canada[72]	320	145/175	26.7	29.2	25.1
Hulkko, Finland[52]	368	271/97	22.4	23.3 ± 7.1	20.0 ± 5.4
Brukner et al., Australia[15]	180	102/78	21.8		
Geyer et al., Germany[36]	70	42/28	22.6 ± 6.6		
Ha et al., South Korea[44]	131	68/63	21.3	22.6	20.2

Table 2   Age and Location of the Athletic Stress Fractures (8 Finnish Studies)

Location	Sample Size	Males/ Females	Average Age (yrs)	Average Age/Males	Average Age, Females
Patella[93]	5	2/3	21.2	23.5	19.7
Tibia[53]	182	139/43	21.1		
Fibula[53]	44	40/4	23.6		
Anterior mid-tibia[90]	17	12/5	25.7 ±7.4	27.6 ±7.6	21.2 ±4.4
Medial malleolus[92]	8	7/1	28.0 ±13.5	23.4 ±4.1	60
Navicular[51]	9	6/3	19.7 ±1.5	19.8 ±1.2	19.3 ±2.3
Fifth metatarsal[49]	11	8/3	24.3		
Sesamoid bones[50]	15	9/6	22.3 ±4.1	24.4 ±3.6	20.1 ±3.7
Toe bones[49]	8	5/3	19.5 ±6.9	21.8 ±7.1	15.7 ±1.4
All cases	299	226/71	21.9		

with history of stress fracture are more likely to have hormonal and nutritional disturbances than those without history of stress fracture (see Chapter 3).

Age and Location of the Stress Fracture

Matheson et al.[72] found significantly more femoral and tarsal stress fractures in older athletes and more tibial and fibular stress fractures in younger athletes; however, an interaction between age and site was not confirmed in another large series.[54] In a review of the literature, Khan[64] found that the mean age of the athletes with stress fracture of the tarsal navicular was 20.5 years. Eight Finnish case series of different stress fracture locations collected from a total material of 600 athletic stress fractures from 1971 to 1995 (Table 2)[93,90,92,51,50,91,53,49] show that stress fractures of the toes, tarsal navicular, and posteromedial tibia are more common in younger athletes. The distribution of these fractures among the various sports events follows a common pattern, i.e., the majority occur in runners. Two Swedish studies indicate that stress fractures of the femoral neck and anterior mid-tibia are more often found in older runners.[56,57] In contrast, the mean age for stress fractures of the anterior mid-tibia in a series of basketball players was only 19 years.[100]

AGE AS A RISK FACTOR FOR STRESS FRACTURES IN SPORTS AND BALLET

Track and Field

An athletic stress fracture study group from Melbourne, Australia has provided us during the last five years with many interesting results about the epidemiology of stress fractures in track and field athletes. In their studies the group has used both retrospective and prospective cohort designs, and their results thus may be epidemiologically more valid than most earlier reports.

In a prospective study over 12 months, the incidence and distribution of stress fractures were evaluated in 53 female and 56 male competitive track and field athletes at club, state, or national levels. The age range was 17 to 26 years; the mean age for women was 20.5 ± 2.2 years and for men 20.3 ± 2.0 years.[6] The incidence of stress fractures was 21.1% during the study. Age of menarche and calf girth were the best independent predictors of stress fractures in women. No risk factor was able to predict the occurrence of stress fractures in men. There was no age difference between female or male stress fracture and non–stress fracture groups.

A prospective study was done to evaluate bone turnover in 46 female and 49 male track and field athletes aged 17 to 26 years (mean age 20.3 ± 2.0), 20 of whom developed a stress fracture. The mean age of the female athletes with stress fractures was 20.6 ± 1.8 years, and the mean age of the male athletes with stress fractures 20.3 ± 1.5 years. There was no significant difference in age in either sex when comparing the group who sustained stress fractures with the group who did not.[10]

In a retrospective cohort study, Bennell and Crossley[7] evaluated the musculo-skeletal injuries in 95 track and field athletes recruited from a number of athletic clubs in the Melbourne metropolitan region. The most common diagnoses were stress fractures (21%) and hamstring strains (14%). There was no association between age and the risk of developing an injury in the 17 to 26 year range. The older athletes were more likely to sustain multiple injuries. Athletes had commenced training for track and field at 10.7 ± 5.7 years of age.

Several studies have shown that the mean age of marathon and long distance runners who sustain stress fractures is significantly higher than the mean age of the sprinters and middle distance runners.[52,68,69]

Running

The term runner refers not only to a competitive runner but also to a recreational runner logging high mileage on a nearly daily basis. In a large Canadian series of running injuries[69] there were 89% recreational runners and only 11% competitive track and field and marathon runners. The more serious recreational runners often take part in marathon or other long distance or terrain races. The term jogger applies to low mileage runners who run more intermittently.[12,55] Most runners are 25 to 44 years of age, but the number of runners 45 and older is increasing.[71]

The mean age of the recreational runners with stress fractures varies in different series from 36 to 46 years.[12,52,56,72] The mean age of males is about 40 years and the mean age of females about 30 years.[17,56,113] Brunet and al.[17] showed in their study that there was not an age–related decline in miles run per week. Women runners tended to increase mileage with age from 21 to 25 miles per week. Running pace showed a steady decline with increasing age for men and women.

Many studies of stress fracture risk in running populations report either no age effect[12,17] or a decreased risk with age.[69,71] Marti et al.[71] suggested that this is a sign of better adaptation to running on the biomechanical and/or biological levels. They also found a decrease of interruptions due to running injuries with increasing years of regular training. In contrast, it has been suggested that injuries in the earlier years select out those athletes not suited to continue training into middle age.[7]

Ballet

Ballet dancers are at a relatively high risk for stress fractures of the metatarsals and tibia.[9,11,62] 30% of female dancers and 20% of male dancers have experienced stress fractures.[46] Ballet and aerobics may cause hormonal disturbances in the same way as endurance running. Increased training time and menstrual irregularities are associated with an increased incidence in stress fractures.[62] Kadel et.al.[62] found no correlation between age and incidence of stress fractures in ballet dancers. In contrast, Hamilton et al.[46] found that stress fracture rates were significantly higher in both male and female dancers who entered the ballet company at a later age.

CONCLUSIONS

Many prospective studies conclude that age is not an important factor in the etiology of stress fractures. Stress fractures may occur at all ages, but the peak incidence is found in late adolescence and early adulthood. The most common stress fractures in all age categories are stress fractures of the tibia and fibula. Reports in the literature indicate that age is an important factor in determining the location of stress fractures in the upper and lower extremities and the spine.

There are a number of factors which may change the current epidemiological picture. Universal military service is disappearing in many countries and the number of stress fractures in military recruits is decreasing at the same time. Professional soldiers are usually well conditioned and their risk for stress fractures is less than the risk in recruits.[61] Prevention techniques are more widely used in military and athletic populations (see Chapters 15 to 17). At the same time, the intensity of training in sports in general, and in top level and professional athletes especially, continues to increase. In many events it is now possible to compete throughout the year, which puts higher demands on bone strength.[36] The participation of children and adolescents in organized, competitive sports is increasing globally,[2,23,44] and in some events the top performers are children or adolescents. There are also sudden trend changes in participation and adoption of new sports events for children, adolescents, and even adults.[70] It takes several years before the picture of overuse injuries in a new event becomes clear. The same applies if the basic style is radically changed, which happened in cross-country skiing in the 1970s.

Participation of middle-aged and older people in recreational and competitive sports is also increasing. There are athletes over 40 in endurance and other events who belong to the absolute world elite. It becomes increasingly difficult to distinguish between stress or fatigue fractures and insufficiency fractures in middle-aged and older people. Osteoporotic insufficiency fractures are a serious threat to aging female athletes, especially runners, if they begin their sports at age 50 or older.[11,75] These athletes should have bone density measurements performed before starting a training regime.

REFERENCES

1. Apple, D.F., Jr., Adolescent runners, *Clin. Sports Med.*, 4, 641, 1985.
2. Backx, F.J.G., Beijer, H.J.M., Bol, E., and Erich, W.B.M., Injuries in high-risk persons and high-risk sports. A longitudinal study of 1818 school children, *Am. J. Sports Med.*, 19, 124, 1991.
3. Banas, M.P. and Lewis, R.A., Nonunion of an olecranon epiphyseal plate stress fracture in an adolescent, *Orthopedics*, 18, 1111, 1995.
4. Beck, T.J., Ruff, C.B., Mourtada, F.A., Shaffer, R.A., Maxwell-Williams, K., Kao, G.L., Sartoris, D.J., and Brodine, S., Dual-energy X-ray absorptiometry derived structural geometry for stress fracture prediction in male U.S. Marine Corps recruits, *J. Bone Miner. Res.*, 11, 645, 1996.
5. Bennell, K.L., Malcolm, S.A., Thomas, S.A., Ebeling, P.R., McCrory, P.R., Wark, J.D., and Brukner, P.D., Risk factors for stress fractures in female track-and-field athletes: a retrospective analysis, *Clin. J. Sport Med.*, 5, 229, 1995.
6. Bennell, K.L., Malcolm, S.A., Thomas, S.A., Wark, J.D., and Brukner, P.D., The incidence and distribution of stress fractures in competitive track and field athletes. A twelve-month prospective study, *Am. J. Sports Med.*, 24, 211, 1996.
7. Bennell, K.L. and Crossley, K., Musculoskeletal injuries in track and field: incidence, distribution and risk factors, *Aust. J. Sci. Med. Sport*, 28, 69, 1996.
8. Bennell, K.L., Malcolm, S.A., Thomas, S.A., Reid, S.J., Brukner, P.D., Ebeling, P.R., and Wark, J.D., Risk factors for stress fractures in track and field athletes, *Am. J. Sports Med.*, 24, 810, 1996.
9. Bennell, K.L. and Brukner, P.D., Epidemiology and site specificity of stress fractures, *Clin. Sports Med.*, 16, 179, 1997.
10. Bennell, K.L., Malcolm, S.A., Brukner, P.D.,Green, R.M., Hopper, J.L., Wark, J.D., and Ebeling, P.R., A 12-month prospective study of the relationship between stress fractures and bone turnover in athletes, *Calcif. Tissue Int.*, 63, 80, 1998.
11. Bennell, K.L., Matheson, G., Meeuwisse, W., and Brukner, P.D., Risk factors for stress fractures, *Sports Med.*, 28, 91, 1999.
12. Blair, S.N., Kohl, H.W., and Goodyear, N.N., Rates and risks for running and exercise injuries: studies in three populations, *Res. Q. Exerc. Sport*, 58, 221, 1987.
13. Boyd, K.T. and Batt, M.E., Stress fracture of the proximal humeral epiphysis in an elite junior badminton player, *Br. J. Sports Med.*, 31, 252, 1997.
14. Brudvig, T.J.S., Gudger, T.D., and Obermeyer, L., Stress fractures in 295 trainees. A one-year study of incidence as related to age, sex and race, *Mil. Med.*, 148, 666, 1983.
15. Brukner, P., Bradshaw, C., Khan, K.M., White, S., and Crossley, K., Stress fractures: a review of 180 cases, *Clin. J. Sport Med.*, 6, 85, 1996.
16. Brukner, P., Stress fractures of the upper limb, *Sports Med.*, 26, 415, 1998.
17. Brunet, M.E., Cook, S.D., Brinker, M.R., and Dickinson, J.A., A survey of running injuries in 1505 competitive and recreational runners, *J. Sports Med. Phys. Fitness*, 30, 307, 1990.
18. Buckley, S.L., Robertson, W.W., Jr., and Shalaby-Rana, E., Stress fractures of the femoral diaphysis in young children. A report of 2 cases, *Clin. Orthop.*, 310, 165, 1995.
19. Caine, D., Roy, S., Singer, K.M., and Broekhoff, J., Stress changes of the distal radial growth plate. A radiographic survey and review of the literature, *Am. J. Sports Med.*, 20, 290, 1992.
20. Caine, D., Howe, W., Ross, W., and Bergman, G., Does repetitive physical loading inhibit radial growth in female gymnasts? *Clin. J. Sports Med.*, 7, 302, 1997.

21. Cahill, B.R., Tullos, H.S., and Fain, R.H., Little League shoulder, *J. Sports Med.*, 2, 150, 1974.

22. Cahill, B.R., Stress fracture of the proximal tibial epiphysis: a case report, *Am. J. Sports Med.*, 5, 186, 1977.

23. Coady, C.M. and Micheli, L.J., Stress fractures in the pediatric athlete, *Clin. Sports Med.*, 16, 225, 1997.

24. Crossley, K., Bennell, K.L., Wrigley, T., and Oakes, B.W., Ground reaction forces, bone characteristics, and tibial stress fracture in male runners, *Med. Sci. Sports Exerc.*, 31, 1088, 1999.

25. DeLee, J. and Farney, W.C., Incidence of injury in Texas high school football, *Am. J. Sports Med.*, 20, 575, 1992.

26. Devas, M.B., Stress fractures in children, *J. Bone Jt. Surg.*, 45(B), 528, 1963.

27. Dixon, M. and Fricker, P., Injuries to elite gymnasts over 10 yr, *Med. Sci. Sports Exerc.*, 25, 1322, 1993.

28. Donati, R.B., Echo, B.S., and Powell, C.E., Bilateral tibial stress fractures in a six-year-old male. A case report, *Am. J. Sports Med.*, 18, 323, 1990.

29. Dowey, K.E. and Moore, G.W., Stress fractures in athletes, *Ulster Med. J.*, 53, 121, 1984.

30. Egol, K.A., Koval, K.J., Kummer, F., and Frankel, V.H., Stress fractures of the femoral neck, *Clin. Orthop.*, 348, 72, 1998.

31. Ekenman, I., The stress fractures in athletes — an investigation of possible predisposing factors, thesis, Karolinska Institutet, Stockholm, 1998.

32. Engh, C.A., Robinson, R.A., and Milgram, J., Stress fractures in children, *J. Trauma*, 10, 532, 1970.

33. Finestone, A., Shlamkovitch, N., Eldad, A., Wosk, J., Laor, A., Danon, Y.L., and Milgrom, C., Risk factors for stress fractures among Israeli infantry recruits, *Mil. Med.*, 156, 528, 1991.

34. Fyhrie, D.P., Milgrom, C., Hoshaw, S.J., Simkin, A., Dar, S., Drumb, D., and Burr, D.B., Effect of fatiguing exercise on longitudinal bone strain as related to stress fracture in humans, *Ann. Biomed. Eng.*, 26, 660, 1998.

35. Gardner, L.I., Dziados, J.E., Jones, B.H., Brundage, J.F., Harris, J.M., Sullivan, G., and Gill, P., Prevention of lower extremity stress fractures: a controlled trial of shock absorbent insole, *Am. J. Publ. Health*, 78, 1563, 1988.

36. Geyer, M., Sander-Beuermann, A., Wegner, U., and Wirth, C.J., Stressreaktionen und stressfrakturen beim leistungssportler. ursachen, diagnostik und therapie, *Unfallchirurg*, 96, 66, 1993.

37. Giladi, M., Ahronson, Z., Stein, M., Danon, Y.L., and Milgrom, C., Unusual distribution and onset of stress fractures in soldiers, *Clin. Orthop.*, 192, 142, 1985.

38. Giladi, M., Milgrom, C., Simkin, A., and Danon Y., Stress fractures. Identifiable risk factors, *Am. J. Sports Med.*, 19, 647, 1991.

39. Godshall, R.W., Hansen, C.A., and Rising, D.C., Stress fractures through the distal femoral epiphysis, *Am. J. Sports Med.*, 9, 114, 1981.

40. Goldberg, B. and Pecora, C., Stress fractures. A risk of increased training in freshmen, *Physician Sportsmed.*, 22, 68, 1994.

41. Goldstein, J.D., Berger, P.E., Windler, G.E., and Jackson, D.W., Spine injuries in gymnasts and swimmers. An epidemiological investigation, *Am. J. Sports Med.*, 19, 463, 1991.

42. Graff, K.H. and Krahl, H., Überlastungschäden im fussbereich beim leichtathleten, *Leichtathletik*, 24, 81, 1984.

43. Gugenheim, J.J., Jr., Stanley, R.F., Woods, G.W., and Tullos, H.S., Little League survey: the Houston study, *Am. J. Sports Med.*, 4, 189, 1976.

44. Ha, K.I., Hahn, S.H., Chung, M., Yang, B.K., and Yi, S.R., A clinical study of stress fractures in sports activities, *Orthopedics*, 14, 1089, 1991.

45. Halvorsen, T.M., Nilsson, S., and Nakstad, P.H., Stress fractures. Spondylolysis and spondylolisthesis of the lumbar vertebrae among young athletes with back pain, *Tidsskr. Nor. Laegeforen.*, 116, 1999, 1996.

46. Hamilton, L.H., Hamilton, W.G., Meltzer, J.D., Marshall, P., and Molnar, M., Personality, stress and injuries in professional ballet dancers, *Am. J. Sports Med.*, 17, 263, 1989.

47. Hickey, G.J., Fricker, P.A., and McDonald, W.A., Injuries of young elite female basketball players over a six-year period, *Clin. J. Sport Med.*, 7, 252, 1997.

48. Hoffman, J.R., Chapnik, L., Shamis, A., Givon, U., and Davidson, B., The effect of leg strength on the incidence of lower extremity overuse injuries during military training, *Mil. Med.*, 164, 153, 1999.

49. Hulkko, A., Orava, S., and Nikula, P., Stress fracture of the fifth metatarsal in athletes, *Ann. Chir. Gyn.*, 74, 233, 1985.

50. Hulkko, A., Orava, S., Pellinen, P., and Puranen, J., Stress fractures of the sesamoid bones of the first metatarsophalangeal joint in athletes, *Arch. Orthop. Trauma Surg.*, 104, 113, 1985.

51. Hulkko, A., Orava, S., Peltokallio, P., Tulikoura, I., and Walden, M., Stress fracture of the navicular bone, *Acta Orthop. Scand.*, 56, 503, 1985.

52. Hulkko, A., Stress fractures in athletes. A clinical study of 368 cases, thesis, University of Oulu, Oulu, 1988.

53. Hulkko, A., Alén, M., and Orava, S., Stress fractures of the lower leg, *Scand. J. Sports Med.*, 9, 1, 1987.

54. Hulkko, A. and Orava, S., Stress fractures in athletes, *Int. J. Sports Med.*, 8, 221, 1987.

55. James, S.L., Bates, B.T., and Osternig, L.R., Injuries to runners, *Am. J. Sports Med.*, 6, 40, 1978.

56. Johansson, C., Ekenman, I., Törnkvist, H., and Eriksson, E., Stress fractures of the femoral neck in athletes. The consequence of a delay in diagnosis, *Am. J. Sports Med.*, 18, 524, 1990.

57. Johansson, C., Ekenman, I., and Lewander, R., Stress fracture of the tibia in athletes: diagnosis and natural course, *Scand. J. Med. Sci. Sports*, 2, 87, 1992.

58. Jones, B.H., Harris, J., Vinh, T.N., and Rubin, C., Exercise induced stress fractures and stress reactions of bone: epidemiology, etiology and classification, *Exerc. Sports Sci. Rev.*, 17, 379, 1989.

59. Jones, B.H., Cowan, D.N., Tomlinson, J.P., Robinson, J.R., Polly, D.W., and Frykman, P.N., Epidemiology of injuries associated with physical training among young men in the army, *Med. Sci. Sports Exerc.*, 25, 197, 1993.

60. Jones, B.H., Bovee, M.W., Harris, J. McA., III, and Cowan, D.N., Intrinsic risk factors for exercise-related injuries among male and female army trainees, *Am. J. Sports Med.*, 21, 705, 1993.

61. Jones, B.H. and Knapik, J.J., Physical training and exercise-related injuries, *Sports Med.*, 27, 111, 1999.

62. Kadel, N.J., Teitz, C.C., and Kronmal, R.A., Stress fractures in ballet dancers, *Am. J. Sports Med.*, 20, 445, 1992.

63. Keller, T.S., Lovin, J.D., Spengler, D.M., and Carter, D.R., Fatigue of immature baboon cortical bone, *J. Biomech.*, 18, 297, 1985.

64. Khan, K.M., Brukner, P.D., Kearney, C., Fuller, P.J., Bradshaw, C.J., and Kiss, Z.S., Tarsal navicular stress fracture in athletes, *Sports Med.*, 17, 65, 1994.

65. Kozlowski, K. and Urbanoviciene, A., Stress fractures of the fibula in the first few years of life (report of six cases), *Australas. Radiol.*, 40, 261, 1996.

66. Letts, M., Smallman, T., Afanasiev, R., and Gouw, G., Fracture of the pars interarticularis in adolescent athletes: a clinical-biomechanical analysis, *J. Ped. Orthop.*, 46, 40, 1986.

67. Lysens, R.J., Ostyn, M.S., Auweele, Y.V., Lefevre, J., Vuylsteke, M., and Renson, L., The accident-prone and overuse-prone profiles of the young athlete, *Am. J. Sports Med.*, 17, 612, 1989.

68. Lysholm, J. and Wiklander, J., Injuries in runners, *Am. J. Sports Med.*, 15, 168, 1987.

69. MacIntyre, J.G., Taunton, J.E., Clement, D.B., Lloyd-Smith, D.R., McKenzie, D.C., and Morrell, R.W., Running injuries: a clinical study of 4,173 cases, *Clin. J. Sports Med.*, 1, 81, 1991.

70. Maitra, R.S. and Johnson, D.L., Stress fractures. Clinical history and physical examination, *Clin. Sports Med.*, 16, 259, 1997.

71. Marti, B., Vader, J.P., Minder, C., and Abelin, T., On the epidemiology of running injuries. The 1984 Bern Grand-Prix study, *Am. J. Sports Med.*, 16, 285, 1988.

72. Matheson, G., Clement, D.B., McKenzie, D.C., Taunton, J.E., Lloyd-Smith, D.R., MacIntyre, J.G., Stress fractures in athletes. A Study of 320 cases, *Am. J. Sports Med.*, 15, 46, 1987.

73. Mauch, M., Currey, J.D., and Sedman, A.J., Creep fractures in bones with different stiffnesses, *J. Biomech.*, 25, 11, 1992.

74. McBryde, A.M., Jr., Stress fractures in runners, *Clin. Sports Med.*, 4, 737, 1985.

75. Menard, D. and Stanish, W.D., The aging athlete, *Am. J. Sports Med.*, 17, 187, 1989.

76. Micheli, L.J., Overuse injuries in children's sports: the growth factor, *Orthop. Clin. N. Am.*, 14, 337, 1983.

77. Micheli, L.J. and Wood, R., Back pain in young athletes. Significant differences from adults in causes and patterns, *Arch. Pediatr. Adolesc. Med.*, 149, 15, 1995.

78. Milgrom, C., Giladi, M., Simkin, A., Rand, N., Kedem, R., Kashtan, H., and Stein, M., An analysis of the biomechanical mechanism of tibial stress fractures among Israeli infantry recruits. A prospective study, *Clin. Orthop.*, 231, 216, 1988.

79. Milgrom, C., Finestone, A., Shlamkovitch, N., Youth is a risk factor for stress fracture: a study of 783 infantry recruits, *J. Bone Jt. Surg.*, 76(B), 20, 1994.

80. Monteleone, G.P., Jr., Stress fractures in the athlete, *Orthop. Clin. N. Am.*, 26, 423, 1995.

81. Moon, B.S., Price, C.T., and Campbell, J.B., Upper extremity and rib stress fractures in a child, *Skeletal Radiol.*, 27, 403, 1998.

82. Mucklow, E.S. and Evans, G., Stress fractures in a hyperactive 3-year-old girl, *Lancet*, 349, 854, 1997.

83. Nattiv, A. and Armsey, T.D., Jr., Stress injury to bone in the female athlete, *Clin. Sports Med.*, 16, 197, 1997.

84. Nielsen, A.B. and Yde, J., Epidemiology and traumatology of injuries in soccer, *Am. J. Sports Med.*, 17, 803, 1989.

85. Ogawa, K. and Yoshida, A., Throwing fracture of the humeral shaft. An analysis of 90 patients, *Am. J. Sports Med.*, 26, 242, 1998.

86. Omey, M.L. and Micheli, L.J., Foot and ankle problems in the young athlete, *Med. Sci. Sports Exerc.*, 31, S470, 1999.

87. Orava, S., Puranen, J. and Ala-Ketola, L., Stress fractures caused by physical exercise, *Acta Orthop. Scand.*, 49, 19, 1978.

88. Orava, S., Exertion injuries due to sports and physical exercise, thesis, University of Oulu, Oulu, 1980.

89. Orava, S., Jormakka, E., and Hulkko, A., Stress fractures in young athletes, *Arch. Orthop. Traumat. Surg.*, 98, 271, 1981.

90. Orava, S., Karpakka, J., Hulkko, A., Väänänen, K., Takala, T., Kallinen, M., and Alén, M., Diagnosis and treatment of stress fractures located at the mid-tibial shaft in athletes, *Int. J. Sports Med.*, 12, 419, 1991.

91. Orava, S., Hulkko, A., Taimela, S., Koskinen, S., Leppävuori, J., Kallio, T., and Karpakka, J., Stress fractures of the toe bones in athletes and military recruits, *Isr. J. Sports Med.*, 1, 151, 1994.

92. Orava, S., Karpakka, J., Taimela, S., Hulkko, A., Permi, J., and Kujala, U., Stress fracture of the medial malleolus, *J. Bone Jt. Surg.*, 77-A, 362, 1995.

93. Orava, S., Taimela, S., Kvist, M., Karpakka, J., Hulkko, A., and Kujala, U., Diagnosis and treatment of stress fracture of the patella in athletes, *Knee Surg. Sports Traumatol. Arthroscopy*, 4, 206, 1996.

94. Orchard, J., Wood, T., Seward, H., and Broad, A., Comparison of injuries in elite senior and junior Australian football, *J. Sci. Med. Sport*, 1, 83, 1998.

95. Pirker, H., Bruch der oberschenkeldiaphyse durch muskelzug, *Arch. Klin. Chir.*, 75, 155, 1934.

96. Pope, R.P., Herbert, R., Kirwan, J.D., and Graham, B.J., Predicting attrition in basic military training, *Mil. Med.*, 164, 710, 1999.

97. Powell, J.W., National High School Athletic Injury Registry, *Am. J. Sports Med.*, 16(1), 134, 1988.

98. Read, M.T.F., Stress fractures of the distal radius in adolescent gymnasts, *Br. J. Sports Med.*, 15, 272, 1981.

99. Rettig, A.C., Stress fracture of the ulna in an adolescent tournament tennis player, *Am. J. Sports Med.*, 11, 103, 1983.

100. Rettig, A.C., Shelbourne, K.D., McCarroll, J.R., et al., The natural history and treatment of delayed union stress fractures of the anterior cortex of the tibia, *Am. J. Sports Med.*, 16, 250, 1988.

101. Roy, S., Caine, D., and Singer, K.M., Stress changes of the distal radial epiphysis in young gymnasts, *Am. J. Sports Med.*, 13, 301, 1985.

102. Saunders, A.J.S., El Sayed, T.F., Hilson, A.J.W., Maisey, M.N., and Grahame, R., Stress lesions of the lower leg and foot, *Clin. Radiol.*, 30, 649, 1979.

103. Scheerlink, T. and De Boeck, H., Bilateral stress fractures of the femoral neck complicated by unilateral displacement in a child, *J. Pediatr. Orthop.*, 7, 246, 1998.

104. Schwendtner, P., Schneider, K., and Dietz, H.G., Stress fractures in childhood and adolescence, *Sportverletz. Sportschaden*, 10, 19, 1996.

105. Segesser, B., Morscher, E., and Goesele, A., Störungen der wachstumsfugen durch sportliche überlastung, *Orthopäde*, 24, 446, 1995.

106. Shaffer, R.A., Brodine, S.K., Almeida, S.A., Williams, K.M., and Ronaghy, S., Use of simple measures of physical activity to predict stress fractures in young men undergoing a rigorous physical training program, *Am. J. Epidemiol.*, 149, 236, 1999.

107. Sheehan, K.M., Gordon, S., and Tanz, R.R., Bilateral fibula fractures from infant walker use, *Pediatr. Emerg. Care*, 11, 27, 1995.

108. Shwayhat, A.F., Linenger, J.M., Hofherr, L.K., Slymen, D.J., and Johnson, C.W., Profiles of exercise history and overuse injuries among United States Navy Sea, Air and Land (SEAL) recruits, *Am. J. Sports Med.*, 24, 835, 1994.

109. St Pierre, P., Staheli, L.T., Smith, J.B., and Green, N.E., Femoral neck stress fractures in children and adolescents, *J. Pediatr. Orthop.*, 15, 470, 1995.

110. Tachdjian, M.O., Stress fractures, in *Pediatric Orthopedics,* Vol. 4, Tachdjian, M.O., Ed., W.B. Saunders, Philadelphia, 1990, 3359.

111. Taimela, S., Hulkko, A., Koskinen, S., and Orava, S., Stressfrakturen bei sportlern und militärrekruten, *Orthopäde,* 24, 457, 1995.

112. Tanabe, S., Nakahira, J., Bando, E., Yamaguchi, H., Miyamoto, H., and Yamamoto, A., Fatigue fracture of the ulna occurring in pitchers of fast-pitch softball, *Am. J. Sports Med.,* 19, 317, 1991.

113. Tomten, S.E., Prevalence of menstrual dysfunction in Norwegian long-distance runners participating in the Oslo Marathon games, *Scand. J. Med. Sci. Sports,* 6, 164, 1996.

114. Toren, A., Goshen, E., Katz, M., Levi, R., and Rechavi, G., Bilateral femoral stress fractures in a child due to in-line (roller) skating, *Acta Paediatr.,* 86, 332, 1997.

115. Torg, J.S. and Moyer, R.A., Non-union of a stress fracture through the olecranon epiphyseal plate observed in an adolescent baseball pitcher, *J. Bone Jt. Surg.,* 59(A), 264, 1977.

116. Torg, J.S., Pavlov, H., Cooley, L.H., Bryant, M.H., Arnoczky, S.P., Bergfeld, J., and Hunter, L.Y., Stress fractures of the tarsal navicular, *J. Bone Jt. Surg.,* 64(A), 700, 1982.

117. Tullos, H.S. and Fain, R.H., Rotational stress fracture of proximal humeral epiphysis, *Am. J. Sports Med.,* 2, 152, 1974.

118. Walker, R.N., Green, N.E., and Spindler, K.P., Stress fractures in skeletally immature patients, *J. Pediatr. Orthop.,* 16, 578, 1996.

119. Wiita, B.G. and Stombaugh, I.A., Nutrition knowledge, eating practices, and health of adolescent female runners: a 3-year longitudinal study, *Int. J. Sport,* 6, 414, 1996.

120. Wiltse, L.L., Widell, E.H., and Jackson, D.W., Fatigue fracture: the basic lesion in isthmic spondylolysis, *J. Bone Jt. Surg.,* 57(A), 17, 1975.

121. Winfield, A.C., Moore, J., Bracker, M., Johnson, C.W., Risk factors associated with stress reactions in female Marines, *Mil. Med.,* 162, 698, 1997.

122. Wood, G.W., II, Other disorders of spine, in *Campbell's Operative Orthopaedics,* Vol. 3, Mosby-Yearbook, St Louis, 1998, 3125.

123. Yngve, D.A., Stress fractures in the pediatric athlete, in *The Pediatric Athlete,* Sullivan, J.A. and Grana, W.A., Eds., American Academy of Orthopedic Surgeons, Park Ridge, IL, 1988, 235.

124. Zweymüller, K. and Frank, W., Ermüdungsbrüche der tibia in kindesalter, *Z. Orthop.,* 112, 450, 1974.

CHAPTER **5**

The Prediction of Stress Fractures

Thomas J. Beck

CONTENTS

Introduction 73
Bone Mineral Density and Stress Fracture 74
Why Are Some Bones Weaker Than Others? 75
    The Case for Bone Geometry 75
    The Case for Measuring Muscle 79
Can Stress Fracture Be Predicted? 80
    Technical Difficulties in Measurement of Bone and Muscle Properties 80
    Where to Measure: 81
Where Do We Go From Here? 81
References 82

INTRODUCTION

One clear message from studies on stress fracture incidence is that most individuals who undergo intense physical training programs will *not* suffer stress fractures. Those who do fracture must certainly have characteristics that increase their susceptibility. If those characteristics are measurable and differentiable from their non-fractured cohorts, then it should be possible to predict who among them is likely to suffer a stress fracture. Furthermore, if susceptibility characteristics are modifiable it may also be possible to prevent them from occurring. The purpose of this chapter is to examine, from a biomechanical perspective, what measurable differences have been demonstrated between fracture cases and controls and how best to measure those differences.

BONE MINERAL DENSITY AND STRESS FRACTURE

It is logical to surmise that stress fracture is a result of weak bones. Because osteoporosis is also a condition of diminished bone strength, similarities in susceptibility factors between stress fractures in young athletes and fragility fractures in the osteoporotic elderly may be relevant. Freidl and Nuovo[8] noted that U.S. Army women with a family history of osteoporosis were more likely to suffer stress fractures. The ethnicity pattern found in stress fractures (more likely among whites and Asians than among African-Americans) is similar to that of osteoporotic fractures in the elderly.[8,16] Bone densitometry, the assessment method used to determine osteoporotic fracture risk, may also be relevant in the exploration of stress fracture susceptibility. Bone densitometry has been used by a number of investigators to characterize strength differences between fracture cases and controls, but with mixed results.

In a prospective study of male Israeli Army recruits, Giladi et al. used single photon absorptiometry to measure bone mineral content (BMC) in the lower leg, 8 cm proximal to the ankle joint.[12] No differences were found between cases and controls at the measured cortical site. Pouilles and colleagues used dual photon absorptiometry (DPA) to measure hip bone mineral density (BMD) in a case/control study on young male military recruits. These authors did find lower BMDs, but only when cases and measurement sites were partitioned. For example, femoral stress fracture cases had lower femoral neck BMDs, and calcaneous fracture cases had lower trochanteric BMDs, but cases and controls with lower leg or metatarsal fractures showed no BMD differences.[23] In a case-control study of female U.S. Army recruits, Cline et al. found no significant differences in hip, spine, or forearm BMD, although the number of controls with BMD measurements was small (n = 13).[7] Bennell and colleagues conducted a retrospective case-control study of female track and field athletes using a total body dual energy x-ray absorptiometry (DXA) scan partitioned into regions to distinguish BMD at the lumbar spine, total lower limb, and tibia-fibula. They found lower BMDs in all regions among athletes with stress fractures, but none reached statistical significance.[5] In a later prospective study of male and female track and field athletes these investigators further refined the total body DXA method to partition the lower limb regions into femur, lower leg, and foot regions, averaged bilaterally. None of the male stress fracture cases had significantly lower BMD at any location, but among females, cases had lower total body BMCs and lower BMDs in the foot and lumbar spine regions. When tibial stress fracture cases were examined separately, lower BMDs were found in lower leg regions, although the differences were significant only in females. Finally, Lauder and colleagues matched 27 fracture cases with 158 controls among female Army recruits using DXA to measure BMD at the hip and spine. Using a multivariate analysis controlling for body size, exercise behavior, age, and other factors they found significantly lower femoral neck BMDs in fracture cases.[17]

Overall, the relationship between BMD and stress fracture incidence is equivocal and difficult to interpret. Some differences in results may be due to variations in measurement methodologies and measurement sites. Body size scaling may play a part, but the case may also be made that apparent strength differences are not reliably measured in a BMD measurement. While it is clear that lower density bones are a hallmark of osteoporotic fracture, it does not automatically follow that bone strength in otherwise healthy young individuals is a function of bone density. Even in the elderly, the relationship between BMD and osteoporotic fracture is entirely dependent upon statistical inference and not on any mechanical property of bone measured by BMD. Why two bones or any two structural members have different strengths is essentially an engineering issue and should be addressed from that context.

WHY ARE SOME BONES WEAKER THAN OTHERS?

Strength of a structure is dependent on its shape and dimensions (geometry), the properties of the material, and the loading conditions. Bone differs from other structures in that it is a live tissue that adapts its geometry over time to accommodate changing loading conditions.[9] In normal physical activities, skeletal loading in long bones is dominated by muscle-mediated bending forces.[6,11] Repetitive bending loads produce stresses that peak on subperiosteal surfaces, where stress fractures are thought to originate. Is there any evidence that stress fracture cases have weaker bone material properties or bone geometries that generate higher stresses? While ultrasonic methods show some theoretical promise, there are currently no reliable methods for measuring bone material properties *in vivo*.[1] Conceivably, dietary extremes or hormonal imbalances might produce exceptions, but there is no reason to suspect that normal young U.S. adults might have deficient bone tissue properties. There is, however, strong evidence showing that bones of stress fracture cases have geometric differences that should generate higher mechanical stresses. This evidence can also aid in explaining why BMD measurements are often equivocal.

The Case for Bone Geometry

Evidence for geometric differences in stress fracture cases was first shown by Giladi et al. These investigators used radiographs of Israeli Army trainees to demonstrate narrower mediolateral bone widths at the tibia and femur in fracture cases compared to controls.[12] Bone width is a component of the cross-sectional moment of inertia I, an index of structural bending strength, i.e., bending stress is inversely dependent on I. A later study of Israeli Army trainees used cortical dimensions from tibial radiographs to compute mediolateral cross-sectional moments of inertia, I_{ml}. This study showed smaller values of I_{ml} in fracture cases, consistent with higher bending stresses.[21] Work in our laboratory adapted a DXA method first described by Martin and Burr[19] to measure I_{ml} at the mid-shaft of the femur and at the distal third of the tibia in male Marine Corps recruits. We found that pooled fracture cases had smaller values of I_{ml} and mediolateral bone widths at both scan locations after correcting for body weight.[2] In a later study on female Marine Corps recruits we made the same measurements but concentrated on section moduli and bone strength indices at tibia and femur scan sites. The section modulus (Z) defines the maximum

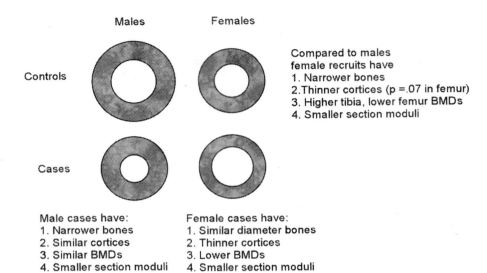

Males   Females

Controls

Compared to males
female recruits have
1. Narrower bones
2. Thinner cortices (p =.07 in femur)
3. Higher tibia, lower femur BMDs
4. Smaller section moduli

Cases

Male cases have:
1. Narrower bones
2. Similar cortices
3. Similar BMDs
4. Smaller section moduli

Female cases have:
1. Similar diameter bones
2. Thinner cortices
3. Lower BMDs
4. Smaller section moduli

Figure 1   Graphic depiction (not to scale) of the cross-sectional differences between cases and controls within sex (vertical comparisons) and between the sexes after adjustment for body size (horizontal comparisons). From Beck, T.J., et al., Bone, 27, 437, 2000. With permission.

stress on the bone surface in bending, and is computed by dividing I by the bone outer radius (half of bone width).* The bone strength index is based on the work of Selker and Carter,[24] who note that animal long bone strength scales as Z/l where $l =$ bone length. In addition to these parameters, we estimated mean cortical thickness at scan sites. In this study we compared results in female recruits to those of the previous male study expanded with 15 additional fracture cases. As shown in Table 1, we found that after correcting for height and weight, both male and female fracture cases had significantly smaller mediolateral section moduli (Z_{ml}) in both tibiae and femora compared to controls within sex.[3] Interestingly, size–adjusted BMD was lower at the femur and tibia in female fracture cases but not in males. This is consistent with the results of Bennell et al.[4] The explanation for the discrepancy between section modulus and BMD is evident in the cortical dimensions. In males, size–adjusted bone diameters were significantly narrower in fracture cases, consistent with the work of Giladi et al.,[12] but mean cortical thicknesses were similar to controls. Since the amount of bone within the periosteal envelope of male cases was similar to that of controls, BMDs were not significantly smaller. In females, however, the dimensional differences underlying their smaller section moduli were dissimilar (Figure 1). Unlike males, adjusted bone diameters were not narrower in female fracture cases, although cortices were significantly thinner. Only in female cases was there a relatively smaller amount of bone within the periosteal envelope and thus a smaller BMD, as also found by Lauder and colleagues.[17]

---

* This is not strictly correct; section modulus is actually computed by dividing I by the distance from the neutral axis to the appropriate surface. The neutral axis is not always in the middle of the bone. In effect, computing Z by dividing I by the outer radius provides an "average" section modulus.

Table 1 Means and standard deviations of tibia and femur geometries, pelvic widths, and muscle size after correction for height and weight. All measurements were recorded at the beginning of training.

Parameter	Males						Females					
	Controls (N = 587)		Cases (N = 38)		Percent Difference	Significance†	Controls (N = 626)		Cases (N = 37)		Percent Difference	Significance†
	Mean	SD	Mean	SD			Mean	SD	Mean	SD		
Pelvic breadth	28.42	±2.09	29.23	±1.98	2.7%	0.026	27.92	±1.61	27.85	±1.62	-0.3%	(0.79)
Thigh length (cm)	52.2	±1.872	53.3	±2.225	2.0%	0.001	50.9	±2.166	51.0	±2.500	0.3%	(0.66)
Thigh muscle CSA (cm²)	204.3	±16.4	196.0	±16.2	-4.0%	0.003	168.9	±16.2	162.7	±11.9	-3.7%	0.047
Tibia BMD* (g/cm²)	1.526	±0.125	1.493	±0.096	-2.2%	(0.22)	1.440	±0.146	1.366	±0.127	-5.2%	0.0033
Subperiosteal diameter* (cm)	2.172	±0.150	2.098	±0.092	-3.4%	0.023	1.886	±0.141	1.860	±0.147	-1.4%	(0.29)
Mean cortical thickness* (cm)	0.353	±0.038	0.346	±0.028	-2.0%	(0.36)	0.342	±0.047	0.320	±0.038	-6.4%	0.0073
Section Modulus* (cm³)	0.718	±0.111	0.662	±0.062	-7.8%	0.018	0.503	±0.089	0.466	±0.086	-7.3%	0.018
Bone Strength Index*ª	1.764	±0.267	1.643	±0.159	-6.9%	0.037	1.350	±0.229	1.261	±0.218	-6.5%	0.029
Femur BMD (g/cm²)	2.155	±0.161	2.137	±0.152	-0.8%	(0.51)	1.937	±0.144	1.852	±0.126	-4.4%	0.0007
Subperiosteal diameter (cm)	2.479	±0.158	2.419	±0.152	-2.4%	0.022	2.201	±0.130	2.159	±0.107	-1.9%	(0.062)
Mean cortical thickness (cm)	0.533	±0.059	0.532	±0.061	-0.2%	(0.97)	0.481	±0.052	0.454	±0.042	-5.7%	0.0033
Section Modulus (cm³)	1.315	±0.178	1.245	±0.144	-5.3%	0.018	0.924	±0.125	0.860	±0.098	-7.3%	0.0019
Bone Strength Indexª	2.509	±0.337	2.334	±0.263	-6.9%	0.0018	1.815	±0.258	1.691	±0.222	-6.9%	0.0060

† Values in parentheses not significant (p > 0.05, two tailed t = test).
* Tibia statistics exclude one male femoral fracture case with BMI in the 99th percentile.
ª Bone Strength Index = Section Modulus/bone length × 100.

Table 2   Bone size-adjusted means and standard deviations of anthropometric dimensions, BMD, and bone geometry compared between male and female Marine Corps recruit subjects. All measurements were recorded at the beginning of training. Also listed are percent differences in the adjusted parameter, expressed as percent difference from male value for females.

Height and Weight Adjusted Parameter	Males Mean	SD	Females Mean	SD	Percent Difference	Significance[†]
Femur bicondylar breadth (cm)	9.945	±0.650	9.563	±0.406	−3.8%	<0.0001
Thigh girth (cm)	52.75	±2.14	54.31	±2.54	3.0%	<0.0001
Calf girth (cm)	35.94	±1.63	36.15	±1.63	0.6%	0.032
Pelvic breadth	27.67	±2.12	28.61	±1.70	3.4%	<0.0001
Tibia length (cm)	38.83	±1.45	38.73	±1.45	−0.3%	(0.23)
Thigh length (cm)	50.85	±1.99	52.18	±2.29	2.6%	<0.0001
Thigh muscle CSA (cm²)	188.4	±16.9	187.9	±15.7	−0.3%	(0.64)
Tibia BMD* (g/cm²)	1.47	±0.124	1.49	±0.145	1.4%	0.036
Subperiosteal diameter* (cm)	2.05	±0.15	1.99	±0.14	−2.9%	<0.001
Mean cortical thickness* (cm)	0.342	±0.038	0.350	±0.046	2.3%	0.0018
Section Modulus* (cm³)	0.618	±0.108	0.591	±0.088	−4.4%	<0.0001
Bone Strength Index*[a]	1.58	±0.267	1.51	±0.230	−4.4%	<0.0001
Femur BMD (g/cm²)	2.05	±0.162	2.03	±0.144	−1.0%	0.008
Subperiosteal diameter (cm)	2.35	±0.154	2.32	±0.126	−1.3%	0.0002
Mean cortical thickness (cm)	0.508	±0.060	0.502	±0.052	−1.2%	(0.067)
Section Modulus (cm³)	1.13	±0.171	1.089	±0.125	−3.6%	<0.0001
Bone Strength Index[a]	2.21	±0.340	2.082	±0.269	−5.8%	<0.0001

[†] Signfiicantly different by unpaired t-test (p < 0.05).
* Tibia statistics exclude one male femoral fracture case with BMI in the 99th percentile.
[a] Bone Strength Index = Section Modulus/bone length × 100.

Because stress fractures are generally acknowledged to occur at higher rates among females,[8,15,16,25] we contrasted skeletal measurements between the sexes in our sex comparison study after adjustment for height and weight. The resulting differences in lower limb geometry are listed in Table 2, and the important bone geometry differences between the sexes and between fracture cases and controls within sex are summarized in Figure 1. Note that if bone strength was adequately described by BMD, one would expect uniformly higher BMDs in males. Femur BMDs were slightly smaller in females than in males but slightly higher in the tibia. We would nevertheless hypothesize that higher stress fracture rates among females would arise from weaker bones in that sex. Indeed, section moduli of both tibia and femur bones are significantly smaller in women (Table 2). When section moduli are scaled to bone length in the strength index, the longer, female femora increase the sex discrepancy in bone strength. This observation may help to explain the higher incidence of above-the-knee stress fractures among females compared to males. Among males (Table 1), a relatively wider pelvis was associated with stress fracture, and females on average have significantly wider pelves than males.

The Case for Measuring Muscle

It is frequently not appreciated that the forces on bones resulting from physical activity are mostly mediated though the actions of muscle.[6,10,11] Muscle may conceivably play an important role in the etiology of stress fracture, and its role may be complex. For example, there is evidence in both animals[26] and humans[20] that muscle fatigue leads to increased bone stress magnitudes. This may be due to a protective role of muscle in limiting some stresses on bone. Possibly the mechanism works by contraction of muscles attached to the terminal ends of long bones during loading activities. Contractions should oppose bending and perhaps torsion as well, converting more harmful tensile and shear stresses to compression. Although compressive stresses would increase, such an adaptation would be advantageous because bone is intrinsically stronger in compression than in tension or shear.[14]

A number of studies on stress fracture have noted that compared to controls, fracture cases show poorer physical condition[3,8,17] or lower prior physical activity.[7] Bennell and colleagues noted that stress fracture cases among female track and field athletes had significantly lower size corrected calf girths and less lean muscle mass in the lower limbs when compared to controls.[4] However, neither these investigators nor Giladi et al.[13] observed this in male fracture cases. In our prospective studies of male and female Marine Corps recruits we used a DXA method combined with thigh girth to estimate the total thigh muscle cross-sectional area.[3] We found that after adjustment for body size, thigh muscles were significantly smaller in both male and female fracture cases compared to controls (Table1). Interestingly, we found no differences in thigh muscle size between the sexes in the pooled sample after correction for sex differences in body size (Table 2) despite apparent differences in bone geometry.

The observation that thigh muscles were smaller in fracture cases, and that the cases were on average less physically fit is important because it is well established that physical fitness influences the size and strength of muscles. The mechanostat of Frost would suggest that physical activity or loading history should also influence bone strength,[10] although the evidence in humans is scant. The smaller section moduli and muscle sizes in fracture cases (Table 1) may be indicative of the level of adaptation prior to physical training. Since muscle hypertrophy occurs with physical training more rapidly than is likely in bone, propensity for stress fracture may also be in part due to a mismatch between the abilities of muscle and bone tissues to adapt to increasing skeletal loads in an intense training period.

Ultimately, it may be shown that measurements of lower limb muscle size or strength are as important as bone measurements in the identification of those at risk for stress fracture.

CAN STRESS FRACTURE BE PREDICTED?

Technical Difficulties in Measurement of Bone and Muscle Properties

We have shown that stress fracture cases have smaller muscles, that their bone cross-sectional properties and linear dimensions are consistent with higher mechanical stresses under repetitive loads, and that these differences are not readily apparent in the conventional BMD measurement. Logically one should be able to use this information to prospectively isolate those at high risk, culling them in advance or intervening with a graduated exercise program. The main problem is that the most successful techniques have technical limitations and are neither standardized nor commercially available. Bone length can be measured reasonably well with tape measures between bony landmarks, or more accurately using calibrated radiographs. Thigh muscle size can be measured using DXA capabilities for measuring lean muscle mass fraction in soft tissue regions. We combined lean mass fraction measured in a narrow thigh region with a measure of the thigh circumference to estimate total muscle cross-sectional area.[3] This relatively simple method could be improved and applied to other lower extremity locations such as the calf.

The main technical difficulty in stress fracture prediction at this point is in measuring bone cross-sectional geometry with sufficient accuracy. The technical demands are considerable, as the underlying dimensional differences can be quite small relative to measurement precision. For example, the average difference in bone widths between male tibia cases and controls in our sex comparison study was 0.07 mm, while our standard deviation *in vivo* averaged 0.03 mm.[2] Our work and the methods used by Milgrom et al.[21] were based on measurements from two-dimensional projections (DXA images or radiographs). However, the information needed is derived from dimensions of bone cross-sections orthogonal to the plane of the image. At best, the DXA or radiographic methods view bone cross-sections "on edge" and provide only those dimensions projected into the image plane. If bones were axially symmetric, then the information provided by DXA or radiographic methods would be equal regardless of the direction of projection (or rotation of bone). Unfortunately, real bones are not axially symmetric, and asymmetry varies between individuals and between locations on the same individual. Changes in position, mostly with respect to axial rotation, or changes in region location result in dimensional differences that may confound results. Some of this uncertainty can be diminished by careful subject positioning with special positioning jigs[2] and may ultimately be soluble with a special purpose rotating DXA scanner. Given currently available technology, however, the ideal method for defining the cross-sectional geometry in lower limb bones may be computed tomography (CT). Since CT directly images the cross-sectional plane, all relevant dimensions are available, although specialized software may be required. Some larger versions of peripheral quantitative (pQCT) scanners designed for osteoporosis assessment have become available and can be used to scan the lower leg and mid-thigh with some size restrictions. Commercial pQCT scanners can also provide software for measuring section geometric properties. Conceivably, such devices could be used to predict stress fracture, although this has not yet been demonstrated. Another advantage of CT methods is that one can also measure muscle size directly from the image. Scans at the mid-thigh using full body CT systems have been shown to be useful in assessing nutritional status and total muscle mass.[18,22]

Where to Measure

In practice, technical issues may make certain sites inaccessible, but it is apparent that measurements should at least be made in the lower extremity where fractures occur. Ideally, the measurement site should correspond to likely fracture locations. Within the pelvis and lower extremities there is significant heterogeneity in the locations of stress fractures between studies and between the sexes. In some male studies, fractures of the foot (calcaneus or metatarsals) are most common, while in others tibial fractures predominate.[16] This type of heterogeneity is probably due to the type of training, and one might use historical perspective to select a measurement site. Although geometric measurements could be made at the metatarsals and calcaneus, most work has concentrated on the larger femur and tibia bones, mainly due to the accessibility of these sites. Generally, measurements are based on the broad supposition that individuals have "weaker bones", so a measurement site based on convenience may be appropriate. This assumption may not always be true, however. For example, a significant fraction of female stress fractures occur in the pelvis, but appropriate geometric methods have not yet been described for measurements at this location. When we looked at these cases separately in our sex comparison study,[3] we found that neither femoral nor tibial geometry was predictive of stress fractures in these cases. However, both male and female cases with fractures at locations in the foot were predicted by reduced geometry at the measured locations. Some compromise in measurement location is inevitable. Our experience would suggest that measurements at the distal 2/3 of the tibia and the mid-shaft of the femur are reasonable sites for depicting generalized lower extremity weakness. Improvements in measurement technologies and further studies with better technologies may better define optimal measurement locations.

WHERE DO WE GO FROM HERE?

At present it appears that successful prediction of stress fracture susceptibility is possible, but the record suggests that the problem should be approached from a biomechanical perspective and that conventional bone mineral analyses have limited value. Stress fracture susceptibility clearly has both bone and muscle components, and it appears that these can be measured. Bones of stress fracture cases have geometric characteristics that lead to higher mechanical stresses under repetitive load. Moreover, they have smaller, apparently weaker muscles that may be important in the etiology of the weaker bone as well as the ability of bone to withstand repetitive loading. Nevertheless, there is considerable room for refinement of measurement methodologies, technologies, and measurement protocols. Current DXA based technologies may not have sufficient precision to measure bone geometry and permit the isolation of a given individual at risk. Improvements in DXA scanners and specialized software may ultimately provide these capabilities. Theoretically, high resolution quantitative CT (qCT), capable of measuring lower limb locations, may be ideal for characterizing both bone geometry and muscle size, though this is yet to be shown. The path toward optimal musculoskeletal measurements that will lead to practical, accurate prediction of stress fracture susceptibility is clear, though much work remains to be done.

REFERENCES

1. Antich, P.P., Anderson, J.A., Ashman, R.B., Dowdey, J.E., Gonzales, J., Murry, R.C., Zerwekh, J.E., and D Pak, C.Y., Measurement of mechanical properties of bone material in vitro by ultrasound reflection: methodology and comparison with ultrasound transmission, *J. Bone Miner. Res.,* 6, 417, 1991.
2. Beck, T., Ruff, C., Mourtada, F., Shaffer, R., Maxwell-Williams, K., Kao, G., Sartoris, D., and Brodine, S., DXA-derived structural geometry for stress fracture prediction in male U.S. Marine Corps recruits, *J. Bone Miner. Res.,* 11, 645, 1996.
3. Beck, T.J., Ruff, C.B., Shaffer, R.A., Betsinger, K., Trone, D.W., and Brodine, S.K., Stress fracture in military recruits: sex differences in muscle and bone susceptibility factors, *Bone,* 27, 437, 2000.
4. Bennell, K.L., Malcolm, S.A., Brukner, P.D., Green, R.M., Hopper, J.L., Wark, J.D., and Ebeling, P.R., A 12-month prospective study of the relationship between stress fractures and bone turnover in athletes, *Calcif. Tiss. Int.,* 63, 80, 1998.
5. Bennell, K.L., Malcolm, S.A., Thomas, S.A., Ebeling, P.R., McCrory, P.R., Wark, J.D., and Brukner, P.D., Risk factors for stress fractures in female track-and-field athletes: a retrospective analysis, *Clin. J. Sports Med.,* 5, 229, 1995.
6. Burr, D.B., Muscle strength, bone mass, and age-related bone loss, *J. Bone Miner. Res.,* 12, 1547, 1997.
7. Cline, A.D., Jansen, G.R., and Melby, C.L. Stress fractures in female army recruits: implications of bone density, calcium intake and exercise, *J. Am. Coll. Nutr.,* 17, 128, 1998.
8. Friedl, K. and Nuovo, J., Factors associated with stress fracture in young army women: Indications for further research, *Mil. Med.,* 157, 334, 1992.
9. Frost, H.M., The mechanostat: a proposed pathogenic mechanism of osteoporosis and the bone mass effects of mechanical and nonmechanical agents, *Bone Miner.,* 2, 73, 1987.
10. Frost. H.M., Why do marathon runners have less bone than weight lifters? A vital biomechanical view and explanation, *Bone,* 20, 183, 1997.
11. Frost, H.M., Ferretti, J.L., and Jee, W.S., Perspectives: some roles of mechanical usage, muscle strength, and the mechanostat in skeletal physiology, disease, and research, *Calcif. Tiss. Int.,* 62, 1, 1998.
12. Giladi, M., Milgrom, C., Simkin, A., Stein, M., Kashtan, H., Margulies, J., Rand, N., Chisin, R., Steinberg, R., Aharonson, R., Kedem, R., and Frankel, V.H., Stress fractures and tibial bone width: a risk factor, *J. Bone Jt. Surg.,* 69(B), 326, 1987.
13. Giladi, M., Milgrom, C., Simkin, A., and Danon, Y., Stress fractures: identifiable risk factors, *Am. J. Sports Med.,* 19, 647, 1991.
14. Hayes, W. and Bouxsein, M., Biomechanics of cortical and trabecular bone: implications for assessment of fracture risk, in *Basic Orthopaedic Biomechanics,* Hayes, W.C. and Mow, V.C., Eds., Lippincott-Raven, Philadelphia, 1997, 69.

15. Jones, B., Manikowski, R., Harris, J., Dziados, J., Norton, S., Ewart, T., and Vogel, J., Incidence of and risk factors for injury and illness among male and female Army basic trainees, in *U.S. ARMY RIEM Tech Report*, 1988, T19.
16. Jones, B.H., Harris, J.M., Vinh, T.N., and Rubin, C.R., Exercise-induced stress fractures and stress reactions of bone: epidemiology, etiology, and classification, in *Exercise and Sports Sciences Reviews,* Williams & Wilkins, Baltimore, 1989, 379.
17. Lauder, T.D., Sameer, D., Pezzin, L.E., and Williams, M.V., The relation between stress fractures and bone mineral density: evidence from active-duty Army women, *Arch. Phys. Med. Rehabil.*, 81, 73, 2000.
18. Lerner, A., Feld, L.G., Riddlesberger, M.M., Rossi, T.M., and Lebenthal, E., Computed axial tomographic scanning of the thigh: an alternative method of nutritional assessment in pediatrics, *Pediatrics*, 77, 732, 1986.
19. Martin, R. and Burr, D., Non-invasive measurement of long bone cross-sectional moment of inertia by photon absorptiometry, *J. Biomech.*, 17, 195, 1984.
20. Milgrom, C., Finestone, A., Ekenman, I., Larrson, B., Millgram, M., Mendelson, S., Simkin, A., Benjuya, N., and Burr, D., Tibial strain rate increases following muscular fatigue in both men and women, *Trans. Orthop. Res. Soc.*, 24, 1999.
21. Milgrom, C., Giladi, M., Simkin, A., Rand, N., Kedem, R., Kashtan, H., Stein, M., and Gomori, M., The area moment of inertia of the tibia: a risk factor for stress fractures, *J. Biomech.*, 22, 1243, 1989.
22. Ohkawa, S., Odamaki, M., Yoneyama, T., Hibi, I., Miyaji, K., and Kumagai, H., Standardized thigh muscle area measured by computed axial tomography as an alternate muscle mass index for nutritional assessment of hemodialysis patients, *Am. J. Clin. Nutr.*, 71, 485, 2000.
23. Pouilles, J.M., Bernard, J., Tremollieres, F., Louvet, J.P., and Ribot, C., Femoral bone density in young male adults with stress fractures, *Bone*, 10, 105, 1989.
24. Selker, F. and Carter, D.R., Scaling of long bone fracture strength with animal mass, *J. Biomech.*, 22, 1175, 1989.
25. Shaffer, R., Brodine, S., Corwin, C., Almeida, S., and Maxwell-Williams, K., Impact of musculoskeletal injury due to rigorous physical activity during U.S. Marine Corps basic training, *Med. Sci. Sports Exerc.*, 26, S141, 1994.
26. Yoshikawa, T., Mori, S., Santiesteban, A.J., Sun, T.C., Hafstad, E., Chen, J., and Burr, D.B., The effects of muscle fatigue on bone strain, *J. Exp. Biol.*, 188, 217, 1994.

CHAPTER 6

Bone Fatigue and Stress Fractures

Scott A. Yerby and Dennis R. Carter

CONTENTS

Introduction...85
Factors Affecting Fatigue Strength...86
Creep and Damage 90
Trabecular Bone..97
Fatigue Damage and Skeletal Adaptation 98
Mathematical Modeling..99
References..100

INTRODUCTION

The repeated loading to which the skeleton is exposed during daily activities can result in accumulation of microscopic damage that can weaken the bones at specific locations. Many contend that this local microdamage triggers a remodeling response that serves to repair the bone tissue. If damage accumulates faster than it can be repaired, however, a fatigue fracture may result. Clinical studies have reported fatigue fractures in many different anatomic locations (see Chapter 2), including the upper and lower extremities, sacrum, vertebrae, and ribs.[1-12]

As a first step to developing a better understanding of the *in vivo* fatigue behavior of bone, investigators have studied the *ex vivo* characteristics of devitalized cortical and trabecular bone. In one of the earliest studies of this kind, Evans and Lebow machined cortical specimens from human femora and tibiae and subjected them to cyclic cantilever bending loads using a single stress range of ±34.5 MPa.[13] The number of cycles to failure varied from 47,000 to 6,541,000. They suggested that the wide range of variability could be partially attributed to the disease state of some specimens; one subject was paraplegic and another had diabetes. This study was followed by a similar study by Evans and Riolo, who also performed cantilever bending fatigue experiments with machined specimens from human tibiae using a single stress range.[14] In this study, all of the specimens were acquired from previously active amputee patients and the goal was to determine a relationship between the fatigue life and the histologic structure of the specimens. They found a positive correlation between fatigue life (the number of cycles to failure) and the area occupied by osteons at the fracture surface of the specimens. Swanson et al. performed a series of fatigue tests at different stress ranges using compact bone specimens machined from human femora.[15] The cylindrical specimens were loaded as rotating cantilevers, thereby subjecting each circumferential location of the specimen surface to repeated cycles of tension and compression. From these data, the first S-N curve (stress or strain level versus cycles to failure) for fresh/frozen cortical bone was generated.

Fatigue tests conducted in fully reversed bending expose the specimen surfaces to cyclic tension and compression loading of equal magnitudes. *In vivo*, however, some local bone regions may be exposed to loading that is primarily compressive or primarily tensile. Gray and Korbacher reported the first study of uniaxial compressive fatigue behavior by applying varying stress ranges to cortical cylinders from bovine femora.[16] Using stress ranges comparable to those of the previously mentioned bending fatigue studies, they found that the number of cycles to failure was 100 times the number of cycles to failure reported by Swanson et al. (1.58×10^6 versus 1.3×10^4 at 84 MPa). The increased fatigue life can be attributed to (1) the differences in microstructure between human and bovine compact bone, and, more importantly, (2) the differences in loading mode, e.g., fully reversed bending loading versus uniaxial compressive loading.

FACTORS AFFECTING FATIGUE STRENGTH

The fatigue life of bone is affected by a number of factors including loading mode, frequency, temperature, microstructure, and density.[17-23] In the first of a series of fatigue studies, Carter and Hayes machined test specimens from bovine femora and tested them as rotating cantilevers at a range of stress amplitudes and temperatures.[18] After testing, measurements of dry density were made and the specimens were sectioned for histological examination of bone microstructure. At a given temperature, there was a strong correlation between the number of cycles to failure and the stress amplitude. Likewise, for a given stress amplitude, there was a strong correlation between the cycles to failure and the temperature. It was also determined that the error between the measured number of cycles to failure and the predicted values from linear regression could be partially explained by the variation in density among the specimens. The following multiple linear regression was formulated to empirically model the number of cycles to failure as a function of stress amplitude, temperature, and density:

$$\log(2N) = H\log\sigma + JT + K\rho + M \tag{1}$$

where H, J, K, and M are constants, $2N$ is the number of cycles to failure, σ is the stress amplitude (MPa), T is the temperature (°C), and ρ is the dry density (g/cm³).

The second paper in this series analyzed the effect of microstructure in addition to the previously mentioned stress amplitude, temperature, and density.[17] The microstructure of each specimen was graded from 1 to 4, where 1 represented fully primary bone and 4 represented fully secondary bone, while grades 2 and 3 were intermediate grades which included different proportions of primary and secondary bone. For a given stress amplitude, temperature, and density, specimens comprised of entirely primary bone had a significantly greater fatigue life than specimens comprised entirely of secondary bone. This result was described by the following multiple regression equation:

$$\log(2N) = -7.789\log\sigma - 0.0206T + 2.364\rho + M_i \tag{2}$$

where i is the microstructural index (1,2,3, or 4). These two reports describe the influence of both external factors (stress and temperature) and material characteristics (structure and density) on the fatigue life of bone. The data suggest that bone remodeling leads to a decrease in fatigue strength. This decrease is most likely caused by a decrease in specimen density (which can be due to changes in both mineralization and porosity) and a change in strucure from primary to secondary bone.

To understand the effect of cyclic loading on the ultimate strength of compact bone, Carter and Hayes subjected cortical bone samples to a predetermined number of cycles and then loaded the specimens to failure to determine the residual strength.[19] They reported that rotating bending fatigue loading of compact bone caused a progressive decrease in the ultimate uniaxial tensile strength of the tissue. For example, when bone was cycled to 31% of the expected fatigue life, the ultimate tensile load decreased from 128 MPa to 118 MPa. A progressive decrease in stiffness and an increase in hysteresis was also observed while the bone was cyclically loaded, further indicating an accumulation of damage in the specimens. Finally, specimens cyclically loaded from zero to tension exhibited a substantial amount of creep during the test — although this was only graphically depicted and not discussed.

Lafferty and Raju determined that the relationship between stress and cycles to failure was dependent on the loading frequency.[24] They loaded compact bone specimens in rotating bending at four different stress amplitudes (60, 70, 95, and 112 MPa) and at two frequencies (30 and 60 Hz), and determined the number of cycles to failure. Earlier it had been shown that the ultimate compressive strength of a bone sample is dependent on the strain rate,[25] and Lafferty and Raju adapted this relationship to rotating beam specimens using the relationship:

$$\sigma = Af^\alpha \tag{3}$$

where σ is the stress amplitude, f is the loading frequency, and A and α are constants. In addition, for a given frequency, temperature, density, and microstructure, the following relationship applies to stress amplitude (σ) and fatigue life (N) of cortical bone:

$$\sigma = BN^{-\beta} \tag{4}$$

where B and β are constants. Combining these two relationships yields a relationship between the applied stress amplitude and the loading frequency and fatigue life:

$$\sigma = Kf^{\alpha}N^{-\beta} \tag{5}$$

where K is a constant. Using data collected by Lafferty and Raju at 30 and 60 Hz, as well as a relationship for data collected by Carter and Hayes[18] at 125 Hz, the following constants were determined: $K = 235.02$, $\alpha = 0.098$, and $\beta = 0.13$. The samples used by Lafferty and Raju and those used by Carter and Hayes were machined from bovine femora and presumably had a similar microstructure (primary bone) and density which makes for a much easier comparison between the data sets.

Carter et al. later examined the influence of uniaxial fatigue of cortical bone using mean strains of –0.2%, 0%, and 0.2%, and strain ranges from 0.5% to 1.0%.[22] Specimens were machined from the mid-diaphysis of human femora and tested uniaxially at 37°C. The data showed that the strain range was a much better predictor of fatigue life than the maximum strain, and the mean strain had no significant influence on the relationship between the strain range and the number of cycles to failure. The number of cycles to failure for all three strain ranges was expressed as:

$$N_f = 2.94 \, \Delta\varepsilon^{-5.342} \times 10^{-9} \tag{6}$$

where N_f is the number of cycles to failure and $\Delta\varepsilon$ is the strain range. Although the number of cycles to failure was not influenced by the mean strain, the stress-strain behavior of the specimens loaded with each of the three mean strains was significantly different. For specimens subjected to a zero mean strain, the peak tensile stress decreased more than the compressive stress, and the tensile hysteresis increased more than the compressive hysteresis (Figure 1A). For specimens tested with a tensile mean strain, the peak tensile stress decreased rapidly, while the compressive stress actually increased initially and then returned to its beginning stress level (Figure 1B). The hysteresis increased under both tensile and compressive strains but was much more pronounced in the tensile strain region of the load curve. Specimens tested with a mean compressive strain exhibited a gradual decrease in both peak compressive and peak tensile stress, but the decrease was slightly more prounouced on the compressive side (Figure 1C). Likewise, the gradual increase of hysteresis was slightly more pronounced on the compressive side than on the tensile side.

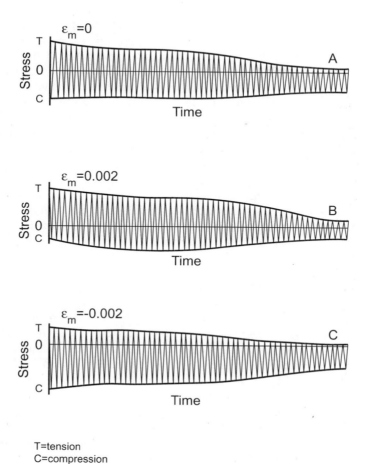

T=tension
C=compression

Figure 1 Stress versus time histories for cortical bone specimens tested under a constant uniaxial strain range (0.006) and three mean strains, ε_m (0, 0.002, and −0.002). (A) With a mean strain of zero, both the peak tensile and compressive stresses decrease over time, but this decrease is much more pronounced for the tensile stress. (B) The mean tensile strain produced a rapid decrease of the peak tensile stress, and an initial increase in compressive stress over time. (C) The mean compressive strain produced gradual decreases of the peak compressive and tensile stresses, but was more pronounced for the compressive stress. From Carter, D.R., Caler, W.E., Spengler, D.M., and Frankel, V.H., *Acta. Orthop. Scand.*, 52, 481, 1981. With permission.

In a similar study by Carter et al., it was shown that strain range is a better predictor of cycles to failure than the initial stress range under strain range-controlled fatigue.[21] It was also shown that the scatter in the initial stress range versus cycles to failure plot could be substantially reduced by normalizing the stress range with the initial elastic modulus of the specimen. This finding is consistent with data from montonic failure tests, which indicate that changes in modulus have little effect on the yield strain yet significantly affect the yield and ultimate stress values.

The results by Carter et al. also indicate that the fatigue life of bone specimens tested in uniaxial fatigue is much lower than reported in the previous studies of specimens tested in cyclic bending.[13-15] In bending fatigue tests only the outer fibers of the specimens are loaded to the peak stress, and the inner fibers are subjected to a gradient of lower stresses. These lower-stressed inner fibers are much less prone to damage, thereby extending the fatigue life relative to that of a uniaxially loaded specimen. Other factors that may contribute to the discrepanices may be the difference in temperature and tissue microstructure. The difference between bending and uniaxial loading results can be related to the "stressed volume" considerations that have been used by Taylor et al. which account for the scatter between experimental data sets.[26,27] These authors state that larger specimens will have shorter fatigue lives than smaller specimens, since larger specimens are more likely to contain larger cracks or voids. Similarly, since uniaxial loading causes a much greater volume of bone to be critically loaded than would be loaded in bending, uniaxial loading would be expected to cause earlier failure than bending loading in specimens of identical size.

One must remember that bone is in a constant state of turnover, and all of the previously mentioned studies were conducted using devitalized tissue with no ability to repair micro– or fatigue fractures. In addition, it is difficult to estimate the magnitudes and directions of the loads that individual bones experience *in vivo*. However, it can be assumed with some certainty that microfractures do occur *in vivo*, and the previously mentioned studies have shown that density, structure, and loading direction all contribute to the fatigue life of bony tissue. For instance, higher density bone is more fatigue resistant than lower density bone, and cortical bone with more osteons and less lamellae is more fatigue resistant than bone with fewer osteons and more lamellae. Also, for a given loading magnitude, bone loaded in tension is less fatigue resistant than the same tissue loaded in compression. Again, all of these relationships were determined from cadaveric tissue in a laboratory setting, yet all of the principles can be applied to an *in vivo* setting; only the magnitudes will change.

CREEP AND DAMAGE

The creep behavior depicted in earlier reports by Carter and Hayes[19,20] was later studied in greater detail by Carter and Caler.[23] Cortical bone specimens were machined from human femora and cyclically tested to failure at constant stress ranges in either zero-tension or tension-compression loading modes. At high cyclic stresses (low cycles to failure), the fatigue life of the zero-tension specimens was substantially less than that of the tension-compression specimens, whereas at low stress levels there was no difference in fatigue life. The zero-tension specimens demonstrated creep characteristics during the cyclic loading. The strain versus time curve of the zero-tension specimens displayed three distinct regions: (1) an initial, primary stage with rapid creep, (2) a secondary stage with low level creep, and (3) a tertiary stage with rapid creep until failure (Figure 2). The following relationship was established to describe the relationship between the time to failure and the stress range for the zero-tension specimens:

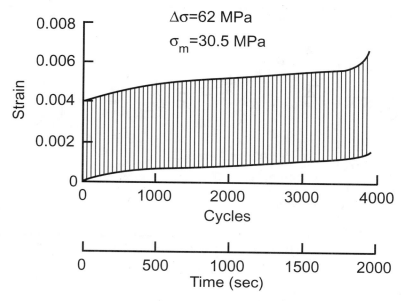

Figure 2 The strain versus loading cycles (and time) plot for cortical bone subjected to zero-tension fatigue loading. The plot shows an initial increase in strain, followed by a steady linear increase in the middle of the loading history. Fracture is preceded by a rapid increase in strain. This load history is representative of time-dependent creep behavior which will be discussed in following sections. $\Delta\sigma$ is the strain range and σ_m is the mean strain. From Carter, D.R. and Caler, W.E., *J. Biomech. Eng.*, 105, 166, 1983. With permission.

$$t_f = KA\Delta\sigma^{-B} \tag{7}$$

where t_f is the time to failure, $\Delta\sigma$ is the stress range, and K, A, and B are empirically determined constants. This relationship suggests that the time to failure for cortical bone cyclically loaded in a zero-tension mode is dependent on the stress range and independent of the loading frequency. Caler and Carter later investigated the time and frequency dependent behavior of cyclically loading cortical bone specimens from human femurs.[28] The specimens were loaded in zero-tension and zero-compression at two different frequencies, 0.02 and 2.0 Hz. The specimens tested in zero-compression exhibited greater fatigue resistance than the zero-tension specimens. As previously suggested by Carter and Caler,[23] the loading frequency affected the number of cycles to failure for both zero-tension and zero-compression loaded specimens (Figure 3A), but had no effect on the time to failure (Figure 3B). The data were well described by the relationship:

$$t_f = F(\Delta\sigma/E^*)^{-G} \tag{8}$$

where t_f is the time to failure, $\Delta\sigma/E^*$ is the stress range normalized by the initial modulus, and F and G are empirically derived constants that differ for zero-compression and

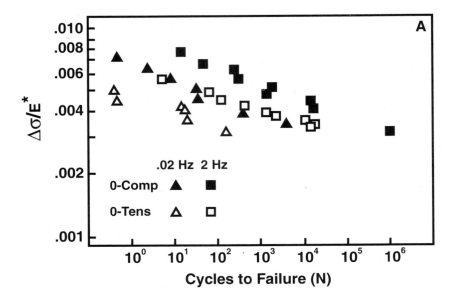

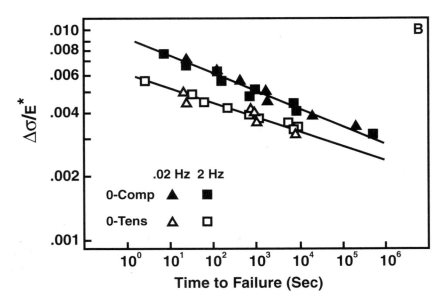

Figure 3 Normalized stress versus cycles to failure (A), and time to failure (B). The loading frequency affects the number of cycles for specimens loaded in zero-compression and those loaded in zero-tension. However, the time to failure is independent of the loading frequency. From Caler, W.E. and Carter, D.R., *J. Biomech.*, 22, 625, 1989. With permission.

zero-tension loading. In addition, it was suggested that damage due to cyclic compression and cyclic tension accumulates in different manners. For example, as shown previously by Carter and Caler,[29] damage due to zero-tension loading is controlled by the time (creep) of loading and can be modeled as follows:

$$D_c(t) = \int_0^t dt \bigg/ A\big(\sigma(t)/E*\big)^{-B} \tag{9}$$

where $D_c(t)$ is the time dependent damage (creep), $\sigma(t)$ is the stress history, E^* is the modulus, and A and B are constants (Figure 4A). Failure occurs at the time when $D_c(t)$ reaches the value of 1.0. On the other hand, zero-compression loading creates primarily cycle-dependent (fatigue) damage and can be modeled as follows:

$$D_f(t) = \omega t \bigg/ K\big(\Delta\sigma/E*\big)^{-N} \tag{10}$$

where $D_f(t)$ is the fatigue dependent damage, ω is the loading frequency, t is the time, $\Delta\sigma$ is the stress range, E^* is the modulus, and K and N are constants (Figure 4B). The term ωt determines the number of loading cycles at time t and gives the relationship its cycle dependency. Similar to the creep damage relationship, failure occurs when $D_f(t)$ reaches a value of 1.0.

During combined loading in tension and compression, a component of the time dependent and cycle dependent relationships will each contribute to the fatigue life. If we assume that there is no interaction between creep and fatigue damage accumulation, a linear superposition model would suggest that:

$$D_s(t) = D_c(t) + D_f(t) \tag{11}$$

where $D_s(t)$ is the summation of the damage caused by creep and the damage caused by fatigue. Failure occurs when $D_s(t)$ reaches a value of 1.0. When Equation 11 was applied to data collected from specimens subjected to tension-compression cyclic loading, however, the model overestimated the time to failure (Figure 4C), suggesting that there probably is an interaction between the time-dependent and cycle-dependent damage accumulation during combined tensile and compressive load histories.[28]

Pattin et al. attempted to further characterize fatigue damage accumulation in compact bone by measuring the energy dissipation and modulus reduction of specimens subjected to uniaxial tension, compression, or fully-reversed tension and compression.[30] Previous research demonstrated that bone stiffness and modulus decreased while the hysteresis increased during cyclic loading.[19,22,31,32] Pattin et al. showed property degradation of cyclically loaded bone, but also reported dramatic differences between the changes of bone loaded in tension and bone loaded in compression. Bone loaded in cyclic tension exhibited a three-phase modulus versus cycle number curve where the secant modulus decreased rapidly in the initial phase, then plateaued to a steady rate of modulus degradation, followed by another region of rapid modulus degradation before failure (Figure 5A). The energy dissipation

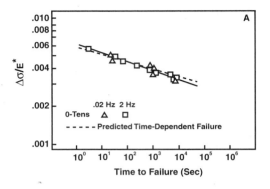

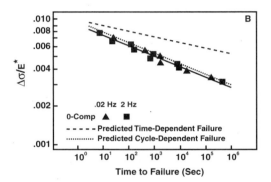

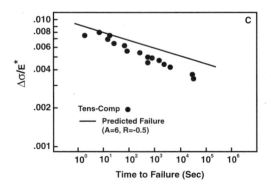

Figure 4 Normalized stress versus time to failure for specimens loaded in zero-tension
(A), zero-compression (B), and combined tension-compression (C). In zero-tension,
the fatigue behavior is best predicted by a time-dependent model (Equation 9),
whereas in zero-compression, the fatigue behavior is best predicted by a cycle-
dependent model (Equation 10). The combined tension-compression behavior was
modeled with a combination of the time– and cycle–dependent models. The discrepancy between the model and the data is likely attributed to an interaction between
the tensile and compressive behavior. (A = stress range/mean stress, R = minimum
stress/maximum stress). From Caler, W.E. and Carter, D.R., *J. Biomech.*, 22, 625,
1989. With permission.

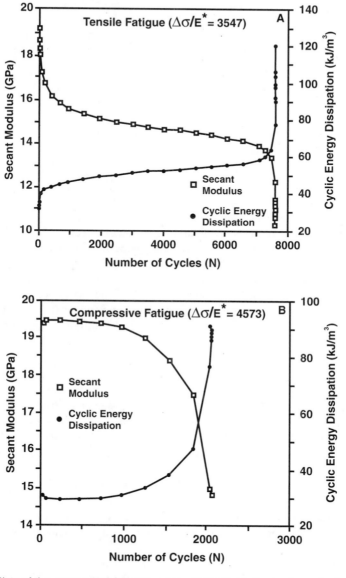

Figure 5 Plots of the secant modulus and energy dissipation behavior for cortical specimens cyclically loaded in (A) tension and (B) compression. During tensile loading, the secant modulus decreased rapidly in the initial stages of loading and then plateaued. Failure was preceded by a rapid decrease in modulus. The energy dissipation followed a similar pattern to that of the secant modulus, except that it increased throughout. Under compressive loading, both the secant modulus and energy dissipation were relatively steady for the first half of fatigue life. During the second half, the secant modulus rapidly decreased and the energy dissipation increased. From Pattin, C.A., Caler, W.E., and Carter, D.R., *J. Biomech.*, 29, 69, 1996. With permission.

followed a similar pattern but increased with greater number of cycles. During compressive loading, the modulus and energy dissipation were relatively constant for the first half of each specimen's life, and then the secant modulus rapidly decreased and energy dissipation rapidly increased during the second half until failure (Figure 5B). For both tensile and compressive loading modes, the initial energy dissipation per loading cycle followed a power law of the effective strain range ($\Delta\sigma/E^*$):

$$H_{Ti} = 5.71 \times 10^{18} \left(\Delta\sigma/E*\right)^{5.81} \qquad (12)$$

and

$$H_{Ci} = 5.69 \times 10^{15} \left(\Delta\sigma/E*\right)^{4.90} \qquad (13)$$

where H_{Ti} and H_{Ci} are, respectively, the initial tensile and compressive dissipation energies per cycle at high effective strains. At lower effective strains, both tensile and compressive dissipation energies correlate with the effective strain range raised to the power of 2.1 (Figure 6). The intersection of the dissipated energies from low and high effective strain ranges suggests that a threshold exists below which bone behaves as a linear viscoelastic material and above which severe degradation occurs. This threshold may also represent a mechanobiologic trigger for remodeling.

Zioupos et al. followed the study by Pattin et al. by introducing another definition for damage[33]:

$$D = 1 - \left(E/E_0\right) \qquad (14)$$

where D is the damage ($D = 0$ represents no damage, and $D = 1.0$ represents complete fracture), E is the modulus at any give cycle, and E_0 is the initial modulus. Zioupos et al. noted that when damage was defined as a reduction in the intial modulus, it increased linearly with the fraction of cycles to failure (N/N_f) up to a damage level of about 0.1· — depending on the stress level. This level was reached at a cycle fraction of about 0.9, after which the damage level dramatically increased to 1. A contour plot of S–N curves for damage levels from 0.01 to 1 (failure) suggests that osteonal bone may indeed have an endurance limit somewhere between 50 and 80 MPa. Also, all damage level curves above 0.2 were coincident with the failure curve ($D = 1$).

The previous data suggest that the mechanism of damage for bone cyclically loaded in tension is drastically different than for the same tissue loaded in compression. Cyclic damage in bone loaded in tension seems to be controlled by the amount of time the bone is loaded and is independent of frequency, whereas bone loaded in compression is controlled by the number of cycles and is frequency dependent. Also, for both modes of loading, there seems to be an effective strain range threshold below which bone behaves as a linear viscoelastic material, and above which severe damage occurs. This suggests that if a given activity exceeds a particular strain range threshold, severe tissue damage may occur and a stress fracture may result. If the resulting strain range from a particular activity does not exceed this threshold, it is

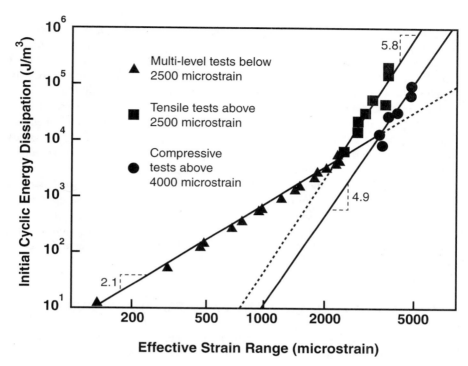

Figure 6 The initial cyclic energy dissipation versus the effective strain range. For combined tensile-compressive loading, the energy dissipation follows a linear viscoelastic behavior with a slope of 2.1 until approximately 2500 microstrain. At 2500 microstrain, the energy dissipation derived from specimens loaded in tension deviates from the viscoelastic behavior and the slope increases to 5.8. At 4000 microstrain, the compressive energy dissipation deviates from the viscoelastic and the slope increases to 4.9. These points of inflection for the specimens loaded in tension and compression indicate that compact bone may indeed have a threshold above which damage occurs and a remodeling response may be initiated. From Pattin, C.A., Caler, W.E., and Carter, D.R., *J. Biomech.*, 29, 69, 1996. With permission.

likely the bone will be able to repair all microfractures without injury. Zioupos et al. have suggested that an endurance stress limit exists for bone, below which no microdamage will occur. However, this limit may be below all typical stresses imparted on bones, and if administered to patients may have detrimental effects such as disuse osteoporosis.

TRABECULAR BONE

The fatigue behavior of trabecular bone has not been investigated as extensively as cortical bone.[34-36] However, there appear to be many common characteristics in the fatigue behavior of these two bone types. Choi and Goldstein fatigue tested extremely small cortical and cancellous bone specimens in 4-point bending to failure. The cortical specimens had a higher fatigue strength than the trabecular specimens, however the microstructure of the two tissue types were substantially different, which may have contributed to the different fatigue lives. The cortical specimens had no cement lines, whereas the trabecular specimens had cement lines throughout. Michel et al. cyclically tested trabecular bone specimens in compression and noted that the specimens exhibited increased nonlinearity and hysteresis throughout the loading. Finally, the slope of the initial strain versus cycles to failure was similar to that of values reported for cortical bone. More recently, Bowman et al. conducted fatigue tests of trabecular specimens and reported both creep and damage components of the tissue during cyclic loading. Similar to the findings in cortical bone, the study also suggests that the cycles to failure, time to failure, and creep rate are all dependent on the temperature and applied loads.

These previous findings suggest that many of the extensively studied principles established for cortical bone may translate to trabecular bone. For example, lower density trabecular tissue may be less fatigue resistant than higher density tissue, and trabecular bone may be more fatigue resistant to compression than tension. Finally, a stress and/or strain threshold may exist, below which repairable damage may occur and above which catastrophic damage may result.

FATIGUE DAMAGE AND SKELETAL ADAPTATION

It is now firmly established that fatigue damage of bone will occur in normal skeletons during rigorous activity and in osteoporotic skeletons during mild to moderate levels of activity. One of the most intriguing aspects of fatigue damage in bone is its relationship to bone modeling and remodeling. Chamay and Tschantz used a canine model to examine the relationships between bone overload, fatigue damage, and bone hypertrophy.[37] In one group of dogs, a small segment of the radius was resected and the animals were allowed to walk on their weakened forepaws, the load being carried only by the ulna. Some animals experienced fatigue fractures of the ulna while others showed massive bone hypertrophy over a nine-month period following the operation. Standard H&E histological examinations demonstrated oblique lesions on the concave ulnar cortex (a region of high compressive stresses) several hours after activity was resumed subsequent to the resection. These lesions were similar to those created by compressive fatigue loading of devitalized bone specimens.[20] Chamay and Tschantz contended that cellular insult resulting from the oblique lesions served as an osteogenic stimulus. However, they also noted hypertrophy in areas where oblique lesions could not be seen and suggested that piezoelectric properties of bone may have provided an osteogenic stimulus in those areas.

The canine radius is much larger than the ulna and it is likely that extremely high, damaging strains were introduced in the radius resection model of Chamay and Tschantz. To examine the influence of mild overload, Carter et al. conducted a canine ulna resection study and examined the histological response of the radius with tetracycline labels for bone formation.[38] Strain gages verified that the strains in the radius were significantly increased, although not to the level where significant fatigue damage could be expected (axial strains increased from approximately 700 to

1500 microstrain). The bone formation in the radius was minimal. Based on these results, Carter proposed that under normal conditions there is a rather broad range of physical activity in which bone is relatively unresponsive to changes in loading history, and it is unlikely that a stress fracture will occur with a mild increase in activity. This general view has since been adopted by several investigators.[39-41] With very low levels of cyclic strain, atrophy can be significant. With high cyclic strain levels, fatigue damage will become significant and hypertrophy or a stress fracture will result. Carter has also suggested that bone atrophy might be affected by a different mechanism than that of bone hypertrophy.[42] Therefore, two (or more) complementary control systems may be involved in the regulation of bone by bone cyclic strain histories and it is probable that mechanical microdamage is one stimulus for increasing bone mass (see Chapter 12). The critical damage cyclic strain magnitudes of 2500 and 4000 microstrain in tension and compression by Pattin et al.[30] are consistent with the concept that bone damage regulates bone hypertrophy in response to mechanical overload.[43] This also suggests that continual loading above these threshold values in either tension or compression is likely to result in either hypertrophy or a stress fracture, depending on the duration and magnitude of the applied stress and/or strain.

MATHEMATICAL MODELING

Carter et al., Whalen et al., and Mikic and Carter introduced formal mathematical representations of daily stress histories, load histories, and strain histories to calculate a daily mechanical stimulus for regulating bone adaptation in response to loading stimuli.[44-46] The equation used to calculate the mechanical stimulus is of the same form as the Miner's rule for calculating fatigue damage accumulation. The implementation of this loading history approach with finite element models has been extremely successful in predicting the morphogenesis of bone structure and functional adaptation of both cancellous bone and cortical bone to changes in the applied stress to the bone.[41,46-49] Although Miner's rule for fatigue life predictions have been demonstrated to not strictly hold for devitalized bone and many other materials, it appears to have some utility as a first order approximation in representing both damage accumulation and a stimulus for bone adaptation.

The considerable evidence suggesting that microdamage is a stimulus for bone functional adaptation has implications to our understanding of mechanobiological regulation in different tissues. For example, Sine's method for predicting multiaxial fatigue in metals assumes that damage is introduced primarily by the octahedral shear stress.[50] That damage is increased by superimposed hydrostatic tensile stress and decreased by hydrostatic compression. In other words, shear loading in addition to tensile stress will promote damage which may lead to a stress fracture, and shear stress in addition to compressive stress will decrease the likelihood of damage and a subsequent fracture. A mathematically equivalent application of Sine's method has been demonstrated to effectively describe the mechanical regulation of cartilage growth and ossification in the developing and aging skeleton in diverse situations.[51-56]

The basic assumption of these studies is that cyclic octahedral shear stress increases cartilage growth and ossification, while cyclic hydrostatic pressure inhibits growth and maintains the cartilage phenotype. It is therefore possible to view the morphogenesis of the post-cranial skeleton as a continuous process of mechanobiological influences upon cartilage and bone within the mathematical framework of a response to local fatigue damage.[49,57-59] However, the growing skeleton is much more metabolically active, has more frequent bone turnover, and has greater fatigue resistance than the aging skeleton, making fatigue fractures much less likely in the growing skeleton.

From an evolutionary standpoint it may be argued that mechanical damage is the ideal parameter for tissues to respond to in order to adapt to their environment during ontogeny. This general view could be extended to virtually every tissue that performs a mechanical function, such as blood vessels, tendons and ligaments, cartilage, and bone. Clearly it is local tissue damage itself that can lead to the mechanical failure of an organ and therefore the demise of the organism. Animals that have an inherent cellular mechanism for responding to local damage by growing and repairing that damage have an obvious advantage in the competition for survival. Although other physicochemical factors related to loading, such as fluid streaming potentials, may also influence the local bone biology, there is no parameter that more directly relates to the function of the organs and survival of the organism than the mechanical damage.

REFERENCES

1. Ahluwalia, R., Datz, F.L., Morton, K.A., Anderson, C.M., and Whiting, J.H., Jr., Bilateral fatigue fractures of the radial shaft in a gymnast, *Clin. Nucl. Med.*, 19, 665, 1994.

2. Albertsen, A.M., Egund, N., and Jurik, A.G., Fatigue fracture of the sacral bone associated with septic arthritis of the symphysis pubis, *Skeletal Radiol.*, 24, 605, 1995.

3. Anderson, E.G., Fatigue fractures of the foot, *Injury*, 21, 275, 1990.

4. Branch, T., Partin, C., Chamberland, P., Emeterio, E., and Sabetelle, M., Spontaneous fractures of the humerus during pitching. A series of 12 cases, *Am. J. Sports Med.*, 20, 468, 1992.

5. Egol, K.A., Koval, K.J., Kummer, F., and Frankel, V.H., Stress fractures of the femoral neck, *Clin. Orthop.*, 348, 72, 1998.

6. Hopson, C.N. and Perry, D.R., Stress fractures of the calcaneus in women marine recruits, *Clin. Orthop.*, 128, 159, 1977.

7. Lord, M.J., Ha, K.I., and Song, K.S., Stress fractures of the ribs in golfers, *Am. J. Sports Med.*, 24, 118, 1996.

8. Mason, R.W., Moore, T.E., Walker, C.W., and Kathol, M.H., Patellar fatigue fractures, *Skeletal Radiol.*, 25, 329, 1996.

9. Matheson, G.O., Clement, D.B., McKenzie, D.C., Taunton, J.E., Lloyd-Smith, D.R., and MacIntyre, J.G., Stress fractures in athletes. A study of 320 cases, *Am. J. Sports Med.*, 15, 46, 1987.

10. Sandrock, A.R., Another sports fatigue fracture. Stress fracture of the coracoid process of the scapula, *Radiology*, 117, 274, 1975.

11. Tanabe, S., Nakahira, J., Bando, E., Yamaguchi, H., Miyamoto, H., and Yamamoto, A., Fatigue fracture of the ulna occurring in pitchers of fast-pitch softball, *Am. J. Sports Med.*, 19, 317, 1991.

12. Wiltse, L.L., Widell, E.H., Jr., and Jackson, D.W., Fatigue fracture: the basic lesion is isthmic spondylolisthesis, *J. Bone Jt. Surg. (Am.)*, 57, 17, 1975.

13. Evans, F. and Lebow, M., Strength of human compact bone under repetitive loading, *J. Appl. Physiol.*, 10, 127, 1957.

14. Evans, F.G. and Riolo, M.L., Relations between the fatigue life and histology of adult human cortical bone, *J. Bone Jt. Surg. (Am.)*, 52, 1579, 1970.

15. Swanson, S.A., Freeman, M.A., and Day, W.H., The fatigue properties of human cortical bone, *Med. Biol. Eng.*, 9, 23, 1971.

16. Gray, R.J. and Korbacher, G.K., Compressive fatigue behavior of bovine compact bone, *J. Biomech.*, 7, 287, 1974.

17. Carter, D.R., Hayes, W.C., and Schurman, D.J., Fatigue life of compact bone. II. Effects of microstructure and density, *J. Biomech.*, 9, 211, 1976.

18. Carter, D.R. and Hayes, W.C., Fatigue life of compact bone. I. Effects of stress amplitude, temperature and density, *J. Biomech.*, 9, 27, 1976.

19. Carter, D.R. and Hayes, W.C., Compact bone fatigue damage. I. Residual strength and stiffness, *J. Biomech.*, 10, 325, 1977.

20. Carter, D.R. and Hayes, W.C., Compact bone fatigue damage: a microscopic examination, *Clin. Orthop.*, 127, 265, 1977.

21. Carter, D.R., Caler, W.E., Spengler, D.M., and Frankel, V.H., Uniaxial fatigue of human cortical bone. The influence of tissue physical characteristics, *J. Biomech.*, 14, 461, 1981.

22. Carter, D.R., Caler, W.E., Spengler, D.M., and Frankel, V.H., Fatigue behavior of adult cortical bone: the influence of mean strain and strain range, *Acta Orthop. Scand.*, 52, 481, 1981.

23. Carter, D.R. and Caler, W.E., Cycle-dependent and time-dependent bone fracture with repeated loading, *J. Biomech. Eng.*, 105, 166, 1983.

24. Lafferty, J. and Raju, P., The influences of stress frequency on the fatigue strength of cortical bone, *J. Biomed. Eng.*, 101, 112, 1979.

25. Carter, D.R. and Hayes, W.C., Bone compressive strength: the influence of density and strain rate, *Science*, 194, 1174, 1976.

26. Taylor, D., Fatigue of bone and bones: an analysis based on stressed volume, *J. Orthop. Res.*, 16, 163, 1998.

27. Taylor, D., O'Brian, F., Prina-Mello, A., Ryan, C., O'Reilly, P., and Lee, T.C., Compression data on bovine bone confirms that a "stressed volume" principle explains the variability of fatigue strength results, *J. Biomech.*, 32, 1199, 1999.

28. Caler, W.E. and Carter, D.R., Bone creep-fatigue damage accumulation, *J. Biomech.*, 22, 625, 1989.

29. Carter, D.R. and Caler, W.E., A cumulative damage model for bone fracture, *J. Orthop. Res.*, 3, 84, 1985.

30. Pattin, C.A., Caler, W.E., and Carter, D.R., Cyclic mechanical property degradation during fatigue loading of cortical bone, *J. Biomech.*, 29, 69, 1996.

31. Gibson, V.A., Stover, S.M., Martin, R.B., Gibeling, J.C., Willits, N.H., Gustafson, M.B., and Griffin, L.V., Fatigue behavior of the equine third metacarpus: mechanical property analysis, *J. Orthop. Res.*, 13, 861, 1995.

32. Schaffler, M.B., Radin, E.L., and Burr, D.B., Long-term fatigue behavior of compact bone at low strain magnitude and rate, *Bone*, 11, 321, 1990.

33. Zioupos, P., Wang, X.T., and Currey, J.D., Experimental and theoretical quantification of the development of damage in fatigue tests of bone and antler, *J. Biomech.*, 29, 989, 1996.

34. Choi, K. and Goldstein, S.A., A comparison of the fatigue behavior of human trabecular and cortical bone tissue, *J. Biomech.*, 25, 1371, 1992.

35. Michel, M.C., Guo, X.D., Gibson, L.J., McMahon, T.A., and Hayes, W.C., Compressive fatigue behavior of bovine trabecular bone *J. Biomech.*, 26, 453, 1993 (published erratum in *J. Biomech.*, 26(9), 1144, 1993.)

36. Bowman, S.M., Guo, X.E., Cheng, D.W., Keaveny, T.M., Gibson, L.J., Hayes, W.C., and McMahon, T.A., Creep contributes to the fatigue behavior of bovine trabecular bone, *J. Biomech. Eng.*, 120, 647, 1998.

37. Chamay, A. and Tschantz, P., Mechanical influences in bone remodeling. Experimental research on Wolff's law, *J. Biomech.*, 5, 173, 1972.

38. Carter, D.R., Harris, W.H., Vasu, R., and Caler, W.E., The mechanical and biological response of cortical bone to in vivo strain histories, in *Mechanical Properties of Bone*, Cowin, S.C., Ed., American Society of Mechanical Engineers, New York, 1981, 81.

39. Cowin, S.C., Bone remodeling of diaphyseal surfaces by torsional loads: theoretical predictions, *J. Biomech.*, 20, 1111, 1987.

40. Frost, H.M., *Intermediary Organization of the Skeleton,* 1986, CRC Press, Boca Raton, 1986, 2v.

41. Huiskes, R., Weinans, H., Grootenboer, H.J., Dalstra, M., Fudala, B., and Slooff, T.J., Adaptive bone-remodeling theory applied to prosthetic-design analysis, *J. Biomech.*, 20, 1135, 1987.

42. Carter, D.R., Mechanical loading histories and cortical bone remodeling, *Calcif. Tissue Int.*, 36, S19, 1984.

43. Levenston, M.E. and Carter, D.R., An energy dissipation-based model for damage stimulated bone adaptation, *J. Biomech.*, 31, 579, 1998.

44. Carter, D.R., Fyhrie, D.P., and Whalen, R.T., Trabecular bone density and loading history: regulation of connective tissue biology by mechanical energy, *J. Biomech.*, 20, 785, 1987.

45. Mikic, B. and Carter, D.R., Bone strain gauge data and theoretical models of functional adaptation, *J. Biomech.*, 28, 465, 1995.

46. Whalen, R.T., Carter, D.R., and Steele, C.R., Influence of physical activity on the regulation of bone density, *J. Biomech.*, 21, 825, 1988.

47. Carter, D.R., Mechanical loading history and skeletal biology, *J. Biomech.*, 20, 1095, 1987.

48. Prendergast, P.J. and Taylor, D., Prediction of bone adaptation using damage accumulation, *J. Biomech.*, 27, 1067, 1994.

49. Carter, D.R. and Beaupré, G.S., *Skeleton Function and Form,* Cambridge University Press, Cambridge, UK, in press.

50. Fuchs, H.O. and Stephens, R.I., *Metal Fatigue in Engineering,* John Wiley & Sons, New York, 1980, xii.

51. Carter, D.R., Orr, T.E., Fyhrie, D.P., and Schurman, D.J., Influences of mechanical stress on prenatal and postnatal skeletal development, *Clin. Orthop.*, 237, 1987.

52. Carter, D.R. and Wong, M., The role of mechanical loading histories in the development of diarthroidal joints, *J. Orthop. Res.*, 6, 804, 1988.

53. Wong, M. and Carter, D.R., Mechanical stress and morphogenetic endochondral ossification of the sternum, *J. Bone Jt. Surg. (Am.),* 70, 992, 1988.

54. Carter, D.R. and Wong, M., Mechanical stresses in joint morphogenesis and mainte-nance, in *Biomechanics of Diarthroidal Joints*, Mow, V., Ratcliffe, A., and Woo, S., Eds., Springer-Verlag, New York, 1990, 155.

55. Wong, M. and Carter, D.R., A theoretical model of endochondral ossification and bone architectural construction in long bone ontogeny, *Anat. Embryol.*, 181, 523, 1990.

56. Heegaard, J.H., Beaupré, G.S., and Carter, D.R., Mechanically modulated cartilage growth may regulate joint surface morphogenesis, *J. Orthop. Res.*, 17, 509, 1999.

57. Wong, M. and Carter, D.R., Theoretical stress analysis of organ culture osteogenesis, *Bone*, 11, 127, 1990.

58. Carter, D.R., Van Der Meulen, M.C., and Beaupré, G.S., Mechanical factors in bone growth and development, *Bone*, 18, 5S, 1996.

59. Stevens, S.S., Beaupré, G.S., and Carter, D.R., Computer model of endochondral growth and ossification in long bones: biological and mechanobiological influences, *J. Orthop. Res.*, 17, 646, 1999.

CHAPTER 7

The Genetic Basis for Stress Fractures

Eitan Friedman, Iris Vered, and Jushua Shemer

CONTENTS

Risk Factors for Stress Fractures 105
Evidence That A Genetic Basis Exists... 106
Candidate Genes 110
The Relationship Between Candidate Genes and Stress Fractures 111
Conclusions.. 112
References... 112

RISK FACTORS FOR STRESS FRACTURES

The exact cause of stress fractures is currently unknown. Strenuous exercise, especially repeated, cyclical, weight bearing activity (as in marching or running on hard surfaces) seems to be an essential prerequisite for development of stress fractures in the lower extremities. Most researchers agree that an inadequate adaptation of the bone to a change in its mechanical environment, involving an imbalance between bone microdamage and remodeling, is the mechanism that underlies stress fractures. However, the fact that only a fraction of soldiers undergoing similar vigorous training programs sustain stress fractures even though they are exposed to similar conditions of fatigue, diet, and weight load, has led to the notion of pre-existing risk factors. Presumably, these risk factors predispose a susceptible individual to developing stress fractures which would become clinically apparent only under the appropriate conditions (i.e., vigorous physical training). Factors reported to be associated with a statistically significant increased risk of developing stress fractures are numerous. Among them are:

- Older age and race (Caucasian more than African American)[1-3]
- Extrinsic factors such as shoe wear, running on hard surfaces, and training errors[2,4,5]
- Biomechanical factors such as tibial bone width[6]
- External rotation of hip[6]
- Arch height[7]
- Genu valgus[8]
- Bodily dimensions such as height,[5,9] higher body mass,[5] body habitus,[10] calf girth,[11] and narrow pelvis.[12]

Additional factors linked to an increased rate of stress fracture occurrence are:

- Current smoking, amenorrhea, and low bone mineral content[13-15]
- Pre-existing levels of physical activity[2,9]
- Increased[16] or decreased[9] motivation.

However, these general predisposing factors were not uniformly confirmed in all studies,[6,12,17,18] and a single unifying hypothesis capable of explaining the underlying mechanisms in all cases has not been formulated.

Female soldiers in the U.S. military are at risk for developing stress fractures during their military training.[2,12,13,19] In fact, in one large study the incidence of stress fractures for female soldiers was about 20% more than for their male counterparts.[13] Other studies noted an even greater propensity for female soldiers to develop stress fractures as compared with their male counterparts, at 10 to 12% versus 1 to 3%, respectively.[19-22] In addition, amenorrhea and family history of osteoporosis have been found to be risk factors for development of stress fractures.[13] Women tend to sustain stress fractures in anatomical locations that are distinct from men, such as the ramus pubis.[23] The reasons for this apparent increased risk in female soldiers are not clear, and hypotheses pertaining to this difference cite bodily dimensions, stride requirements, the effects of sex hormones, and biomechanical factors.[12,19]

EVIDENCE THAT A GENETIC BASIS EXISTS

Several observations suggest a genetic component that contributes to stress fracture predisposition. In 1990, Singer and co-workers described multiple stress fractures in monozygotic twins.[24] Remarkably, both affected individuals, who served in the same unit, sustained stress fractures at the same anatomical sites, and the onset of symptoms was traced to the sixth week of basic training in both. No mention is given in that report to family history of stress fractures, and it remains the sole reported case of bona fide familial stress fractures. This report probably provides the best indirect link to genetic factors in stress fracture pathogenesis. Meurman and Elfving[25] report two soldiers with six stress fractures and one with seven stress fractures. Milgrom and co-workers, report the occurrence of 11 simultaneous stress fractures in a single individual in a span of six weeks, and later the same individual developed two additional fractures.[26] Others also report the occurrence of multiple lower limb stress fractures in individuals.[27-29] Having more than one stress fracture may indicate that bone composition is defective overall, and thus genetic factors would be implicated as the underlying cause. Similarly, recurrence of stress fractures at different anatomical loci in the same individual may imply an inherent bone structure abnormality that is genetically determined. Indeed, among 66 Israeli soldiers who sustained stress fractures, seven (10.6%) developed an additional stress fracture at a different anatomical site within a year.[30]

Stress fractures are primarily diagnosed in the second or third decade of life. The occurrence of stress fractures in the pediatric age group may imply an inherited predisposition. Table 1 summarizes the majority of reports in English of pediatric cases (under 10 years of age) with lower limb stress fractures.[31-52] Family history of stress fracture or bone disease is not mentioned in any report. In the majority of cases, there are no obvious associated medical conditions known to predispose to increased bone fragility (e.g., osteogenesis imperfecta). Stress fracture can be related to a specific cause in only a minority of the cases. Thus, these cases provide more credence to the genetic component notion in stress fractures.

Additional lines of indirect evidence of genetic factors in stress fracture pathogenesis are the variations in stress fracture incidence given the similar training load among soldiers the same unit.[53-55] Furthermore, the anthropometric differences between soldiers with stress fractures as compared with controls (e.g., narrower tibiae,[7,56] genu varus[8]), can also be explained by predetermined genetic factors. Lastly, stress fractures were reported to occur in the context of known genetic disorders such as adult hypophosphatasia[57] and rare cases of Marfan syndrome.[58]

Thus, it seems logical that in a subset of patients with stress fractures, the underlying cause is a predisposing genetic susceptibility in the form of a mutation within a gene involved in bone formation, remodeling, or bone matrix formation. Exposing a genetically susceptible individual to strenuous exercise unmasks this otherwise clinically subtle mutation and results in stress fracture.

In most studies relating to predisposing factors of stress fractures, little or no mention is made of family history of bone disease or stress fracture. However, in one study, known family history of osteoporosis was significantly associated with increased risk of stress fractures in females.[13] Our preliminary data also indicate that 51 of 307 (16.6%) soldiers with stress fractures diagnosed and treated during 1995 to 1996 in the Israeli Defense Forces (IDF) reported the occurrence of bone disease in an immediate (first- or second-degree) family member. Moreover, 26 of 307 (8.5%) also reported the occurrence of stress fracture in a sibling.[59] Even though the differences in the reported occurrence of familial bone disease and/or stress fracture between soldiers with stress fractures and an asymptomatic control group were statistically insignificant, this provides strong support for the notion of a genetic basis. In order to characterize and identify the genes that are putatively involved, two approaches may be employed: the candidate gene approach and the whole genome scanning approach. The latter approach requires at least one but preferably several multigenerational families with a clear-cut mode of trait transmission, unifying criteria for diagnosing stress fractures, and sufficient numbers of affected and unaffected individuals, to attain linkage or even association with a defined genomic region. Presently, these resources are not available, so to assess the putative genes that contribute to stress fracture pathogenesis, the candidate gene approach has been adopted.

Table 1 Femoral, Tibial, and Fibular Stress Fractures in the First Decade of Life Reported in the English Literature*

Reference	Age/Sex	Cause	Site	Associated Conditions	Diagnosis
Roberts 1939	6½/F	??	Tibia	None	X ray
	6½/F	??	Tibia	None	X ray
	8½/M	??	Tibia	None	X ray
	9½/M	??	Tibia	None	X ray
	4/F	??	Tibia	None	X ray
**Siemens 1942	16 Mo./M	??	Tibia	None	X ray
Ingersoll 1943	9/M	Skating	Fibula	None	X ray
	9/M	Skating	Fibula	None	X ray
	9/M	Skating	Fibula	None	X ray
Griffiths 1952	4½/M	Jumping	Fibula	None	X ray
	5/F	Jumping	Fibula	None	X ray
	3/M	Jumping	Fibula	None	X ray
	5/M	??	Fibula	None	X ray
	5/F	??	Fibula	None	X ray
	2/F	??	Fibula	None	X ray
	8/F	??	Fibula	None	X ray
	3½/F	??	Fibula	None	X ray
Devas 1963	5/M	??	Tibia	None	X ray
	5/F	??	Tibia	None	X ray
	9/M	??	Tibia	None	X ray
	9/F	??	Tibia	None	X ray
	8/F	??	Tibia	None	X ray
	2/F	??	Bil Fibula	None	X ray
	3/F	??	Fibula	None	X ray
	5/M	??	Fibula	None	X ray
	5/M	??	Fibula	None	X ray
	6/M	??	*Pelvis	None	X ray
	8/M	??	*Pelvis	None	X ray
	5/M	??	*Pelvis	None	X ray
	5/F	??	*Pelvis	None	X ray
	5/M	??	*Pelvis	None	X ray
Engh 1970	4/M	??	Tibia	None	X ray
	21 Mo./M	??	Tibia	None	X ray
	2/M	??	Tibia	None	X ray
	7/M	??	Tibia	None	X ray
	9/F	??	Tibia	None	X ray
Wolfgang 1977	10/F	Jungle gym	Femur	None	X ray
Burks 1984	4½/M	Hyperactive	Femur	None	X ray
	3/M	Hiking	Femur	None	X ray
Horev 1990	9/F	??	Tibia	None	CT, MRI
Kozlowski 1991	17 Mo./F	Hyperactive	Fibula	None	X ray
	3/M	??	Fibula	None	X ray
	3½/F	Hyperactive	Fibula	None	X ray
	5/M	Skating No trauma	Fibula	None	X ray
	6/F	??	Fibula	None	X ray
	8/F	Hyperactive	Fibula	None	X ray
	8⁷⁄₁₂/M	??	Fibula	None	X ray
	9/F	??	Fibula	None	X ray

Table 1 (continued)   Femoral, Tibial, and Fibular Stress Fractures in the First Decade of Life Reported in the English Literature*

Reference	Age/Sex	Cause	Site	Associated Conditions	Diagnosis
Meany 1992	5/F	??	Femur	None	X ray
	9/M	??	Femur	Perthes' dis.	X ray
Buckley 1995	3/F	??	Femur	None	Tc Scan
	5/M	??	Femur	None	X ray
St. Pierre 1995	9/F	Trampoline use	Femur	None	X ray
	7/F	Scooter use	Femur	Obesity	X ray
	8/F	??	Femur	CDH hydrocephalus	X ray
Sheehan 1995	10 Mo./F	Infant walker	Bil Fibula	None	X ray
Hitchen 1996	9/F	Roller Blading	Tibia	None	X ray
Kozlowski 1996	15 Mo./F	??	Fibula	None	X ray
	15 Mo./F	??	Fibula	None	X ray
	16 Mo./F	??	Fibula	None	X ray
	2/M	??	Fibula	None	X ray
	2/F	Hyperactive	Fibula	None	X ray
	3/M	??	Fibula	None	X ray
Walker 1996	4/M	??	Fibula	None	X ray
	7/F	??	Femur	Fibrous cortical defect	X ray
	9/M	??	Tibia	None	X ray
	8/F	??	Tibia	None	X ray
	2/M	??	Tibia	None	X ray
	8/M	??	Tibia	None	X ray
	30 Mo./F	??	Fibula	None	X ray
	8/M	??	Tibia	None	X ray
	7½/F	??	Femur		
	6/M	??	Tibia/Femur	None	X ray
	4/M	??	Fibula	Osteopenia (steroid induced)	X ray
	8/F	??	Fibula	None	X ray
	3/M	??	Tibia	None	X ray
	6/M	??	Femur	None	X ray
	6/M	??	Tibia	None	X ray
	7/F	??	Fibula	None	X ray
	35 Mo./F	??	Tibia	None	X ray
	4/F	??	Tibia	None	X ray
Toren 1997	5/M	Roller blading	Bil Femur	None	X ray
Mucklow 1997	3/F	Hyperactive	Tibia/Fibula	None	X ray
Ariyoshi 1997	8/M	??	Tibia (multiple)	None	X ray, Tc Scan, MRI
Scheerlinck 1998	8/F	??	Bil Femur	None	Tc scan

Bil denotes bilateral; Tc scan — 99m Tc scintigraphy.

• Pelvic stress fracture is at the ischiopubic junction

** Quoted by Devas.[34]

Additional pediatric cases are described by Walter,[37] Hulkko,[39] and Donati.[41]

CANDIDATE GENES

Several candidate genes may harbor mutations associated with stress fracture susceptibility. The common denominator of these genes is that each one was either shown to be involved in abnormal bone formation, or to be involved in in genetic disorders that lead to a variety of bone pathologies with resultant increased bone fragility. Alternatively, these may be putative candidate genes in stress fracture predisposition, based on tissue expression pattern and/or known protein function. These candidates include, among others, the genes encoding for procollagen type 1 (COL1A1 and COL1A2), vitamin D receptor (VDR), estrogen receptor (ER), calcitonin receptor (CTR), insulin-like growth factor 1 (IGF1), and glucocerebrosidase (Gaucher disease gene). Admittedly, most of these genes have been associated with low peak bone mass and/or osteoporosis, whereas low peak bone mass has never been conclusively related to stress fracture predisposition. However, the undisputed pivotal role these genes play in maintaining bone integrity and bone formation makes them at least attractive candidates.

Mutations within *COL1A1* and *COL1A2* have been shown to be the major underlying cause of Osteogenesis Imperfecta (OI).[60,61] Mutations in these genes have also been noted in other, more common bone diseases.[62-64] Indeed, 3 of 26 patients with no clinically apparent bone disease but with a positive family history of osteopenia or osteoporosis displayed mutations within one of these genes.[65] Using a mouse model to genetically recreate the mutations, the phenotype of the mutant mouse is highly suggestive of a causal role for these mutations in the pathogenesis of bone diseases.[66,67] Moreover, an Sp1 polymorphism in the 5' untranslated region of the *COL1A1* was found to be correlated with bone mineral density and osteoporosis risk in pre– and postmenopausal women.[68-70] These theoretical considerations, taken together with the known phenotypic variability of OI that at times may be nearly asymptomatic, have led us to speculate that these two genes are intimately involved in stress fracture predisposition. Consequently, mutational analysis of these genes in Israeli soldiers with high-grade stress fractures has been undertaken (see below).

Another strong candidate gene involved in bone mass determination is the VDR gene. Morrison and co-workers[71] showed the existence of a specific pattern of alleles of the VDR gene in healthy individuals in Australia, and a close relationship between these allelic patterns and serum osteocalcin. This pioneering work suggested that genetic variations in the VDR gene could underlie some of the physiologic variations in circulating osteocalcin, and hence may also play a role in determining bone mass. Moreover, analysis of the VDR alleles in asymptomatic individuals could potentially be used as a genetic marker for identifying a predisposition to low bone mass, and predict fracture risk. Thus, VDR alleles are attractive candidates for the genetic determinants of bone mass. Despite initial enthusiasm and duplication of the Australian data by independent investigators from England[72] and Japan,[73] no association between VDR allelic pattern and bone mass or osteoporosis was demonstrated in North American[74] and Scandinavian[75] women. Thus, the contribution of VDR polymorphism to bone mass variance in healthy persons and its possible use as a predictor of osteoporosis is a subject of controversy.[76] It was suggested that VDR genotypes determine adaptability to low calcium intake: subjects with the bb genotype have more efficient intestinal calcium absorption, which may serve as a protective mechanism from bone loss.[77] In summary, the contribution of the VDR genotype to bone mass determination and osteoporosis is an intriguing area of research of yet undefined significance and applicability to the general population. However, more studies concentrating on well-defined populations with a common ethnic background may help to shed light on this controversial issue. Despite its questionable role in osteoporosis, the VDR gene also seems suitable for a subtle modification of bone structure in a way that would make it more susceptible to stress fractures.

Clinically, osteoporosis has been intimately associated with estrogen deficiency in females, so that ER inactivation (by point mutations), decreased expression, or uncoupling from intracellular effectors are likely to contribute to osteoporosis susceptibility. Indeed, a germline mutation in the ER gene in a 28 year old male that resulted in failure of epiphyseal closure, reduced bone mass, and increased bone turnover underscores the relevance of ER to bone mass status in male osteoporosis.[78] More recently, an association was reported between genetic variations (i.e., polymorphisms) of the ER gene with postmenopausal osteoporosis in Japan[79] and bone mineral density in Australia.[80] Gross alterations in the ER gene are unlikely to play a major role in stress fracture pathogenesis in male soldiers, for obvious reasons. However, subtle alterations even at the tissue expression level may contribute to stress fracture predisposition in females. Indeed, in female world class athletes, especially long distance runners, stress fractures have been related to amenorrhea or disturbed menstrual cycle.[11,13,15]

An additional candidate gene that may be relevant to genetic susceptibility to osteoporosis is the glucocerebrosidase gene, which is mutated in Gaucher's disease.[81] Several reports show that enzyme replacement therapy of homozygous patients with Gaucher's disease results in increased bone mass and reduction of fracture incidence.[82-84] These reports give rise to the notion that some cases of unexplained low bone mass may be attributable to an otherwise asymptomatic heterozygous gene carrier. This gene may have special significance in the IDF, as the rate of heterozygous mutation carriers among Ashkenazi Jews is appreciably high (1:25-30).

Two other candidate genes are IGF1 and calcitonin receptor. Both genes have been shown in some studies to be associated with osteoporosis or its prevention,[85] and in the case of the calcitonin receptor, a novel polymorphism has also been correlated with an altered bone mineral content.[86]

THE RELATIONSHIP BETWEEN CANDIDATE GENES AND STRESS FRACTURES

Ongoing work in the IDF, with funding from the U.S. military, has resulted in analyses of the status of some of the above-mentioned candidate genes in a subset of IDF soldiers with high grade stress fractures. These analyses were performed using two mutually non-exclusive approaches: direct mutational analysis of the COL1A1 and COL1A2 genes, and association studies using known and novel polymorphisms within the candidate genes. More complete results are not available at this time. However, one interesting observation that emanated from these studies is the relationship between OI and stress fractures. Among the 60 OI patients clinically and genetically evaluated by us over the past four years, there were three individuals with type 1 OI who served the full three-year compulsory military service in the IDF without sustaining stress fractures. Moreover, in a single soldier who sustained multiple stress fractures, protein-based analyses failed to reveal any alterations in the *COL1A1* or *COL1A2* proteins (Friedman et al., unpublished observations). These latter data may indicate that abnormal *COL1A1* and *COL1A2* contribute little, if any, to stress fracture predisposition.

CONCLUSIONS

There is a mounting body of indirect evidence that genetic factors play a role in stress fracture predisposition. Deciphering the genes that are involved is an ongoing task that should proceed along several paths. First, all presumed candidate genes should be evaluated in individuals with stress fractures. This can be accomplished by direct mutational analyses or by comparing the rates of known polymorphisms within these genes in stress fracture patients with the rates in asymptomatic, healthy controls. For this approach to be successful, large numbers of both patients and controls have to be recruited and genotyped. Even so, the risk of being forced to choose from the rather limited pool of known genes, with several *a priori* assumptions about protein function and pathogenic mechanisms, severely detracts from this approach. An alternative is to perform a genome-wide search for regions that harbor genes involved in stress fracture predisposition. This approach does not assume a known function, and using a brute force technique, analyzes for regions in the human genome that are associated with stress fracture predisposition. For this approach to succeed, families with more than one affected individual in a generation should be identified, where the mode of transmission can be precisely assigned and then used for genotyping. In addition, the sibling pair analysis approach may be employed, where a more limited number of individuals within a family may be sufficient to give a meaningful result.

Regardless of the approach used to characterize the putative genes conferring an increased risk for developing stress fractures, it is clear that future research into stress fracture pathogenesis should incorporate the genetic aspect, and more attention should be paid to eliciting family history of stress fractures by military physicians.

REFERENCES

1. Brudvig, T.J.S., Gudger, T.D., and Obermeyer, L., Stress fractures in 295 trainees: a one year study of incidence as related to age, sex, and race, *Mil. Med.*, 148, 666, 1983.
2. Gardner, L., Dziados, J.E., Jones, B.H., Brundage, J.F., Harris, J.M. and Grill, R., Prevention of lower extremity stress fractures: a controlled trial of shock absorbent insole, *Am. J. Public Health*, 78, 1563, 1988.
3. Milgrom, C., Finestone, A., Shlamkovitch, N., Rand, N., Lev, B., Simkin, A., and Wiener, M., Youth is a risk factor for stress fracture. A study of 783 infantry recruits, *J. Bone Jt. Surg. (Br.)*, 76, 20, 1994.

4. Schwellnus, M.P., Jordaan, G., and Noakes, T.D., Prevention of common overuse injuries by the use of shock absorbing insoles. A prospective study, *Am. J. Sports Med.*, 18, 636, 1990.

5. Jones, B.H., Bovee, M.W., Harris, J.M., III, and Cowan, D.N., Intrinsic risk factors for exercise-related injuries among male and female army trainees, *Am. J. Sports Med.*, 21, 705, 1993.

6. Giladi, M., Milgrom, C., Simkin, A., and Danon, Y., Stress fractures: identifiable risk factors, *Am. J. Sports Med.*, 19, 647, 1991.

7. Giladi, M., Milgrom, C., Stein, M., and Danon, Y., The low arch, a protective factor in stress fractures. A prospective study of 295 military recruits, *Orthop. Rev.*, 14, 81, 1985.

8. Cowan, D.N., Jones, B.H., Frykman, P.N., Polly, D.W., Jr., Harman, E.A., Rosenstein, R.M., and Rosenstein, M.T., Lower limb morphology and risk of overuse injury among male infantry trainees, *Med. Sci. Sports Exerc.*, 28, 945, 1996.

9. Taimela, S., Kujala, U.M., and Osterman, K., Stress injury proneness: a prospective study during a physical training program, *Int. J. Sports Med.*, 11, 162, 1990.

10. Gilbert, R.S. and Johnson, H.A., Stress fractures in military recruits. A review of twelve years' experience, *Mil. Med.*, 131, 716, 1968.

11. Bennell, K.L., Malcolm, S.A., Thomas, S.A., Reid, S.J., Brukner, P.D., Ebeling, P.R., and Wark, J.D., Risk factors for stress fractures in track and field athletes. A twelve-month prospective study, *Am. J. Sports Med.*, 24, 810, 1996.

12. Winfield, A.C., Moore, J., Bracker, M., and Johnson, C.W., Risk factors associated with stress reactions in female Marines, *Mil. Med.*, 162, 698, 1997.

13. Friedl, K.E., Nuovo, J.A., Patience, T.H., and Dettori, J.R., Factors associated with stress fracture in young Army women: indications for further research, *Mil. Med.*, 157, 334, 1992.

14. Myburgh, K.H., Hutchins, J., Fataar, A.B., Hough, S.F., and Noakes, T.D., Low bone density is an etiologic factor for stress fractures in athletes, *Ann. Intern. Med.*, 113, 754, 1990.

15. Bennell, K.L., Malcolm, S.A., Thomas, S.A., Ebeling, P.R., McCrory, P.R., Wark, J.D., and Brukner, P.D., Risk factors for stress fractures in female track-and-field athletes: a retrospective analysis, *Clin. J. Sport Med.*, 5, 229, 1995.

16. Hallel, T., Amit, S., and Segal, D., Fatigue fractures of tibial and femoral shaft in soldiers, *Clin. Orthoped.*, 118, 35, 1976.

17. Ekenman, I., Tsai-Fetlander, L., Westblad, P., Turan, I., and Rolf, C., A study of intrinsic factors in patients with stress fractures of the tibia, *Foot Ankle Int.*, 17, 477, 1996.

18. Jones, B.H. and Knapik, J.J., Physical training and exercise-related injuries. Surveillance, research and injury prevention in military populations, *Sports Med.*, 27, 111, 1999.

19. Bijur, P.E., Horodyski, M., Egerton, W., Kurzon, M., Lifrak, S., and Friedman, S., Comparison of injury during cadet basic training by gender, *Arch. Pediatr. Adolesc. Med.*, 151, 456, 1997.

20. Protzman, R.R., Physiologic performance of women compared to men: observations of cadets at the United States Military Academy, *Am. J. Sports Med.*, 7, 191, 1979.

21. Reinker, K.A. and Ozburne, S., A comparison of male and female orthopedic pathology in basic training, *Mil. Med.*, 144, 532, 1979.

22. Jones, B.H., Harris, J.M., Vinh, T.N., and Rubin, C., Exercise-induced stress fractures and stress reactions of bone: epidemiology, etiology, and classification, *Exerc. Sports Sci. Rev.*, 17, 379, 1989.

23. Hill, P.F., Chatterji, S., Chambers, D., and Keeling, J.D., Stress fracture of the pubic ramus in female recruits, *J. Bone Jt. Surg. (Br.)*, 78, 383, 1996.

24. Singer, A., Ben-Yehuda, O., Ben-Ezra, Z., and Zaltzman, S., Multiple identical stress fractures in monozygotic twins, *J. Bone Jt. Surg.*, 72, 444, 1990.

25. Meurman, K.O. and Elfving, S., Stress fracture in soldiers: a multifocal bone disorder. A comparative radiological and scintigraphic study, *Radiology*, 134, 483, 1980.

26. Milgrom, C., Chisin, R., Giladi, M., Stein, M., Kashtan, H., Marguiles, J., and Atlan, H., Multiple stress fractures. A longitudinal study of a soldier with 13 lesions, *Clin. Orthop.*, 192, 174, 1985.

27. Nielens, H., Devogelaer, J.P., Malghem, J. Occurrence of a painful stress fracture of the femoral neck simultaneously with six other asymptomatic localizations in a runner, *J. Sports Med. Phys. Fitness*, 34, 79, 1994.

28. Lambros, G. and Alder, D., Multiple stress fractures of the tibia in a healthy adult, *Am. J. Orthop.*, 26, 687, 1997.

29. Ariyoshi, M., Nagata, K., Kubo, M., Sato, K., and Inoue, A., Three stress fractures at different sites in the same tibia — a case report, *Acta Orthop. Scand.*, 68, 406, 1997.

30. Giladi, M., Milgrom, C., Kashtan, H., Stein, M., Chisin, R., and Dizian, R., Recurrent stress fractures in military recruits, *J. Bone Jt. Surg.*, 68, 1090, 1986.

31. Roberts, S.M. and Vogt, E.C., Pseudofracture of the tibia, *J. Bone Jt. Surg.*, 21, 891, 1939.

32. Ingersoll, C.F., Ice skater's fracture, *Am. J. Roentgenol.*, 50, 469, 1943.

33. Griffiths, A.L., Fatigue fractures of the fibula in childhood, *Arch. Dis. Child.* 27, 552, 1952.

34. Devas, M.B., Stress fractures in children, *J. Bone Jt. Surg. (Br.)*, 45, 528, 1963.

35. Engh, C.A., Robinson, R.A., and Milgram, J., Stress fractures in children, *J. Trauma*, 10, 532, 1970.

36. Wolfgang, G.L., Stress fracture of the femoral neck in a patient with open capital femoral epiphyses, *J. Bone Jt. Surg. (Am.)*, 59, 680, 1977.

37. Walter, N.E. and Wolf, M.D., Stress fractures in young athletes, *Am. J. Sports Med.*, 5, 165, 1977.

38. Burks, R.T. and Sutherland, D.H., Stress fracture of the femoral shaft in children: Report of two cases and discussion, *J. Pediatr. Orthoped.*, 4, 614, 1984.

39. Hulkko, A. and Orava, S., Stress fractures in athletes, *Int. J. Sports Med.*, 8, 221, 1987.

40. Horev, G., Korenreich, L., Ziv, N., and Grunebaum, M., The enigma of stress fractures in the pediatric age: clarification or confusion through the new imaging modalities, *Pediatr. Radiol.*, 20, 469, 1990.

41. Donati, R.B., Echo, B.S., and Powell, C.E., Bilateral tibial stress fractures in a six-year-old male. A case report, *Am. J, Sports Med.*, 18, 323, 1990.

42. Kozlowski, K., Azouz, M., and Hoff, D., Stress fracture of the fibula in the first decade of life. Report of eight cases, *Pediatr. Radiol.*, 21, 381, 1991.

43. Meany, J.E.M. and Carty, H., Femoral stress fractures in children, *Skeletal Radiol.*, 21, 173, 1992.

44. St Pierre, P., Staheli, L.T., Smith, J.B., and Green, N.E., Femoral neck stress fractures in children and adolescents. *J. Pediatr. Orthop.*, 15, 470, 1995.

45. Buckley, S.L., Robertson, W.W., Jr., and Shalaby-Rana, E., Stress fractures of the femoral diaphysis in young children. A report of 2 cases, *Clin. Orthop.*, 310, 165, 1995.

46. Sheehan, K.M., Gordon, S., and Tanz, R.R., Bilateral fibula fractures from infant walker use, *Pediatr. Emerg. Care*, 11, 27, 1995

47. Hitchen, P.R. and Lyons, W.J., Fatigue fracture of the medial malleolus in a junior roller skater, *Aust. N. Z. J. Surg.*, 66, 265, 1996.

48. Walker, R.N., Green, N.E., and Spindler, K.P., Stress fractures in skeletally immature patients, *J. Pediatr. Orthop.*, 16, 578, 1996.

49. Kozlowski, K. and Urbonaviciene, A., Stress fractures of the fibula in the first few years of life (report of six cases), *Australas. Radiol.*, 40, 261, 1996.

50. Toren, A., Goshen, E., Katz, M., Levi, R., and Rechavi, G., Bilateral femoral stress fractures in a child due to in-line (roller) skating, *Acta Paediatr.*, 86, 332, 1997.

51. Mucklow, E.S. and Evans, G., Stress fractures in a hyperactive 3-year-old girl, *Lancet*, 349(9055), 854, 1997.

52. Scheerlinck, T. and De Boeck, H., Bilateral stress fractures of the femoral neck complicated by unilateral displacement in a child, *J. Pediatr. Orthop. (Br.)*, 7, 246, 1998.

53. Milgrom, C., Giladi, M., Stein, H., Kashtan, H., Marguiles, J., Chisin, R., Steinberg, R., and Aharonson, Z., Stress fractures in military recruits: a prospective study showing an unusually high incidence, *J. Bone Jt. Surg.*, 67B, 732, 1985.

54. Gill, R.M.F. and Hopkins, G.O., Stress fractures in parachute regiment recruits, *J. R. Army Med. Corps.*, 134, 91, 1988.

55. Linenger, J.M. and Shwayhat, A.F., Epidemiology of podiatric injuries in U.S. Marine recruits undergoing basic training, *J. Amer. Pod. Med. Soc.*, 82, 269, 1992.

56. Milgrom, C., Giladi, M., Simkin, A., Randi, N., Kedem, R., Kashtan, H., Stein, M., and Gomori, M., The area moment of inertia of the tibia: a risk factor for stress fractures, *J. Biomech.*, 22, 1243, 1989.

57. Whyte, M.P., Teitelbaum, S.L., Murphy, W.A., Bergfeld, M.A., and Avioli, L.V., Adult hypophosphatasia. Clinical, laboratory, and genetic investigation of a large kindred with review of the literature, *Medicine (Baltimore)*, 58, 329, 1979.

58. Kharrazi, F.D., Rodgers, W.B., Coran, D.L., Kasser, J.R., and Hall, J.E., Protrusio acetabuli and bilateral basicervical femoral neck fractures in a patient with Marfan syndrome, *Am. J. Orthop.*, 26, 689, 1997.

59. Givon, U., Friedman, E., Reiner, A.,Vered, I., Finestone, A., and Shemer, J., Stress fractures in the Israeli Defense Forces in 1995 to 1996, *Clin. Orthopaed. Relat. Res.*, (in press), 2000.

60. Prockop, D.J., Mutations that alter the primary structure of Type 1 collagen, *J. Biol. Chem.*, 265, 15349, 1990.

61. Prockop, D.J., Mutations in collagen genes as a cause of connective tissue diseases, *N. Engl. J. Med.*, 326, 540, 1992.

62. Kuivaniemi, H., Tromp, G., and Prockop, D.J., Mutations in collagen genes: causes of rare and some common diseases in humans, *FASEB J.*, 5, 2052, 1991.

63. Spotila, L.D., Constantinou, C.D., Sereda, L., Ganguly, A., Riggs, B.L., and Prockop, D.J., Mutation in the gene for type I procollagen (COL1A1) in a woman with post menopausal osteoporosis: evidence for phenotypic and genotypic overlap with mild osteogenesis imperfecta, *Proc. Natl. Acad. Sci. USA*, 88, 5423, 1991.

64. Hampson, G., Evans, C., Petitt, R.J., Evans, W.D., Woodhead, S.J., Peters, J.R., and Ralston, S.H., Bone mineral density, collagen type 1 alpha 1 genotypes and bone turnover in premenopausal women with diabetes mellitus, *Diabetologia*, 41, 1314, 1998.

65. Spotila, L.D., Colige, A., Sereda, L., Constantinou-Deltas, C.D., Whyte, M.P., Riggs, B.L., Shaker, J.L., Spector, T.D., Hume, E., Olsen, N., Attie, M., Tenenhouse, A., Shane, E., Briney, W., and Prockop, D.J., Mutation analysis of coding sequences for type 1 procollagen in individuals with low bone density, *J. Bone Miner. Metab.*, 9, 923, 1994.

66. Stacey, A., Bateman, J., Choi, T., Mascara, T., Cole, W., and Jaenisch, R., Perinatal lethal osteogenesis imperfecta in transgenic mice bearing an engineered mutant pro-α1(I) collagen gene, *Nature,* 332, 131, 1988.

67. Khillan, J.S., Olsen, A.E., Kontussari, S., Sokolov, B., and Prockop, D.J., Transgenic mice that express a mini-gene version for type I procollagen (COL1AI) developed a phenotype resembling a lethal from of osteogenesis imperfecta, *J. Biol. Chem.,* 266, 23373, 1991.

68. Grant, S.F.A., Reid, D.M., Blake, G., Herd, R., Fogelman, I., and Ralston, S.H., Reduced bone density and osteoporosis associated with a polymorphic Sp1 binding site in the collagen type 1a1 gene, *Nat. Genet.,* 14, 203, 1996.

69. Uitterlinden, A.G., Burger, H., Huang, Q., Yue, F., McGuigan, F.E., Grant, S.F., Hofman, A., van-Leeuwen, J.P., Pols, H.A., and Ralston, S.H., Relation of alleles of the collagen type 1alpha1 gene to bone density and the risk of osteoporotic fractures in postmenopausal women, *N. Engl. J. Med.,* 338, 1016, 1998.

70. Langdahl, B.L., Ralston, S.H., Grant, S.F.A., and Eriksen, E.F., An Sp1 binding site polymorphism in the COL1A1 gene predicts osteoporotic fractures in men and women, *J. Bone Miner. Res.,* 13, 1384, 1998.

71. Morrison, N.A., Qi, J.C., Tokita, A., Kelly, P.J., Crofts, L., Nguyen, T.V., Sambrook, P.N., and Eisman, J.A., Prediction of bone density from vitamin D receptor alleles, *Nature,* 367, 284, 1994.

72. Spector, T.D., Keen, R.W., Arden, N.K., Morrison, N.A., Major. P.J., Nguyen, T.V., Kelly, P.J., Baker, J.R., Sambrook, P.N., and Lanchbury, J.S., Influence of vitamin D receptor genotype on bone mineral density in postmenopausal women: a twin study in Britain, *Br. Med. J.,* 310(6991), 1357, 1995.

73. Yamagata, Z. Miyamura, T., Iijima, S., Asaka, A., Sasaki, M., Kato, J., and Koizumi, K., Vitamin D receptor gene polymorphism and bone mineral density in healthy Japanese women, *Lancet,* 344, 1027, 1994.

74. Husmyer, F.G., Peacock, M., Hui, S., Johnston, C.C., and Christian, J., Bone mineral density in relation to polymorphism at the vitamin D receptor gene locus, *J. Clin. Invest.,* 94, 2130, 1994.

75. Melhus, H., Kindmark, A., Amer, S., Wilen, B., Lindh, E., and Ljunghall, S., Vitamin D receptor genotypes in osteoporosis, *Lancet,* 344, 919, 1994.

76. Parfitt, A.M., Vitamin D receptor genotypes in osteoporosis, *Lancet,* 344, 1580, 1994.

77. Hayes, J.C., Nguyen, T.V., and Need, A.G., Vitamin D receptor genotypes and functional gut calcium absorption, *J. Bone Miner. Res.,* 10, S188, 1995.

78. Smith, E.P., Boyd, J., Franck, G.R., Takahashi, H., Cohen, R.M., Specker, B., Williams, T.C., Lubahn, D.B., and Korach, K.S., Estrogen resistance caused by a mutation in the estrogen-receptor gene in a man, *N. Engl. J. Med.,* 331, 1056, 1994.

79. Sano, M., Inoue, S., Hosoi, T., Ouchi, Y., Emi, M., Shiraki, M., Orimo, H., Association of estrogen receptor dinucleotide repeat polymorphism with osteoporosis, *Biochem. Biophys. Res. Commun.,* 217, 378, 1995.

80. Koboyashi, S., Inoue, S., Hosoi, T., Ouchi, Y., Shiraki, M., and Orimo, H., Association of bone mineral density with polymorphism of the estrogen receptor gene, *J. Bone Miner. Metab.,* 11, 306, 1996.

81. Mankin, H.J., Doppelt, S.H., Rosenberg, A.E., and Barranger, J.A., Metabolic bone disease in patients with Gaucher's disease, in *Metabolic Bone Disease and Clinically Related Disorders,* Avioli, L.V. and Krane, S.M., Eds., WB Saunders, Philadelphia, 1990, 730.

82. Bembi, B., Agosti, E., Boehm, P., Nassimbeni, G., Zanatta, M., and Vidoni, L., Aminohydroxypropylidene biphosphonate in the treatment of bone lesions in a case of Gaucher's disease type 3, *Acta Paediatr.,* 83, 122, 1994.

83. Ostlere, L., Warner, T., Meunier, P.J., Hulme, P., Hesp, R., Watts, R.W., and Reeve, J., Treatment of type 1 Gaucher's disease affecting bone with aminohydroxypropylidene bisphosphonate (pamidronate), *Q. J. Med.,* 79(290), 503, 1991.

84. Pastores, G.M., Wallenstein, S., Desnick, R.J., and Luckey, M.M., Bone density in type 1 Gaucher's disease, *J. Bone Miner. Res.,* 11, 1801, 1996.

85. Langlois, J.A., Rosen, C.J., Visser, M., Hannan, M.T., Harris, T., Wilson, P.W., and Kiel, D.P., Association between insulin-like growth factor 1 and bone mineral density in older women and men: The Framingham Heart Study, *J. Clin. Endocrinol. Metab.,* 83, 4257, 1998.

86. Taboulet, J., Frenkian, M., Frendo, J.L., Feingold, N., Jullienne, A., and de Vernejoul, M.C., Calcitonin receptor polymorphism is associated with a decreased fracture risk in post-menopausal women, *Hum. Mol. Genet.,* 7, 2129, 1998.

CHAPTER 8

The Role of Strain and Strain Rates in Stress Fractures

Charles Milgrom

CONTENTS

Introduction..119
Ex Vivo Studies of Strain and Strain Rate 120
In Vivo Studies of Strain and Strain Rate 120
    Strains and Strain Rates in the Human Tibia 121
    Strains and Strain Rates in the Human Metatarsal...................................124
    The Role of Muscle Fatigue on Strain and Strain Rates..........................124
The Role of Gender and Age in Developing High Strains and Strain Rates 126
Conclusion 127
References..127

INTRODUCTION

Most people are first introduced to the role of strain and strain rate in the fatigue failure of material inadvertently. As a child I can remember wanting to break a tree branch. I grabbed the ends of the branch and bent it in a direction against the thinnest cross section with as much force as I could generate. When it did not break, I quickly learned that if I repeated the bending motion multiple times I could cause cracks in the branch. I persisted with the bending motions and eventually broke the branch. When breaking the next branch I observed that if I bent it more quickly the branch would break sooner. I then observed that while I could easily fatigue and break a pine branch, it was much harder or impossible to do the same with an oak branch. Without knowing it, I had learned much about the role of strain and strain rate in the pathophysiology of stress fracture. It, would, however, take me many years of formal education, epidemiological observations, and experiments before I appreciated the lesson.

EX VIVO STUDIES OF STRAIN AND STRAIN RATE

Historically, the first steps in our understanding of the role of bone strain and strain rates in pathogenesis of stress fracture began with *ex vivo* testing (see Chapter 6). At strains later found to be usually higher than physiological, (5,000–10,000 µε), cortical bone fails within 10^3 to 10^5 loading cycles.[1] At strains of 3000 µε in uniaxial tension cortical bone fails in 10^6 cycles. When uniaxial tensile strains within the physiological range (~1200–1500 µε) are applied, the stiffness of bone is decreased (i.e., fatigue occurs, which is defined as loss of elastic stiffness in the bone). However, even after one million loading cycles, which is approximately equivalent to 1000 miles of walking, cortical bone failure (defined as a 30% loss of stiffness) does not occur.[2] It was also found that during loading of the cortical bone specimens using the same strain parameters, but at a strain rate equivalent to that of running, much greater bone fatigue occurred.[2] In an additional experiment, Schaffler et al. loaded cortical bone in uniaxial tension between 0 and 1200 µε and between 0 and 1500 µε for 13-20 million load cycles.[3] All specimens exhibited fatigue during the first several million loading cycles, evidenced by a 6% decrease in specimen modulus. After that, however, the modulus stabilized and did not change for the duration of the loading. This indicates that fatigue can be expected in the normal bone loading environment, but this does not lead to fatigue failure within a physiological, reasonable number of load cycles.

IN VIVO STUDIES OF STRAIN AND STRAIN RATE

Extrapolating from these experiments and ignoring the possibility of a bone remodeling response, bone fatigue and eventual stress fracture are a mathematical function of strain magnitude and/or strain rate multiplied by the number of load cycles (see Chapter 6). This function is complicated by the viscoelastic nature of bone, according to which there is a strain rate dependency for its mechanical properties. Loading at higher strain rates will cause a relative increase in bone stiffness.[4] It is well known that the relationship between strain magnitude and cycles to failure *ex vivo* is not linear.[5] The number of loading cycles necessary to produce stress fracture *in vivo* is unknown, but can be calculated from epidemiologic data.

Probably the most studied and best characterized stress fracture model is the Israeli infantry recruit.[6] During 14 weeks of intensive basic training the stress fracture incidence is consistently between 20 and 31%. Peak incidence, defined by the time of onset of bone pain, is during the third and fourth weeks of training. It can be estimated that by the fourth week of training recruits have already walked, marched, and/or run 250 miles, or about 210,000 loading cycles. This is much fewer than predicted by *ex vivo* tests to lead to a fracture unless the strains at the stress fracture site are much higher than usual physiologic strains or strain rates.

Strains and Strain Rates in the Human Tibia

The first human *in vivo* bone strain measurements were reported by Lanyon et al.[7] in 1975. In their experiment a strain gage was bonded to the tibia of one of the members of the research staff using cyanoacrylate glue. Technologically, their experiment was limited to direct access of gage output by a cable connection. Therefore their recordings were only taken during walking and treadmill running. Lanyon et al. found principal strains in the range of 400-600 µɛ during treadmill walking; these were doubled during running. Strains were not recorded in this experiment during activities that parallel those of competitive athletes or infantry recruits. Because of a concern about possible carcinogenicity of the cyanoacrylate glue, no additional *in vivo* human bone strain gage experiments were reported for many years.

Some twenty years later, Hoshaw et al.[8] developed and validated an alternative technique for bonding strain gages to bone. They used polymethylmethacrylate, a substance used for years in total joint replacements. Burr et al.[9] employed their technique in a subsequent *in vivo* strain gage study, reported in 1996. They hypothesized that the extremely high incidence of stress fractures observed among Israeli infantry recruits was secondary to the development of high bone strain and strain rates during training. Because the most prevalent stress fracture in the Israeli infantry is in the middle third of the tibia, *in vivo* tibial strain gage recordings during vigorous activities that mimicked infantry training were made at this site in a single subject. The maximum strains generated were 2000 µɛ in shear during zig-zag downhill running. Similar to the study of Lanyon et al.,[7] principal compressive and tensile strains during running were two to three times those of walking, but still never rose above 2000 microstrain. Figure 1 is adapted from the work of Burr et al.[9] It illustrates the principal *in vivo* tibial strains of some of the activities they studied. Strain rates also doubled or tripled in the human tibia during strenuous physical activity, reaching 50,000/sec (Figure 2). These strain rates are higher than previously recorded in humans but are within the range of strain rates reported for running horses[10] and dogs,[11] which can range up to 80,000/sec. The biggest differences found between walking and vigorous activities were in strain rates and not strain magnitudes. This implies an association between the elevation of strain rate and subsequent development of a stress fracture.

An obvious limitation to this study is that measurements are specific to the site of the strain gage. Ekenman et al. recorded concomitantly *in vivo* tibial strains in one volunteer subject using two uniaxial strain gaged bone staples, one mounted at the posteromedial distal third and the other at the anterior mid-diaphysis of the tibia.[12] Neither of these sites was measured in the previous Lanyon et al. and Burr et al. studies. Measurements were made while walking, running, drop landing on a force plate from 45 cm, and during forward jumps, landing on either the heel or the forefoot. During the drop landing, the peak axial tension was 2128 µɛ and peak

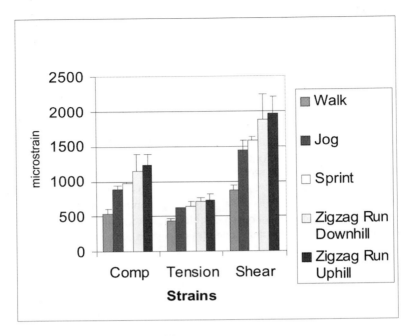

Figure 1 Principal strains versus activity.

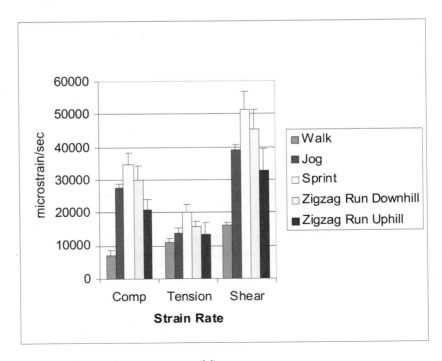

Figure 2 Principal strain rates versus activity.

compression −23 με at the mid-diaphysis, compared to a peak tension of 436 με and a peak compression −970 με at the distal third diaphysis. During walking the peak axial tension was 334 μs and peak compression −14 με, compared to a peak tension of 950 με and peak compression of −1065 με at the distal third diaphysis. During 30 cm forward jumping, the landing technique was found to greatly influence strains. Peak tension ranged from 2700–4200 με at the distal tibia during five successive forefoot landings, compared to an average of 1500 με during heel landing. However, at the mid-diaphysis only a minimal elevation during forefoot landing was observed.

Although the experiment of Burr et al.[9] does not support the hypothesis that the high incidence of tibial stress fractures in Israeli infantry recruits is secondary to their developing very high tibial strains during training, the experiment of Ekenman et al.[12] indicates that there may be anatomical sites on the tibia where high strain magnitudes may be reached. Bone fails in 35,000-50,000 cycles when strains of 4000-5000 microstrain are generated. While the maximal tension strain value recorded by Ekenman et al. during forefoot jumping approaches this range, forefoot jumping is not an activity that anyone repeats for 100,000 cycles of loading. Milgrom et al.[13] reported on four subjects who had tibial strains measured by a rosette cluster of three strain gaged staples implanted at the medial border of the mid-tibial diaphysis. This configuration allowed them to calculate principal and shear strains. Their measuring site was at the same tibial diaphyseal level as the Burr et al. measurements, but was slightly more anterior. They compared the strains and strain rates of running with those of drop-jumps (Figure 3). The compression and tension strains they reported during running were slightly higher than those of Burr et al. However, the

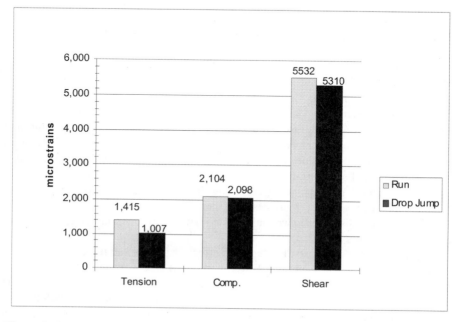

Figure 3 Principal strains during running and drop jumping from 52 cm.

shear strains for both running and drop jumping from 52 cm were about 5000 µε, more than 2.5 times those reported by Burr. As human bone is only about one third as strong in shear as in tension, these data implicate high shear strains as possibly responsible for the pathogenesis of tibial stress fractures.

Strains and Strain Rates in the Human Metatarsal

The epidemiology of metatarsal stress fractures in the Israeli Army is very different from that of tibial stress fractures. In infantry basic training a long night march (from 10 to 90 kilometers) is done once a week. It is not uncommon to find a recruit who was completely asymptomatic before the march present with a frank fracture of one or both cortices of a metatarsal at the end of the march. This suggests the possibility that metatarsal strains during marching may far exceed those reported for the mid-tibia. Milgrom et al. have recorded simultaneously *in vivo* strains using strain gaged bone staples placed in the dorsal surface of the second metatarsal, and in the medial border of the middle and distal tibial diaphysis.[14] They have found metatarsal compression strains of −2500–3000 µε during treadmill walking at a rate of five km/hr. These increased to −5600 µε during treadmill running at 11 km/hr. These values were about three times higher than strains generated in the distal tibia during similar activities. Strains in the middle tibia were less than in the distal tibia. Israeli infantry recruits march typically at a seven km/hr pace or faster and carry 10 to 20 kg packs. Because they march over uneven terrain at night they are also likely to generate much higher impact than during treadmill recordings. It seems likely that the strain magnitude for the metatarsal is sufficient to cause both bone fatigue and bone failure during the 14 weeks of Israeli infantry training.

The Role of Muscle Fatigue on Strain and Strain Rates

In vivo strain measurements of Burr et al.[9] and Ekenman et al.,[12] although valuable, do not duplicate what actually happens in the real training situation of the athlete or military recruit. One major factor they ignore is the possible effect of muscle fatigue on strain and strain rates. Yoshikawa et al. studied the effect of muscle fatigue on bone strain in a foxhound model.[15] In their experiment, they found that a 20 minute exercise program with dogs running on two legs on an inclined treadmill produced quadriceps fatigue as judged by myoelectrical activity. Concomitantly, peak principal and shear strains increased on both compressive and tensile cortices of the tibia. The largest changes were along the anterior and anterolateral surfaces of the tibia, where peak principal strain increased by an average of 26 to 35%. Changes in strain distribution were also found with fatigue. Strain rate changes were not reported in this study.

Fyhrie et al. were the first to study the effect of muscle fatigue on *in vivo* tibial strains in humans.[16] They measured strains using an extensometer mounted on two k-wires placed in the medial cortex of the middle third of the tibia in seven male subjects. The extensometer was chosen to measure strains because it was felt to be a relatively noninvasive alternative to the highly invasive technique of bonding a strain gage to the tibia. Subjects in this study ran at a rate of 11 km/hr on a treadmill until voluntary exhaustion. The data from this study show that strain magnitude does not change significantly after fatiguing exercise, but strain rate is significantly increased, at least in individuals under the age of 35. Strain rates are actually decreased following fatiguing exercise in individuals older than 35 years. Although not conclusive, these data suggest that it is strain rate rather than strain magnitude that may be causal for stress fractures. However, the experiment was complicated by a heel strike artifact that represented direct vibration of the extensometer at heel strike. The data also suggest an age dependence for changes in strain rate following fatiguing exercise, perhaps because the loss of muscle strength and endurance with age prevents forceful contractions when synergistic control of muscles is lost following fatigue.[17,18]

Realizing the limitations of the extensometer, Milgrom et al.[19] examined the effect of muscle fatigue on tibial strains using a strain gaged bone staple. Three strain gaged staples were mounted in a 30° rosette pattern in the tibias of eight subjects. This configuration allowed calculation of all principal and shear strains and strain rates. A fatigue protocol was followed in which *in vivo* tibial strains were measured before and after a fatiguing 2 km run for all subjects, and before and after a 20 km forced fast-paced desert march in four of the subjects. This protocol differed from the fatigue protocol of Fyhrie et al.,[16] in which subjects ran on a treadmill until voluntary exhaustion. It was found that tibial axial tension strains and strain rates increased significantly by about 25% after a 2 km run (Table 1). Four subjects in this study also had measurements made before and after a forced fast-paced 20 kilometer desert march during the summer heat. After the march there was a statistically significant increase in tension strain and compression and tension strain rates (Table 2). Compression strain, however, decreased. Muscular fatigue is shown by a decrease in the maximum torque that the subjects' gastrocnemius could generate on a Biodex (Table 3).

We conclude from these animal and human experiments that mild muscular fatigue can result in significant increases in bone strain and strain rate, but severe muscular fatigue may reduce strain and strain rate, particularly in older subjects.

Table 1   Axial Strain and Strain Rates Pre and Post 2 Km Run for All Subjects

Trial	Strain ($\mu\varepsilon$)		Strain Rate ($\mu\varepsilon$/sec)	
	Tension	Compression	Tension	Compression
Pre run	386.2	533.2	3967.2	3544.5
Post run	524.9	542.0	4905	4635.3
P value	*0.001*	*0.436*	*0.001*	*0.013*

Table 2   Axial Strain and Strain Rates Pre and Post Run and Post March

Trial	Strain ($\mu\varepsilon$)		Strain Rate ($\mu\varepsilon$/sec)	
	Tension	Compression	Tension	Compression
Pre run	436.2	683.1	4754.6	3857.2
Post run	527.8	545	5271.7	4193
Post march	570	506.8	5319.1	4693.5

Table 3   Peak Gastrocnemius Torque as Measured
           by Biodex Pre and Post 2 Km Run and Post
           30 Km March

| Trial | Peak Gastrocnemius Torque (Nm) | |
	All Subjects	Subjects who Marched
Pre Run	97	111.8
Post Run	94	104.6
Post March		81.3

Table 4   Percentage Change of the Axial Strain and Strain Rates
           Pre and Post Run According to Gender

| Gender | % Change Axial Strain | | % Change Axial Strain Rate | |
	Tension	Compression	Tension	Compression
Men	18.9%	4.9%	19.3%	34.7%
Women	71.4%	−6.3%	39.9%	11.2%

THE ROLE OF GENDER AND AGE IN DEVELOPING
HIGH STRAINS AND STRAIN RATES

Strain and strain rate are also associated with other identified risk factors for stress fractures. Women have a higher risk for stress fracture than men (Chapter 3). In a study at West Point, women who underwent the same training as men sustained a ten times higher incidence of stress fractures.[20] Milgrom et al., in a preliminary study, measured tibial strains in five males and three females during common exercise activities. The women on average had higher strains than males for many of the activities. They also had greater increases in tension strains and principal tensile strain rates after fatiguing exercises than men (Table 4). These two factors partially explain women's increased susceptibility for stress fractures.

Age has also been shown to be associated with stress fracture risk. Milgrom et al. found in the Israeli infantry recruit model that for every year increase in recruit age between 17 to 26 years old, stress fracture risk decreased by 28%.[21] Other studies either support[22] or refute[23,24] the reduced risk with aging, but most studies have shown some association (Chapters 2 and 4). Although there is no *in vivo* strain gage data encompassing the 17 to 26 age bracket, there is parallel strain gage data from racehorses, another species prone to stress fracture. Young racehorses, 1 to 3 years old, have extremely high incidences of stress fractures (Chapter 13), and fractures may occur after only 35,000-50,000 cycles of loading. Compressive strain in young horses may be 4,000–5,000 microstrain, much higher than reported in humans, and about twice as high as the third metacarpal strains in older horses doing the same activities.[25] The reason for this age difference in strain is that young bone turns over more rapidly than bone in older animals and there is some lag in the time required for full mineralization, so bone in young animals has not reached its full stiffness. Loads on this immature bone therefore produce higher bone strains and lead to increased risk for stress fracture. A logical conclusion from these data would be that to lower stress fracture incidence in military populations, recruits should be inducted at a later age. General sociological considerations, however, may make this recommendation impractical.

Humans also demonstrate age-associated differences in the development of strain and strain rate during exercise. As indicated previously, tibial strain rates after fatiguing exercise increased in younger subjects but decreased in older subjects, whereas strain magnitude was unchanged in younger subjects but tended to increase in older subjects.[16] This at first seems inconsistent with data from horses, but subjects in the human studies were all mature adults at least 23 years of age. These adults have achieved, or nearly achieved, their maximum bone mineral density,[26] and stiffness of the bone is therefore expected to be greater than it would be in adolescents. These human data are consistent, however, with other human studies that examined age effects[21] and strain rate.[9] They suggest that the age dependence of stress fractures may result from the age dependence of changes in strain and strain rate after fatiguing exercise. They also implicate strain rate as the primary mechanical factor in the etiology of stress fractures in younger subjects.

CONCLUSION

There are still many gaps in our knowledge of the relationship between strain, strain rate, and the occurrence of stress fractures. Our most complete knowledge from an epidemiological standpoint comes from studies of military recruits. Our most complete strain gage data are for the tibia, although some data now exist for the metatarsal and the femur.[28] We lack a good database of strain gage data for women, the young, and the elderly, and we do not know the strain variability that exists in these subpopulations. Nevertheless, we can see the unity between *in vitro*, *in vivo* human, and *in vivo* animal strain measurements and the observed epidemiology of stress fracture. There is evidence that strains are high enough to produce bone fatigue as well as failure in the racehorse and in the human second metatarsal. For the human tibia and femur, the paradox is that bone fails *in vivo* at strain levels which do not produce failure *in vitro*.

REFERENCES

1. Carter, D.R., Caler, W.E., Spengler, D.M., and Frankel, V.H., Fatigue behavior of adult cortical bone. The influence of mean strain and strain rate, *Acta Orthop. Scand.*, 52, 481, 1981.
2. Schaffler, M.B., Burr, D.B., and Radin, E.L., Mechanical and morphological effects of strain rate on fatigue of compact bone, *Bone*, 10, 207, 1989.
3. Schaffler, M.B., Radin, E.L., and Burr, D.B., Long-term fatigue behavior of compact bone at low strain magnitude and rate, *Bone*, 10, 321, 1990.
4. Carter, D. R. and Hayes, W. C., Fatigue life of compact bone-1. Effects of stress amplitude, temperature and density, *J. Biomech.*, 9, 27, 1976.
5. Pattin, C.A., Caler, W.E., and Carter, D.R., Cyclical mechanical property degradation during fatigue loading of cortical bone, *J. Biomech.*, 29, 69, 1996.

6. Milgrom, C., Giladi, M., Stein, M., Kashtan, H., Margulies, J., Chisin, R., Steinberg, R., and Aharonson, Z., Stress fractures in military recruits. A prospective study showing an unusually high incidence, *J. Bone Jt. Surg.*, 67(B), 732, 1985.

7. Lanyon L.E., Hampson G.J., Goodship A.E., and Shan J.S., Bone deformation recorded *in vivo* from strain gages attached to the human tibial shaft, *Acta Orthop. Scand.*, 46, 256, 1975.

8. Hoshaw, S., Fyhrie, D.P., Takano, Y., Burr, D.B., and Milgrom, C., A method suitable for *in vivo* measurement of bone strains in humans, *J. Biomech.*, 30, 521, 1997.

9. Burr, D.B, Milgrom, C., Fyhrie, D., Forwood, M., Nyska, M., Finestone, A., Hoshaw, S., Saiag, E., and Simkin, A., *In vivo* measurement of human tibial strains during vigorous activity, *Bone*, 18, 405, 1996.

10. Davies, H.M.S., McCarthy, R.N., and Jeffcott, L.B., Surface strain on the dorsal metacarpus of thoroughbreds at different speeds and gaits, *Acta Anat.*, 146, 148, 1993.

11. Rubin C.T. and Lanyon, L.E., Limb mechanics as a function of speed and gait: a study of funtional strains in the radius and tibia of horse and dog, *J. Exp. Biol.*, 102, 197, 1982.

12. Ekenman, I., Halvorsen K., Westblad, P., Fellander-Tsai, L, and Rolf, C., Local bone deformation at two predominate sites for stress fracture of the tibia: an *in vivo* study, *Foot Ankle*, 19, 479, 1998.

13. Milgrom, C., Finestone, A., Levi, Y., Simkin, A., Ekenman, I., Mendelson, S., Milligram, M., Nyska, M., Benjuya, N., and Burr, D., Do high impact exercises produce higher tibial strains than running, *Br. J. Sports Med.*, 34, 195, 2000.

14. Milgrom, C., Finestone, A., and Ekenman, I., personal communication, 2000.

15. Yoshikawa, T., Mori, S., Santiesteban, A.J., Sun, T.C., Hafstad, E., Chen, J., and Burr, D.B., The effects of muscule fatigue on bone strain, *J. Exp. Biol.*, 188, 217, 1994.

16. Fyhrie, D.P., Milgrom, C., Hoshaw, S. J., Simkin, A., Dar, S., Drumb, D., and Burr D. B., Effect of fatiguing exercise on longitudinal bone strains as related to stress fracture in humans, *Ann. Biomech. Eng.*, 26, 660, 1998.

17. Schwender, K.I., Mikesky, A. E., Holt, W. S., Peacock, M., and Burr, D.B., Differences in muscle endurance and recovery between fallers and nonfallers, and between young and older women, *J. Gerontol.*, 52A, M155, 1997.

18. Burr, D.B., Muscle strength, bone mass, and age-related bone loss, *J. Bone Min. Res.*, 12, 1547, 1997.

19. Milgrom, C., Finestone, A., Ekenman, I., Larsson, E., Nyska, M., Millgram, M., Mendelson, S., Simkin, A., Benjuya, N., and Burr, D., Tibial strain rate increases in both males and females following muscular fatigue, *Trans. Orthop. Res. Soc.*, 24, 234, 1999.

20. Protzman, R.R. and Griffis, C.G., Stress fractures in men and women undergoing military training, *J. Bone Jt. Surg.*, 59A, 825, 1977.

21. Milgrom, C., Finestone, A., Shlamkovitch, N., Rand, N., Lev, B., Simkin, A., and Weiner, M., Youth: a risk factor for stress fractures, *J. Bone Jt. Surg.*, 76(A), 20, 1994.

22. Friedl, K.E. and Nuovo, J.A., Factors associated with stress fracture in young army women. Indications for further research, *Mil. Med.*, 157, 334, 1992.

23. Brudvig, T.J.S., Gudger, T.D., and Obermeyer, L., Stress fractures in 295 trainees. A one year study of incidence as related to age, sex and race, *Mil. Med.*, 148, 666, 1983.

24. Gardner, L., Dziados, J.E., Jones, B.H., Brundage, J.F., Harris, J.M., Sullivan, R., and Gill, P., Prevention of lower extremity stress fractures; a controlled trial of a shock absorbent sole, *Am. J. Public Health*, 78, 1563, 1988.

25. Nunamaker, D.M., Butterweck, D.M., and Provost, M.T., Fatigue fractures in thoroughbred racehorses: relationship with age, peak bone strain, and training, *J. Orthop. Res.*, 8, 604, 1990.

26. Tegarden. D., Proulx, W.R., Martin, B. R., Zhao, J., McCabe, G.P., Lyle, R.M., Peacock, M., and Slemenda, C., Peak bone mass in young women, *J. Bone Miner. Res.*, 10, 711, 1996.

27. Burr, D.B., Bone, exercise, and stress fractures, *Exerc. Sport Sci. Rev.*, 25, 171, 1997.

28. Aamodt, A., Lund-Larsen, J., Eine, J., Andersen, E., Benum, P. and Schnell Husby, O., *In vivo* measurements show tensile axial strain in the proximal lateral aspect of the human femur, *J. Orthop. Res.*, 15, 927, 1997.

CHAPTER 9

The Role of Muscular Force and Fatigue in Stress Fractures

Seth W. Donahue

CONTENTS

Introduction.. 132
    Mechanics of Muscular Contraction 132
    Molecular Mechanisms of Muscular Contraction and Fatigue 133
Muscular Fatigue and Stress Fractures 134
    Muscular Force in Musculoskeletal Energy Absorption........................... 134
    Relationship between Muscular Conditioning and Stress Fractures 135
    Relationships between Muscular Fatigue, Bone Strain, and Stress
        Fractures.. 136
        The Metatarsal Paradigm.. 137
        The Humerus Paradigm... 140
Muscular Force and Stress Fractures 140
    The Fibula Paradigm 140
    The Femur Paradigm 140
    The Tibia Paradigm 141
    The Patella Paradigm... 141
    The Humerus Paradigm... 141
    The Ulna Paradigm.. 142
    The Rib Paradigm.. 142
Concluding Remarks 144
References... 145

0-8493-0317-6/01/$0.00+$.50
© 2001 by CRC Press LLC

INTRODUCTION

Muscles exert large forces on bones.[1-3] For a strenuous activity such as running, muscular forces in the lower extremity may be more than 20 times body weight.[1] Even for an everyday activity such as walking, muscular forces in the lower extremity may be close to two body weights.[2] External forces, such as ground reaction forces during gait, also act on bones. Muscular and external forces create a complex loading milieu in bones: axial forces, bending moments, and torsion. This loading milieu is responsible for the strains and strain rates engendered by bones; strain and strain rate are ultimately responsible for the damage and failure of bone. Bones are believed to adapt to the strains they experience during habitual activities so that a normal amount of fatigue damage can develop and be repaired.[4] Muscular forces, or lack of muscular forces due to muscular fatigue, may contribute to development of stress fractures by altering the strain environment in bones to a level that exceeds the physiologic processes of adaptation and repair.

Both muscular forces and muscular fatigue have been implicated in the etiology of stress fractures. Some of the earliest clinical investigations into the pathomechanics of rib stress fractures implicated repetitive large muscular forces.[5] In contrast, early clinical studies of metatarsal stress fractures suggested that impaired muscular support due to fatigue was responsible for metatarsal stress fractures.[6] Which line of reasoning is correct? It is likely that they both are. Biomechanical models have provided support for the theories that excessive repetitive muscular forces cause stress fractures of the ribs,[7] and the loss of muscular forces contributes to the development of metatarsal stress fractures.[8-10] The role of muscular forces or muscular fatigue in the etiology of stress fractures most likely depends on the activity, muscles, and bone involved in the injury. V.H. Frankel suggested that "… there are many etiologies for the production of fatigue fractures. One is simple overload brought about by muscle contraction, … Another may be an altered stress distribution in the bone, brought about by continued activities in the presence of muscle fatigue."[11]

Following a brief review of muscle mechanics and physiology, three important concepts of the role muscles play in the development of stress fractures will be discussed. They are (1) the ability of muscles to absorb energy, (2) bone loading due to muscular fatigue, and (3) bone loading due to muscular forces.

Mechanics of Muscular Contraction

The force-generating capability of muscle is dependent on its length and its velocity of shortening or lengthening. Research on isolated muscle fibers has produced the well-known force-length[12,13] and force-velocity[14,15] relationships; Lieber gives a good review.[16] Muscles generate maximum isometric force at muscle lengths where there are a maximum number of myosin molecules overlapped with actin filaments. *In vivo,* muscles may operate on the ascending or descending regions of the force-length curve or centered around the plateau region, depending on muscle function and the level of training.[17] *In vivo* experiments have demonstrated that muscles can generate constant force over the functional joint range of motion, while lengthening by as much as 31%.[18]

Experiments on isolated muscles have shown that muscular force decreases in a parabolic fashion for increasing speeds of concentric (muscle shortening) contractions.[14,15] In healthy human subjects there is a similar relationship between joint torque and speed of muscular shortening: joint torque gradually decreases with increasing muscular shortening speeds.[19-22] This relationship can vary for different muscle groups.[20] Eccentric (muscle lengthening) contractions are relatively independent of contraction velocity and tensions are higher than for isometric contractions.[16] In other words, if a muscle shortens quickly it can develop very little force, but if it lengthens quickly it can develop a very large force. Muscle force-length and force-velocity relationships are important considerations when performing biomechanical analyses to calculate the forces exerted on bones by muscles for a particular activity. Additional considerations for calculating muscular force output are the muscle's architecture, specific tension, and level of activation.[23]

Molecular Mechanisms of Muscular Contraction and Fatigue

Individual myosin "molecular motors" can generate forces of about 5 picoNewtons by utilizing energy derived from ATP hydrolysis.[24-26] Because muscles contain billions of myosin containing thick filaments,[27] whole muscles are able to generate maximum tensions of 35 to 137 Newtons (N) per square centimeter of muscle.[28] This parameter is often referred to as specific tension. Maximum muscular force production can be estimated by multiplying the specific tension by the muscle's cross-sectional area. This simple calculation can be used to illustrate the potential muscles have for generating the enormous forces that act on bones. For example, the quadriceps muscles of a 91 kg man have a physiologic cross-sectional area of about 256 square centimeters[29] and can therefore generate 8,960 to 35,072 N of peak force, depending on the specific tension value for this muscle group. A biomechanical model of running estimated muscular forces to be 22 times bodyweight in the quadriceps and 7 times bodyweight in the gastrocnemius.[1] A more recent experimental investigation calculated peak muscular forces to be 7,700 N in the quadriceps and 4,900 N in the triceps surae during running.[30]

Muscular fatigue reduces the ability of muscles to produce force.[31] The mechanisms that cause fatigue may occur in the central or peripheral nervous systems, at the neuromuscular junction, or within the muscle.[16,31] Many biochemical factors have been implicated in muscular fatigue but the exact mechanisms may be multiple, and are still in dispute. These factors include alterations in intracellular calcium exchange,[32] decreased voluntary neural activation,[33] impairment of high frequency action potential propagation,[34] and a decrease in ATP concentration.[35] Muscular fatigue in marathon runners can decrease maximal isometric knee extension by as much as 35%.[36,37] Indeed, muscles can generate large forces that act on bones, but muscular force generation can be impaired by muscular fatigue.

MUSCULAR FATIGUE AND STRESS FRACTURES

Muscular Force in Musculoskeletal Energy Absorption

Physical activities result in impact forces acting on the musculoskeletal system. Good examples are the ground reaction forces acting on the foot during running or jumping. The musculoskeletal system must absorb the energy put into the system by impact forces. Passive soft tissues contribute little to energy absorption; bones and muscles absorb most of the energy.[38] When bones are loaded, they absorb energy by deforming. Muscles absorb energy by doing negative work (i.e., generating force while lengthening, known as eccentric contraction).[39] Muscular work done to absorb energy may be as important for locomotion as the work done to generate motion.[40] It has been shown that some muscles control movement by absorbing energy,[41] and some function exclusively as energy absorbers.[42] However, it is likely that most mammalian muscles serve a dual function: produce and absorb energy at different times during a cycle of motion.[43] A lack of muscular shock absorption has been suggested to play a role in stress fractures.[44,45]

Energy is the product of force times distance. It is easy to demonstrate that muscles can absorb energy more easily than bones. Even though bones can withstand extremely large loads, they can withstand very little deformation or strain (about 0.031 strain at failure).[46] *In vivo* strain gage experiments have shown that peak functional bone strains are around 3,000 microstrain (0.003 strain).[47] Muscles, on the other hand, can strain about 30% (0.3 strain) of their resting length while generating functional forces.[18] Thus, for a given force of physiologic magnitude, a muscle has the ability to absorb about 100 times as much energy as a bone of the same length.

The concept of how muscles and bones absorb energy can be understood by examining how a person lands from a jump. When a person jumps from an elevation, his legs bend upon landing. While the legs are bending the knee flexor muscles are absorbing energy by contracting eccentrically. Now imagine jumping off your desk and landing without bending your legs, letting your bones absorb most of the energy. The resulting pain would be a good indication that bones are not as efficient at absorbing energy as muscles. This of course is an extreme example, but it demonstrates how the energy-absorbing burden is shifted to the bones when the ability of muscles to absorb energy is compromised. This might also happen when muscles become fatigued.

Shifting the energy-absorbing burden from the muscles to the bones is demonstrated in Figure 1. Imagine holding your arm bent at the elbow so your forearm is perpendicular to the ground and dropping a heavy ball onto your wrist. In experiment 1 you allow your elbow flexor muscles to lengthen while developing force so that the muscles absorb most of the energy put into the musculoskeletal system. Thus, there is little bending of the bones (Figure 1a). In experiment 2 you allow your muscles to develop a force, but do not allow them to lengthen. By doing this most of the energy put into the musculoskeletal system is absorbed by bending the forearm bones, causing larger bending strains than the bones are accustomed to (Figure 1b).

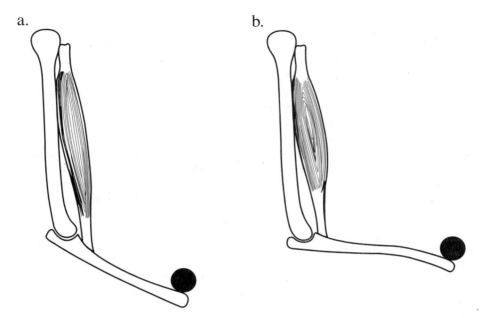

Figure 1   a. When a heavy ball impacts the musculoskeletal system at the wrist, the arm flexor muscles can effectively absorb the energy by contracting eccentrically. b. Isometric contractions of the arm flexor muscles result in energy being absorbed by bending the bones of the forearm.

When muscles develop forces while lengthening they can absorb substantial amounts of energy. This reduces the energy-absorbing burden on the bones. With the onset of muscular fatigue and reduced force-generating capabilities, bones are forced to absorb more energy, resulting in higher bone strains and greater risk for damage accumulation.[38] Thus, the role of muscular fatigue in the development of stress fractures may involve increasing the repetitive energy-absorbing burden of bones during cyclic loading, resulting in accelerated damage accumulation.

Relationship between Muscular Conditioning and Stress Fractures

A low level of physical conditioning and poor muscular development at the commencement of a training regime are considered by many to be risk factors for developing lower extremity injuries, including stress fractures.[48-56] Individuals with poor physical conditioning are believed to be at a higher risk for injury because they lack muscular strength and are more susceptible to muscular fatigue.[52] Stress fractures have been reported to be more prevalent in American military trainees with a lack of running experience.[50,51,57] Winfield et al.[58] found that women who ran fewer miles prior to military training were at greater risk for developing stress fractures. In another study, recruits who were more active prior to basic training were at less risk for developing stress fractures.[59]

There are, however, studies which suggest that prior physical activity does not influence the risk of stress fractures in military recruits.[60,61] Mustajoki et al.[60] found that the amount of running and other physical activities performed 1 to 4 months prior to induction was not related to the incidence of stress fracture in men from the Finnish Defense Forces. Swissa et al.[61] found no correlation between prior sports participation or aerobic fitness and stress fractures in male Israeli infantry recruits. They suggested that the disparity between these studies and the American studies may be attributed to the study design or the methods of determining physical fitness levels.

Besides muscular fatigue, there are other factors that can influence muscular force output. Sudden and large increases in training activity can cause muscular tissue damage.[62,63] Like fatigue, damaged muscular tissue may reduce the force-generating capacity of muscles. Unaccustomed prolonged exercise has been shown to reduce the aerobic performance of muscles by reducing the oxygen-carrying capacity of the blood.[62] Oxygen is needed for oxidative phosphorylation, which is the most efficient mechanism for creating muscular energy supplies (i.e., ATP).[16] Therefore, compromised aerobic performance caused by unaccustomed physical training may also impair muscular force output by limiting the muscle's energy supply.

Relationships between Muscular Fatigue, Bone Strain, and Stress Fractures

Several authors suggest that muscular fatigue causes stress fractures.[6,8-10,44,45,64-66] However, little experimental research has been done on the role of muscular forces in bone loading because of the difficulty of quantifying *in vivo* muscular forces, fatigue, and bone strains. Yoshikawa et al.[67] measured bone strain in the tibiae of dogs that performed exhaustive treadmill running. After twenty minutes of exercise, a frequency shift in the electromyographic signal indicated that the quadriceps muscles were fatigued. Muscular fatigue increased peak principal and shear strains; the peak principal strain increased by an average of 26 to 35%. Fyhrie et al.[68] measured axial strain in the tibiae of military personnel before and after exhaustive exercise. Strains were recorded while the subjects walked on a treadmill before the exhaustive exercise, and again after two hours of strenuous activity followed by treadmill running until voluntary exhaustion. Following exhaustive exercise, strain only increased in half of the subjects, and slightly decreased in the others. The authors suggested that high strain rate due to muscular fatigue may be involved in tibial stress fractures. Milgrom et al.[69] measured *in vivo* tibial strains in humans during normal walking before and after a 2-km run. After running, the tensile strain and tensile and compressive strain rates were significantly greater than the pre–run values. Strains were also recorded in four subjects after attempting a 30 km march at a forced rate of 6 km/hr; the tensile strain and tensile and compressive strain rates were significantly greater than the pre-run and post-run values. Taken together, the findings from these studies suggest that both increased strain and strain rate following muscular fatigue may contribute to an increased risk for stress fracture.

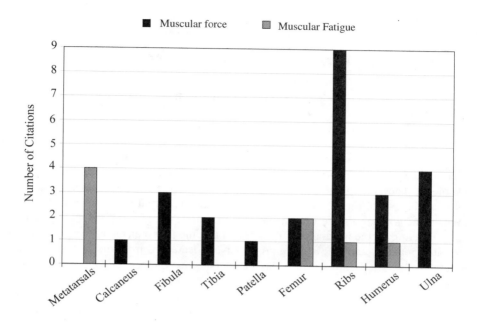

Figure 2 The number of literature citations that implicate either muscular forces or muscular fatigue in the development of stress fractures. A comparison of the results of an extensive Medline search and references prior to 1966 cited therein.

The etiology of stress fractures in the femoral neck has been attributed to lack of shock absorbing capability due to muscular fatigue.[44,45] Lord et al.[64] thought that stress fractures of the ribs in golfers were caused by fatigue of the serratus anterior muscle on the leading side of the golfers. Muscular fatigue has also been implicated in the etiology of stress fractures in the humerus[66] and the metatarsals.[6,8-10] The number of studies that implicate either muscular forces or muscular fatigue in the development of stress fractures is depicted in Figure 2. Most of these studies only postulate the role of muscular forces and fatigue in the development of stress fractures and do not provide experimental verification. Biomechanical analyses of how muscular forces load bones at stress fracture sites have been done for few bones: the rib,[7] fibula,[70] and metatarsals.[8-10] These biomechanical studies suggest that muscular forces contribute to stress fractures in the ribs and fibula, and muscular fatigue contributes to metatarsal stress fractures by increasing bone stresses and strains.

The Metatarsal Paradigm

The German military surgeon J. Briethaupt likely gave the first report on stress fractures in 1855.[71] He described how soldiers developed pain and swelling in their feet following long marches. However, he incorrectly diagnosed the condition as an inflammatory response in the tendon sheaths. It was not until 1897, after the advent of roentgenography, that Stechow discovered that the condition was due to metatarsal fractures.[72] Today the metatarsal bones are still a common stress fracture location, and until recently were the most common sites.[73] Therefore, much attention has been given to the study of the pathomechanics of metatarsal stress fractures.

Muscular fatigue is believed to play a role in metatarsal stress fractures. Strauss stated in 1932 that, "Insidious fractures of the metatarsal bones may occur after exhaustion of the normal muscle and tendon support to the foot. Such fractures occur without obvious trauma...".[6] There is some experimental evidence to support this hypothesis.[8-10]

Stokes et al.[10] studied the role of muscular forces on metatarsal loading during the stance phase of normal walking, using data collected from healthy human subjects. They measured vertical ground reaction forces, bony geometry, and the kinematics of the foot during stance. These data were used for a static analysis of metatarsal loading. Some reasonable assumptions were made about the muscular forces acting on the metatarsals. They found that the first metatarsal engendered the greatest loading, and that loading progressively decreased from the first to the fifth metatarsals. They showed that the metatarsals experience an upward bending moment during the period when the forefoot is in contact with the ground. The pull of the toe flexor muscles (flexor hallucis longus and flexor digitorum longus) was found to counteract the upward bending moment that was caused by the vertical ground reaction force (Figure 3). They concluded that inactivity of the toe flexor musculature causes excessive metatarsal bending, which may be responsible for metatarsal stress fractures.

Sharkey and co-workers have developed static and dynamic gait simulators to study the influence of muscular forces on metatarsal loading.[9,74] These cadaver models apply physiologic muscular forces to the tendons of the ankle plantar flexors and generate ground reaction force profiles representative of healthy human subjects. Sharkey et al.[9] used the static model to study the effect of simulated muscular fatigue

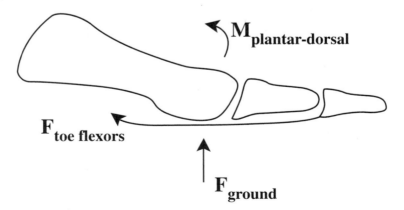

Figure 3 The vertical component of ground reaction force (F_{ground}) causes metatarsal bones to bend in the plantar-to-dorsal direction. Forces ($F_{toe\ flexors}$) in the tendons of toe flexor muscles counteract this bending moment ($M_{plantar-dorsal}$). (Adapted from Stokes et al., *J. Anat.*, 129(3), 579, 1979. With permission.)

on second metatarsal loading during the heel-rise instant of the stance phase of walking. They found that simulated fatigue of the toe flexors significantly increased peak axial strain in the second metatarsal by 35%. This increase in bone strain is consistent with *in vivo* values for tibial strains that have been reported for dogs[67] and humans[69] who performed exhaustive exercise. Sharkey et al.[9] also found that simulated muscular fatigue significantly increased the plantar-to-dorsal bending moment in the second metatarsal by 26%, supporting the hypothesis of Stokes et al.[10]

Similar experiments on simulated muscle fatigue were performed with a dynamic gait simulator that loaded cadaver feet over the entire stance phase of gait.[8] Second and fifth metatarsal axial strains were measured for simulations of normal walking and various levels of muscular fatigue. Peak strains in the mid-diaphyses of second and fifth metatarsals coincided with the peak vertical ground reaction force and peak Achilles tendon tension near the end of the stance phase. For normal walking conditions peak second metatarsal strain (−1897 microstrain) was twice the peak fifth metatarsal strain (−908 microstrain). Simulated muscular fatigue significantly increased the peak strain in second metatarsals by 8% but did not increase peak strain in fifth metatarsals.

The fatigue life of cortical bone exponentially decreases with increasing strains.[75-77] In other words, small increases in bone strain can substantially reduce the number of loading cycles a bone can withstand before failure. An empirically derived equation for the fatigue life of cortical bone and the bone strains recorded during dynamic gait simulations were used to predict the fatigue life of the second and fifth metatarsals (Table 1).[78] These estimations for the number of cycles that a bone can withstand before failure do not account for the *in vivo* repair process of bone remodeling, but they are useful for evaluating the relative risk of muscular fatigue on bone failure. It was estimated that the second metatarsal can withstand about one million cycles before failure with the strains engendered during normal walking. The 8% increase in second metatarsal strain caused by simulated muscular fatigue reduced the estimated fatigue life by 33%. For normal walking, the estimated fatigue life of the fifth metatarsal was 51 times greater than second metatarsal fatigue life due to the lower strains in the fifth metatarsal. Fifth metatarsal fatigue life was relatively unaffected by simulated muscular fatigue. These estimations of metatarsal fatigue life suggest that muscular fatigue may increase the risk of stress fracture in the second metatarsal but not in the fifth. These predictions fit well with clinical observations on stress fractures: second metatarsal stress fractures are much more common than fifth metatarsal stress fractures in runners and military cadets.[79-81]

Table 1 The predicted number of cycles to failure (N_f) for the second and fifth metatarsal bones. Predictions based on the peak bone strains (ε_p) recorded during simulations of normal walking and walking with muscular fatigue. Strains are reported in microstrain ($\mu\varepsilon$).

Metatarsal Bone	Normal Walking		Muscular Fatigue	
	ε_p ($\mu\varepsilon$)	N_f (# of cycles)	ε_p ($\mu\varepsilon$)	N_f (# of cycles)
Second	−1897	1.02×10^6	−2044	6.85×10^5
Fifth	−908	5.22×10^7	−839	7.97×10^7

The Humerus Paradigm

Sterling et al.[66] reported a stress fracture in the humeral shaft of a 14 year old competitive swimmer and baseball pitcher. They believed that muscular fatigue was involved in the development of the fracture. They suggested that muscular fatigue disrupts the balance between antagonistic and agonistic muscular forces, leading to excessive stresses in the humerus during swimming and throwing. Gregersen also believed that when muscular actions become uncoordinated, the humerus is at increased risk for fracture.[82] Rettig and Beltz reported a humeral stress fracture in a 15 year old tennis player.[83] They suggested that the boy fractured his humerus because he possessed insufficient muscular strength to protect it from the repetitive loading incurred while playing tennis.

MUSCULAR FORCE AND STRESS FRACTURES

Repetitive muscular forces have been implicated in causing stress fractures in the calcaneus,[84] fibula,[70,84,85] tibia,[86,87] femur,[44,88] patella,[89] ribs,[5,7,90,91-96] humerus,[97-99] and ulna.[100-103] However, very few biomechanical studies have been done to support these hypotheses.[7,70] Devas stated that, "the cause of stress fractures is muscular pull."[84] He suggested that stress fractures occur because muscles can adapt much faster than bones. For example, he reasoned that when a military recruit begins a new training regime, muscular strength increases and greater muscular forces are exerted on the bones. He proposed that muscular strength increases before the bones can adapt, and therefore the overstressed bones experience stress fractures.

The Fibula Paradigm

Devas reported 50 fibular stress fractures in 49 athletes (46 were runners).[70] He postulated that the fractures were caused by recurrent contraction of the muscles that originate on the fibula. The mechanism by which muscular forces might cause fibular stress fractures was demonstrated by radiographing legs with relaxed and contracted musculature. It was shown that muscular contraction bends the fibula by drawing the shaft of the fibula toward the tibia while the ends remained fixed. Therefore, he proposed that increasing the intensity of the muscular pull on the fibula by performing intense activities may cause a stress fracture before the bone has time to adapt to the increased bending.[84] DiFiori reported a proximal fibular stress fracture in a 14 year old soccer player.[85] He believed that injury was caused by a combination of eccentric contractions of the plantar flexors and external rotation of the proximal tibiofibular joint.

The Femur Paradigm

Stress fractures of the femoral shaft often occur on the medial aspect at the junction of the proximal and middle thirds of the diaphysis.[44] This site is coincident with the attachments of the vastus medialis and adductor brevis muscles. Forces in these muscles are believed to play a role in the development of femoral stress fractures at this location.[44] Large bony excavations have been described at the origins of the gastrocnemius and adductor magnus muscles on the femoral condyles.[88] It was postulated that improved muscular tone led to increased stresses at these muscular attachment sites and that the degree of osteoclastic resorption was related to the intensity of the stress concentration. Bony excavations due to increased muscular forces were postulated to propagate into stress fractures when bone remodeling could not repair these bony defects in a timely fashion.

The Tibia Paradigm

Devas documented tibial stress fractures in 16 athletes (12 runners).[86] He postulated that these fractures might be caused by the repetitive forces of the muscles that attach on the middle to upper region of the posterior aspect of the tibia. He believed these muscular forces caused stress fractures by causing tibial bending, similar to the mechanism he proposed for fibular stress fractures. Stanitski et al. reported 21 lower limb stress fractures in 17 athletes.[87] They believed that the tibial stress fractures in a diver and a basketball player were also consequences of the forces from the posterior muscles that attach to the tibia.

The Patella Paradigm

Teitz and Harrington documented patellar stress fractures in a sailboarder and a belly dancer.[89] Both of the activities involved in the injury require prolonged isometric contractions of the quadriceps muscles. The authors suggested that prolonged quadriceps forces may cause damage to the patella by a creep mechanism, which has been previously described for the failure of bone.[104] It was suggested that the patellar stress fractures may have been caused by creep damage, or creep damage superimposed on damage caused by cyclic loading.

The Humerus Paradigm

Three reports suggest the involvement of strong muscular forces in the etiology of humeral stress fractures. Allen reported a midshaft humeral stress fracture in a 13 year old baseball pitcher.[97] The boy was a side-arm curve ball pitcher. He did not heed the gradual onset of pain, and the humerus eventually fractured midpitch during a game. Repeated muscular forces on the humerus were presumed responsible for the injury. Horwitz and DiStefano reported a humeral stress fracture in a competitive weight lifter.[99] They found tenderness at the bony insertion site of the pectoralis major muscle and confirmed the diagnosis with radiography and bone scan. They assumed that repeated muscular force from this muscle caused the fracture. DiCicco et al.[98] reported a midshaft humeral fracture in a 30 year old baseball pitcher. They believed that humeral torsion induced by muscular forces was responsible for the fracture.

The Ulna Paradigm

Several reports on ulnar stress fractures in athletes implicate repetitive muscular forces in the etiology. Koskinen et al.[101] reported a stress fracture in the distal ulna of a recreational golfer. They proposed that the mechanism of injury was supination combined with overuse of the hand flexor muscles. Escher reported a stress fracture in a bowler at the junction of the proximal and middle thirds of the ulna.[100] He believed the fracture was most likely caused by repeated muscular stress on the ulna at the origin of the flexor profundus muscle. Pascale and Grana suggested that heavy overuse of the flexor muscles was responsible for an ulnar stress fracture in a fastpitch softball pitcher.[103] Nuber and Diment reported two stress fractures of the olecranon process of the ulna in baseball pitchers.[102] They proposed the injuries were caused by repeated pull of the triceps muscles.

The Rib Paradigm

More reports implicate repetitive muscular forces in the etiology of stress fractures of the rib than any other bone (Figure 2). Fractures caused by coughing have been reported in every rib, most frequently in the central ribs.[7] Rib fractures due to coughing are believed to be stress fractures that result from repetitive muscular action, not from a single exceptionally strong cough.[7] In 1936, Oechsli proposed that the forces in the serratus anterior and external oblique muscles were responsible for rib fractures because he found the fracture location to be near the attachment sites of these muscles.[5] In 1954, Debres and Haran performed a detailed biomechanical analysis on the sixth rib.[7] They used a free body diagram to solve for the reaction forces at the costochondral junction and vertebral column, caused by muscular forces (Figure 4a). Subsequently, they calculated bending stresses in the rib at intervals along the length of the rib (Figure 4b). They discovered that rib fractures are most common where stress is the greatest.

More recently, rib stress fractures have been documented in athletes,[90-96] especially rowers.[90,93-95] Holden and Jackson reported rib stress fractures in four Olympic caliber female rowers.[93] They believed that the serratus anterior, major and minor rhomboid, and the trapezius muscles were responsible for the forces that caused the ribs to bend during rowing and training exercises (bench press and pulls). They thought that these stress fractures of the ribs were caused by the repetitive bending stresses generated by muscular pull. McKenzie reported a rib stress fracture in an elite male rower.[95] The fracture occurred along the anterolateral aspect of the rib where the serratus anterior muscle originates. This muscle was believed to be a major contributor to the repetitive stresses that caused the fracture. Karlson studied 14 rib fractures in 10 elite rowers.[94] Fractures were found in ribs 5 through 9. She proposed that rib fractures in rowers are caused by the same mechanism responsible for rib stress fractures due to coughing (i.e., repetitive contraction of the serratus anterior and external oblique muscles). She suggested that the external oblique muscles are near maximum tension at the end of the stroke, and during the "drive" phase of the stroke the serratus anterior muscles generate large forces through

a.

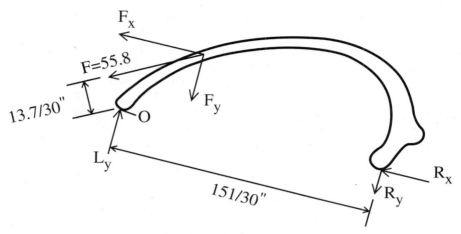

Figure 4a   Free body diagram for calculating the forces acting on the sixth rib. F is the resultant muscle force, R_x and R_y are the reaction forces at the vertebral column, and L_y is the reaction force at the costachondral junction. (Adapted from Debres, V. J. and Haran, T., *Surgery*, 35(2), 294, 1954. With permission.)

b.

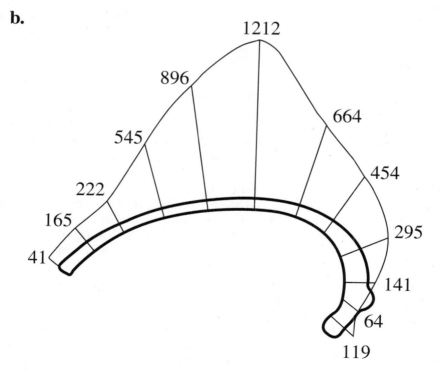

Figure 4b   Stresses (psi) in the sixth rib due to muscular pull. (Adapted from Debres, V. J. and Haran, T., *Surgery*, 35(2), 294, 1954. With permission.)

eccentric contractions. Bojaniac and Desnica also reported a stress fracture in the sixth rib of an Olympic caliber rower that they believed was due to muscular forces.[90]

Gurtler et al.[92] reported a stress fracture in the first rib of a baseball pitcher. They pointed out that a vascular groove in the first rib, which lies between the opposing muscular forces of the scalene and the intercostal and serratus anterior muscles, is the most common stress fracture site in the first rib. Naturally occurring bony architectural features may function as stress fracture nucleation sites by acting as stress concentrators. Mintz et al.[96] suggested that downward pull of the serratus anterior muscle on the first rib was responsible for the stress fracture in a 19 year old male weight lifter. Goyal et al.[91] suggested a possible mechanism for duffer's fracture (i.e., rib stress fractures in golfers caused by repetitively hitting the ground with their club). They postulated that the high impact forces caused by striking the ground cause the serratus anterior muscle to forcefully contract, placing high stress on the ribs.

CONCLUDING REMARKS

Muscles are able to exert forces on bones that are as large as several times body-weight. Impact forces caused by collisions with objects external to the body also act on bones. The musculoskeletal system must absorb the energy put into the system by impact forces; muscles are better designed to absorb energy than bones. Muscular forces can cause bones to bend; however, they can also counteract external forces to resist bone bending. During the initiation of a new exercise or training regime, muscles may adapt faster than bones. This may result in larger muscular forces and higher bone strains. When muscular force production is compromised by muscular fatigue, bones may be required to absorb more energy than they are accustomed to. Excessive muscular force and muscular fatigue may cause bones to bend and strain more than they are adapted to. This unaccustomed straining may result in the damage that causes stress fractures. It is unclear if the level of pre-induction muscular conditioning influences the incidence of stress fractures in military recruits.

Both excessive muscular pull and decreased muscular forces due to fatigue have been implicated in the etiology of stress fractures. There is evidence from biomechanical studies that supports both of these hypotheses. Reduced muscular force has been shown to increase metatarsal bending and strains, whereas muscular forces have been shown to cause bending of the ribs and fibula. The role of muscular forces or muscular fatigue in the etiology of stress fractures most likely depends on the activity, muscles, and bone involved in the injury. The role of muscles in stress fractures may even vary within a given bone. For example, repetitive muscular forces are believed to cause stress fractures in the femoral shaft, but muscular fatigue is thought to cause stress fractures in the femoral neck.

Several clinical studies postulate that repetitive large muscular forces are involved in upper limb stress fractures. However, many of these injuries occur in racket and throwing activities, in which external forces act on the arm (e.g., balls, rackets, oars, and hand grenades). These external forces may cause the arm bones to bend during athletic activity, and normal muscular forces may prevent bone bending from becoming excessive. Therefore, it is possible that muscular fatigue may cause upper limb stress fractures by increasing repetitive bone bending. Biomechanical analyses of how muscular forces act on bones to cause stress fractures have only been done for the rib, fibula, and metatarsals. The role of muscular forces in the development of stress fractures in other bones is generally speculative. Analytical and experimental models can be helpful in elucidating the roles of muscular forces and fatigue in the development of stress fractures.

REFERENCES

1. Harrison, R. N., Lees, A., McCullagh, P. J., and Rowe, W. B., A bioengineering analysis of human muscle and joint forces in the lower limbs during running, *J. Sports Sci.*, 4(3), 201, 1986.
2. McLeish, R. D. and Charnley, J., Abduction forces in the one-legged stance, *J. Biomech.*, 3(2), 191, 1970.
3. Scott, S. H. and Winter, D. A., Internal forces of chronic running injury sites, *Med. Sci. Sports Exerc.*, 22(3), 357, 1990.
4. Frost, H. M., Some ABC's of skeletal pathophysiology. 5. Microdamage physiology (editorial), *Calcif. Tissue Int.*, 49(4), 229, 1991.
5. Oechsli, W. R., Rib fractures from cough, report of 12 cases, *J. Thoracic Surg.*, 5, 530, 1936.
6. Strauss, F. H., Marching fractures of metatarsal bones, *Surg. Gynec. Obstet.*, 54, 581, 1932.
7. Debres, V. J. and Haran, T., Rib fractures from muscular effort with particular reference to cough, *Surgery*, 35(2), 294, 1954.
8. Donahue, S. W. and Sharkey, N. A., Strains in the metatarsals during the stance phase of gait: implications for stress fractures, *J. Bone Jt. Surg. (Am.)*, 81(9), 1236, 1999.
9. Sharkey, N. A., Ferris, L., Smith, T. S., and Matthews, D. K., Strain and loading of the second metatarsal during heel-lift, *J. Bone Jt. Surg.*, 77(7), 1050, 1995.
10. Stokes, I. A. F., Hutton, W. C., and Strott, J. R. R., Forces acting on the metatarsals during normal walking, *J. Anat.*, 129(3), 579, 1979.
11. Frankel, V. H., editorial comment, *Am. J. Sports Med.*, 6(6), 396, 1978.
12. Edman, K. A. P., The relation between sarcomere length and active tension in isolated semitendinosous fibers of the frog, *J. Physiol.*, 183, 407, 1966.
13. Gordon, A. M., Huxley, A. F., and Julian, F. J., The variation in isometric tension with sarcomere length in vertebrate muscle fibres, *J. Physiol. London*, 184(1), 170, 1966.
14. Hill, A. V., The heat of shortening and the dynamic constants of muscle, *Proc. R. Soc. London Ser. B*, 126, 136, 1938.
15. Katz, B., The relation between force and speed in muscular contraction, *J. Physiol.*, 96, 45, 1939.
16. Lieber, R. L., *Skeletal Muscle Structure and Function*, Wiliams and Wilkins, Baltimore, 1992, chap. 2.
17. Rassier, D. E., MacIntosh, B. R., and Herzog, W., Length dependence of active force production in skeletal muscle, *J. Appl. Physiol.*, 86(5), 1445, 1999.
18. Hawkins, D. and Bey, M., Muscle and tendon force-length properties and their interactions in vivo, *J. Biomech.*, 30(1), 63, 1997.
19. Baron, R., Normative data for muscle strength in relation to age, knee angle and velocity, *Wien. Med. Wochenschr.*, 145(22), 600, 1995.

20. Prietto, C. A. and Caiozzo, V. J., The in vivo force-velocity relationship of the knee flexors and extensors, *Am. J. Sports Med.,* 17(5), 607, 1989.

21. Thorstensson, A., Grimby, G., and Karlsson, J., Force-velocity relations and fiber composition in human knee extensor muscles, *J. Appl. Physiol.,* 40(1), 12, 1976.

22. Wickiewicz, T. L., Roy, R. R., Powell, P. L., Perrine, J. J., and Edgerton, V. R., Muscle architecture and force-velocity relationships in humans, *J. Appl. Physiol.,* 57(2), 435, 1984.

23. Kaufman, K. R., An, K. W., Litchy, W. J., and Chao, E. Y., Physiological prediction of muscle forces. I. Theoretical formulation, *Neuroscience,* 40(3), 781, 1991.

24. Ishijima, A., Kojima, H., Funatsu, T., Tokunaga, M., Higuchi, H., Tanaka, H., and Yanagida, T., Simultaneous observation of individual ATPase and mechanical events by a single myosin molecule during interaction with actin, *Cell,* 92(2), 161, 1998.

25. Ishijima, A., Kojima, H., Higuchi, H., Harada, Y., Funatsu, T., and Yanagida, T., Multiple- and single-molecule analysis of the actomyosin motor by nanometer-piconewton manipulation with a microneedle: unitary steps and forces, *Biophys. J.,* 70(1), 383, 1996.

26. Yanagida, T. and Ishijima, A., Forces and steps generated by single myosin molecules, *Biophys. J.,* 68(Suppl. 4), 312S, 1995.

27. Bagshaw, C. R., *Muscle Contraction,* Chapman and Hall, London, 1982, Appendix.

28. Buchanan, T. S., Evidence that maximum muscle stress is not a constant: differences in specific tension in elbow flexors and extensors, *Med. Eng. Phys.,* 17(7), 529, 1995.

29. Frederich, J. A. and Brand, R. A., Muscle fiber architecture in the human lower limb, *J. Biomech.,* 23(1), 91, 1990.

30. Thorpe, S. K., Li, Y., Crompton, R. H., and Alexander, R. M., Stresses in human leg muscles in running and jumping determined by force plate analysis and from published magnetic resonance images, *J. Exp. Biol.,* 201(1), 63, 1998.

31. Gandevia, S. C., Some central and peripheral factors affecting human motoneuronal output in neuromuscular fatigue, *Sports Med.,* 13(2), 93, 1992.

32. Williams, J. H. and Klug, G. A., Calcium exchange hypothesis of skeletal muscle fatigue: a brief review, *Muscle Nerve,* 18(4), 421, 1995.

33. Heakkinen, K., Neuromuscular fatigue in males and females during strenuous heavy resistance loading, *Electromyogr. Clin. Neurophysiol.,* 34(4), 205, 1994.

34. Strojnik, V. and Komi, P. V., Neuromuscular fatigue after maximal stretch-shortening cycle exercise, *J. Appl. Physiol.,* 84(1), 344, 1998.

35. de Haan, A. and Koudijs, J. C., A linear relationship between ATP degradation and fatigue during high-intensity dynamic exercise in rat skeletal muscle, *Exp. Physiol.,* 79(5), 865, 1994.

36. Nicol, C., Komi, P. V., and Marconnet, P., Fatigue effects of marathon running on neuromuscular performance. I. Changes in muscle force and stiffness characteristics, *Scand. J. Med. Sci. Sports,* 1, 10, 1991.

37. Sherman, W. M., Armstrong, L. E., Murray, T. M., Hagerman, F. C., Costill, D. L., Staron, R. C., and Ivy, J. L., Effect of a 42.2-km footrace and subsequent rest or exercise on muscular strength and work capacity, *J. Appl. Physiol.,* 57(6), 1668, 1984.

38. Radin, E. L. and Paul, I. L., Does cartilage compliance reduce skeletal impact loads? The relative force-attenuating properties of articular cartilage, synovial fluid, periarticular soft tissues and bone, *Arthritis Rheum.,* 13(2), 139, 1970.

39. Hill, A. V., Production and absorption of work by muscles, *Science,* 131, 897, 1960.

40. Cavagna, G. A., Storage and utilization of elastic energy in skeletal muscle, *Exerc. Sport Sci. Rev.,* 5, 89, 1977.

41. Tu, M. S. and Dickinson, M. H., The control of wing kinematics by two steering muscles of the blowfly (Calliphora vicina), *J. Comp. Physiol. (A),* 178(6), 813, 1996.

42. Full, R. J., Stokes, D. R., Ahn, A. N., and Josephson, R. K., Energy absorption during running by leg muscles in a cockroach, *J. Exp. Biol.,* 201,997, 1998.

43. Biewener, A. A., Konieczynski, D. D., and Baudinette, R. V., In vivo muscle force-length behavior during steady-speed hopping in tammar wallabies, *J. Exp. Biol.,* 201(11), 1681, 1998.

44. Boden, B. P. and Speer, K. P., Femoral stress fractures, *Clin. Sports Med.,* 16(2), 307, 1997.

45. Fullerton, L. R., Jr., Femoral neck stress fractures, *Sports Med.,* 9(3), 192, 1990.

46. Reilly, D. T. and Burstein, A. H., The elastic and ultimate properties of compact bone tissue, *J. Biomech.,* 8(6), 393, 1975.

47. Rubin, C. T., Skeletal strain and the functional significance of bone architecture, *Calcif. Tissue Int.,* 36 (Suppl. 1), S11, 1984.

48. Bennell, K., Matheson, G., Meeuwisse, W., and Brukner, P., Risk factors for stress fractures, *Sports Med.,* 28(2), 91, 1999.

49. Deuster, P. A., Jones, B. H., and Moore, J., Patterns and risk factors for exercise-related injuries in women: a military perspective, *Mil. Med.,* 162(10), 649, 1997.

50. Garcia, J. E., Grabhorn, L. L., and Franklin, K. J., Factors associated with stress fractures in military recruits, *Mil. Med.,* 152(1), 45, 1987.

51. Gilbert, R. S. and Johnson, H. A., Stress fractures in military recruits — a review of twelve years experience, *Mil. Med.,* 131, 716, 1966.

52. Jones, B. H., Overuse injuries of the lower extremities associated with marching, jogging, and running: a review, *Mil. Med.,* 148(10), 783, 1983.

53. Jones, B. H., Bovee, M. W., Harris, J. M. D., and Cowan, D. N., Intrinsic risk factors for exercise-related injuries among male and female Army trainees, *Am. J. Sports Med.,* 21(5), 705, 1993.

54. Jones, B. H., Cowan, D. N., Tomlinson, J. P., Robinson, J. R., Polly, D. W., and Frykman, P. N., Epidemiology of injuries associated with physical training among young men in the Army, *Med. Sci. Sports Exerc.,* 25(2), 197, 1993.

55. Matheson, G. O., Clement, D. B., McKenzie, D. C., Taunton, J. E., Lloyd-Smith, D. R., and MacIntyre, J. G., Stress fractures in athletes. A study of 320 cases, *Am. J. Sports Med.,* 15(1), 46, 1987.

56. Neely, F. G., Intrinsic risk factors for exercise-related lower limb injuries, *Sports Med.,* 26(4), 253, 1998.

57. Greaney, R. B., Gerber, F. H., Laughlin, R. L., Kmet, J. P., Metz, C. D., Kilcheski, T. S., Rao, B. R., and Silverman, E. D., Distribution and natural history of stress fractures in U.S. Marine recruits, *Radiology,* 146(2), 339, 1983.

58. Winfield, A. C., Moore, J., Bracker, M., and Johnson, C. W., Risk factors associated with stress reactions in female Marines, *Mil. Med.,* 162(10), 698, 1997.

59. Gardner, L. I., Jr., Dziados, J. E., Jones, B. H., Brundage, J. F., Harris, J. M., Sullivan, R., and Gill, P., Prevention of lower extremity stress fractures: a controlled trial of a shock absorbent insole, *Am. J. Public Health,* 78(12), 1563, 1988.

60. Mustajoki, P., Laapio, H., and Meurman, K., Calcium metabolism, physical activity, and stress fractures [letter], *Lancet,* 2(8353), 797, 1983.

61. Swissa, A., Milgrom, C., Giladi, M., Kashtan, H., Stein, M., Margulies, J., Chisin, R., and Aharonson, Z., The effect of pretraining sports activity on the incidence of stress fractures among military recruits. A prospective study, *Clin. Orthop.,* 245, 256, 1989.

62. Dressendorfer, R. H., Wade, C. E., Claybaugh, J., Cucinell, S. A., and Timmis, G. C., Effects of 7 successive days of unaccustomed prolonged exercise on aerobic performance and tissue damage in fitness joggers, *Int. J. Sports Med.,* 12(1), 55, 1991.

63. Hikida, R. S., Staron, R. S., Hagerman, F. C., Sherman, W. M., and Costill, D. L., Muscle fiber necrosis associated with human marathon runners, *J. Neurol. Sci.*, 59(2), 185, 1983.

64. Lord, M. J., Ha, K. I., and Song, K. S., Stress fractures of the ribs in golfers, *Am. J. Sports Med.*, 24(1), 118, 1996.

65. Scully, T. J. and Besterman, G., Stress fracture — a preventable training injury, *Mil. Med.*, 147(4), 285, 1982.

66. Sterling, J. C., Calvo, R. D., and Holden, S. C., An unusual stress fracture in a multiple sport athlete, *Med. Sci. Sports Exerc.*, 23(3), 298, 1991.

67. Yoshikawa, T., Mori, S., Santiesteban, A. J., Sun, T. C., Hafstad, E., Chen, J., and Burr, D. B., The effects of muscle fatigue on bone strain, *J. Exp. Biol.*, 188, 217, 1994.

68. Fyhrie, D. P., Milgrom, C., Hoshaw, S. J., Simkin, A., Dar, S., Drumb, D., and Burr, D. B., Effect of fatiguing exercise on longitudinal bone strain as related to stress fracture in humans, *Ann. Biomed. Eng.*, 26(4), 660, 1998.

69. Milgrom, C., Finestone, A., Ekenman, I., Larsson, E., Nyska, M., Millgram, M., Mendelson, S., Simkin, A., Benjuya, N., and Burr, D., Tibial strain rate increases following muscular fatigue in both men and women, *Transactions of the Forty-Fifth Annual Meeting of the Orthopaedic Research Society,* Anaheim, CA, 1999, 234.

70. Devas, M. B., Stress fractures of the fibula, *J. Bone Jt. Surg.*, 38 B(4), 818, 1956.

71. Breithaupt, J., Zur pathologie des menschlichen fusses, *Med. Ztg.*, 24, 169, 1855.

72. Stechow, Fussoedem und rontrenstrahlen, *Deutsch Mil. Aerztl. Z.*, 26, 465, 1897.

73. Burr, D. B., Bone, exercise, and stress fractures, *Exerc. Sport Sci. Rev.*, 25, 171, 1997.

74. Sharkey, N. A. and Hamel, A. J., A dynamic cadaver model of the stance phase of gait: performance characteristics and kinetic validation, *Clin. Biomech.*, 13, 420, 1998.

75. Caler, W. E. and Carter, D. R., Bone creep-fatigue damage accumulation, *J. Biomech.*, 22(6-7), 625, 1989.

76. Carter, D. R., Caler, W. E., Spengler, D. M., and Frankel, V. H., Fatigue behavior of adult cortical bone: the influence of mean strain and strain range, *Acta Orthop. Scand.*, 52(5), 481, 1981.

77. Carter, D. R., Caler, W. E., Spengler, D. M., and Frankel, V. H., Uniaxial fatigue of human cortical bone. The influence of tissue physical characteristics, *J. Biomech.*, 14(7), 461, 1981.

78. Donahue, S. W., *Bone Strain and Microdamage at Stress Fracture Sites in Human Metatarsals*, Ph.D. dissertation, University of California, Davis, 1999.

79. McBryde, A. M., Jr., Stress fractures in runners, *Clin. Sports Med.*, 4(4), 737, 1985.

80. Meurman, K. O., Less common stress fractures in the foot, *Br. J. Radiol.*, 54(637), 1, 1981.

81. Sullivan, D., Warren, R. F., Pavlov, H., and Kelman, G., Stress fractures in 51 runners, *Clin. Orthop.*, 187, 188, 1984.

82. Gregersen, H. N., Fractures of the humerus from muscular violence, *Acta Orthop. Scand.*, 42(6), 506, 1971.

83. Rettig, A. C. and Beltz, H. F., Stress fracture in the humerus in an adolescent tennis tournament player, *Am. J. Sports Med.*, 13(1), 55, 1985.

84. Devas, M., *Stress Fractures*, Churchill Livingstone, New York, 1975, Chap. 1, 12.

85. DiFiori, J. P., Stress fracture of the proximal fibula in a young soccer player: a case report and a review of the literature, *Med. Sci. Sports Exerc.*, 31(7), 925, 1999.

86. Devas, M. B., Stress fractures of the tibia in athletes or "shin soreness", *J. Bone Jt. Surg.*, 40 B(2), 227, 1958.

87. Stanitski, C. L., McMaster, J. H., and Scranton, P. E., On the nature of stress fractures, *Am. J. Sports Med.*, 6(6), 391, 1978.

88. Hyman, A. A., Heiser, W. J., Kim, S. E., and Norfray, J. F., An excavation of the distal femoral metaphysis: a magnetic resonance imaging study. A case report, *J. Bone Jt. Surg. (Am.)*, 77(12), 1897, 1995.

89. Teitz, C. C. and Harrington, R. M., Patellar stress fracture, *Am. J. Sports Med.*, 20(6), 761, 1992.

90. Bojaniac, I. and Desnica, N., Stress fracture of the sixth rib in an elite athlete, *Croat. Med. J.*, 39(4), 458, 1998.

91. Goyal, M., Kenney, A. J., 3rd, and Hanelin, L. G., Golfer's rib stress fracture (Duffer's fracture). Scintigraphic appearance, *Clin. Nucl. Med.*, 22(7), 503, 1997.

92. Gurtler, R., Pavlov, H., and Torg, J. S., Stress fracture of the ipsilateral first rib in a pitcher, *Am. J. Sports Med.*, 13(4), 277, 1985.

93. Holden, D. L. and Jackson, D. W., Stress fracture of the ribs in female rowers, *Am. J. Sports Med.*, 13(5), 342, 1985.

94. Karlson, K. A., Rib stress fractures in elite rowers. A case series and proposed mechanism, *Am. J. Sports Med.*, 26(4), 516, 1998.

95. McKenzie, D. C., Stress fracture of the rib in an elite oarsman, *Int. J. Sports Med.*, 10(3), 220, 1989.

96. Mintz, A. C., Albano, A., Reisdorff, E. J., Choe, K. A., and Lillegard, W., Stress fracture of the first rib from serratus anterior tension: an unusual mechanism of injury, *Ann. Emerg. Med.*, 19(4), 411, 1990.

97. Allen, M. E., Stress fracture of the humerus. A case study, *Am. J. Sports Med.*, 12(3), 244, 1984.

98. DiCicco, J. D., Mehlman, C. T., and Urse, J. S., Fracture of the shaft of the humerus secondary to muscular violence, *J. Orthop. Trauma*, 7(1), 90, 1993.

99. Horwitz, B. R. and DiStefano, V., Stress fracture of the humerus in a weight lifter, *Orthopedics*, 18(2), 185, 1995.

100. Escher, S. A., Ulnar diaphyseal stress fracture in a bowler, *Am. J. Sports Med.*, 25(3), 412, 1997.

101. Koskinen, S. K., Mattila, K. T., Alanen, A. M., and Aro, H. T., Stress fracture of the ulnar diaphysis in a recreational golfer, *Clin. J. Sport Med.*, 7(1), 63, 1997.

102. Nuber, G. W. and Diment, M. T., Olecranon stress fractures in throwers. A report of two cases and a review of the literature, *Clin .Orthop.*, 278, 58, 1992.

103. Pascale, M. S. and Grana, W. A., Answer please. Stress fracture of the ulna, *Orthopedics*, 11(5), 829, 1988.

104. Carter, D. R. and Caler, W. E., A cumulative damage model for bone fracture, *J. Orthop. Res.*, 3(1), 84, 1985.

CHAPTER **10**

The Histological Appearance
of Stress Fractures

Satoshi Mori, Jiliang Li, and Yoji Kawaguchi

CONTENTS

Introduction 151
Staining Microdamage 153
    The Bulk Stain Technique 153
    Types of Microdamage 153
Evidence for Microdamage Accumulation Associated with Stress Fracture 154
    Biopsy of Stress Fracture 154
    Cytokines and Bone Remodeling at the Stress Fracture Site 157
Summary 158
References 158

INTRODUCTION

Fatigue occurs in materials subjected to repetitive loading.[1] Progressive loss of strength and stiffness are attributed to various levels of material damage; molecular debonding, the initiation, propagation, and coalescence of microdamage, finally resulting in failure.[2,3] Fatigue failure occurs at loads well below those that cause fracture. Physiological repetitive loading imposed during daily activity also causes fatigue in bone.[4,5] While nonbiological materials may fail after many cycles of loading, biological materials often do not fail, because of the biological system's ability to repair microdamage (Figure 1). As long as production and repair of microdamage are balanced, fatigue is a subclinical issue. However, once there is an imbalance, bone fragility progresses and may lead to a stress fracture.[6] Excessive

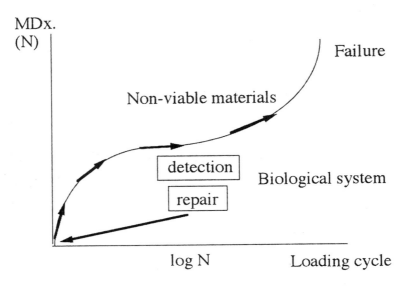

Figure 1 Biological Repair of Microdamage. The biological system can detect and repair microdamage, which prevents accumulation of microdamage and eventual failure.

production of microdamage, impaired repair resulting from failure to detect microdamage, or inhibition of normal remodeling can cause microdamage accumulation (Figure 2).[7] Stress fractures in athletes, dancers, and military recruits may occur by excessive production of microdamage, but this has never been demonstrated

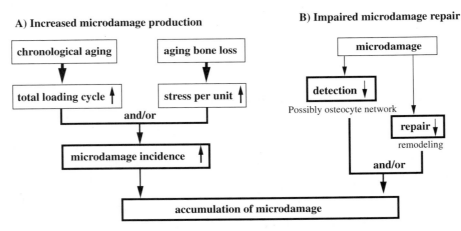

Figure 2 Mechanisms in accumulation of microdamage. Increased microdamage production and impaired microdamage repair cause accumulation of microdamage in bone. Chronological aging and/or bone loss increase microdamage incidence. Microdamage may be detected by the osteocyte network which starts the biological repair action. Remodeling repairs microdamage. (Redrawn from Mori, S., *Mechanical Loading of Bones and Joints,* Springer-Verlag, Tokyo, 1999. With permission.)

histologically. The mechanisms of some pathological fractures such as collapse caused by avascular necrosis of the femoral head,[8] asymptomatic vertebral fractures or femoral neck fractures[9] in osteoporosis, or insufficiency fractures of the pelvis in the elderly can be partly explained by microdamage accumulation. Microdamage accumulation may underlie the pathogenesis of degenerative changes or diseases including osteoporosis[10-12] and osteoarthrosis.[13] However, the role of microdamage in such fractures has not been widely accepted because of lack of histological evidence. One reason may be the difficulty of evaluating microdamage following fracture in clinical cases. Because most stress fractures can be treated conservatively, there is little medical justification for obtaining biopsy specimens from stress fractures other than to rule out tumor. The usual processing technique would obliterate any evidence of microdamage *in vivo*. Biopsy specimens must be taken en bloc and stained by basic fuchsin before processing in order to evaluate microdamage. It is also difficult to produce stress fractures in animal models because substantial cycles of controlled loading are necessary before failure.

STAINING MICRODAMAGE

The Bulk Stain Technique

It has been considered difficult to separate microdamage produced *in vivo* from artifactual cracking caused by tissue preparation. Frost first demonstrated microdamage in human ribs[14] and proposed a technique to distinguish the source of microdamage based on bulk staining of bone with 1.0% basic fuchsin in a graded series of ethanols. Because the specimen is stained en bloc before preparation, only cracks that are present in the bone before sectioning are stained with basic fuchsin. The validity of the bulk staining method was later verified and modified by Burr.[15,16] Microcracks are defined as having sharp borders with a halo of increased basic fuchsin stain surrounding them. Cracks are larger than canaliculi but smaller than vascular canals, running about 50 to 100 µm in cross–section and 200 to 300 µm longitudinally.[17,18] Deeply stained edges can be observed by changing the depth of focus.

Types of Microdamage

Various microcrack types have been found in addition to single linear microcracks. Wenzel et al.[18] have defined multiple linear microcracks near the trabecular surface and cross-hatched microcracks surrounded by diffuse staining within trabeculae. More recently, the confocal microscope has allowed three-dimensional analysis of microcracks.[19,20] Fazzalari et al.[19] showed in their study of vertebral trabecular bone that cross-hatched and diffuse microdamage includes small cracks about 10 µm in length. Boyce et al.[20] found in *ex vivo* bending of human compact bone that diffuse microdamage is located on the tensile side of the bone and consists of a fine network of cracks at sublamellar to submicron levels, linear microdamage is located on the compressive side, and tearing-type (wispy-appearing) microdamage appears near the neutral axis, indicating microdamage morphologies are dependent on local strain mode. The bulk staining technique allows histological evaluation of bone fatigue from either experimental specimens or clinical biopsies.

EVIDENCE FOR MICRODAMAGE ACCUMULATION ASSOCIATED WITH STRESS FRACTURE

Because diagnosis of a clinically suspected stress fracture can be confirmed by a combination of physical examination, x-ray, and a technetium 99m methylene diphosphonate bone scan, a biopsy is unnecessary except for the cases in which tumor must be ruled out.[21] Although microdamage has been demonstrated in experimental fatigue studies[6,22,23] and human cadaveric studies,[10,17-19,24,25] the presence of microdamage in clinical stress fractures[26] has never been demonstrated histologically.

Biopsy of Stress Fracture

We have treated a case of stress fracture necessary to rule out tumor. A 12 year old boy who was in high school baseball club had pain in his left lower leg after training, stronger at night for about 6 months before visiting the hospital. He stopped training for two months but the pain gradually increased. Stress fractures of the tibia are the most prevalent site in athletes and soldiers. These usually involve the medial cortex, and much less frequently the anterior cortex. X-ray examination showed a radiolucent nidus in the anterior mid-shaft region with thickening of the anterior medial tibial cortex (Figure 3a). Tc^{99m} bone scan showed increased uptake (Figure 3b). T$_2$ weighted MRI showed high intensity, indicating edema or hypervascularity in the region (Figure 3c). Because clinical examination could not rule out osteoid osteoma or osteoblastoma, excisional biopsy was performed. The anterior tibial cortex was excised en bloc in surgery. H&E stained decalcified sections showed periosteal woven bone formation and highly porous cortical bone, indicating high remodeling activity (color Figure 4*). Undecalcified bulk stained sections showed extensive microdamage in association with active cutting cones, indicating initiation of damage repair by remodeling (color Figure 5a*, 5b*). A diffuse microcrack lay between two active osteons (color Figure 5c*). Note that these two resorption cavities are spreading into the microdamage, providing indirect evidence that osteonal remodeling does not randomly repair microdamage. Martin[34] (Chapter 12) has developed a mathematical model for repair of fatigue damage and stress fracture by bone remodeling, predicting that (1) fatigue half life of a bolus damage is several months, and is substantially reduced if the amount of damage is increased or the remodeling is well directed at foci of damage; (2) porosity associated with remodeling to remove damage can produce a mechanically unstable state; and (3) periosteal bone formation increases the tolerance of bone but does not prevent stress fracture. Because multicellular unit (BMU) based bone remodeling employs the remodeling space at least

* See color insert following page 182.

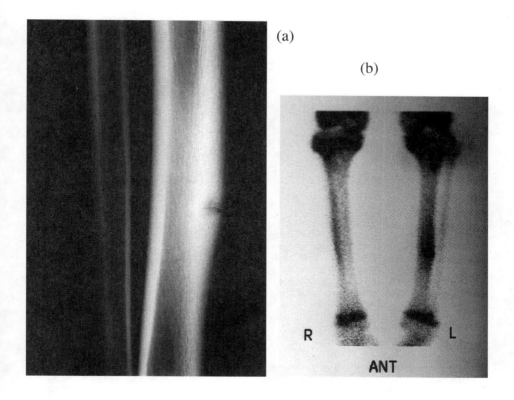

(a)

(b)

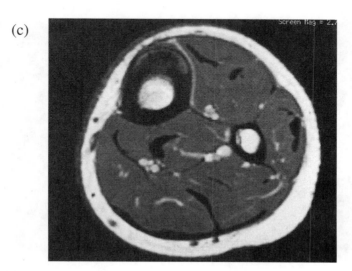

(c)

Figure 3 A case of stress fracture (12 year old male). a. lateral view x-ray of the tibia, b. Tc^{99m} bone scan of lower legs, c. MRI (T$_2$ weighted) axial view of the tibia.

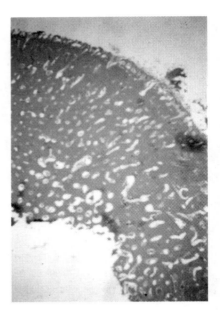

Figure 4 Cross-sectional photomicrograph of stress fracture (H&E stained, ×15.6). New woven bone was formed on the periosteal envelope, and cortical bone was highly porous with a number of cutting cones. No inflammatory changes such as infiltration of neutrophils were observed. See color insert following p. 182.

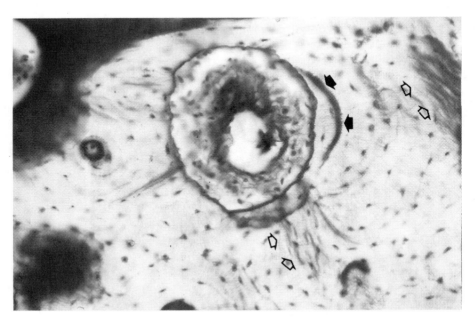

Figure 5 Photomicrographs of microdamage in the bulk stained sections (×62.5). a. Debonding microdamage on the cement line (black arrow), and diffuse microdamage in interstitial bone (white arrow) are associated with resorption cavity.

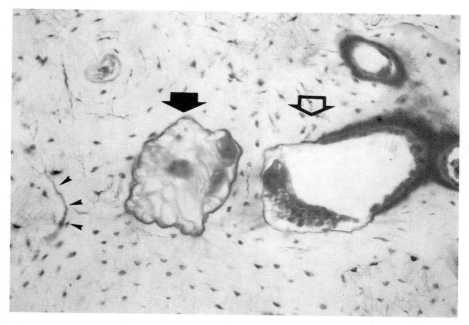

Figure 5 b. An osteon in active resorption phase (black arrow) and another osteon showing both resorption and formation (white arrow) in association with a linear microcrack (black triangle).

transiently, remodeling could temporarily decrease the mechanical properties of the bone during repair of microdamage. This may underlie stress fracture pathogenesis. Our histological finding of microdamage accumulation associated with active remodeling supports the idea that stress fracture is related to positive feedback between damage and repair.

Cytokines and Bone Remodeling at the Stress Fracture Site

Reverse transcription–polymerase chain reaction (RT-PCR) analysis of a fractured bone showed that messenger ribonucleic acid (mRNA) of cyclooxygenase-2 (COX-2), bone morphogenic protein 2 (BMP2), basic fibroblast growth factor (b-FGF), interleukin-6 (IL-6), and osteocalcin (OC) were overexpressed at the fracture site compared to the control bone. It was suggested that IL-6 and b-FGF are related to bone resorptive functions, and BMP2 and osteocalcin are related to bone formative functions. The histotological findings of increased osteonal remodeling support this idea. COX-2 expression in this case suggests two possibilities: (1) inflammation secondary to stress fracture, and/or (2) osteogenesis. While no inflammatory changes were observed histologically in our case, further investigation is needed to understand the relationship of COX-2 with mechanical loading.

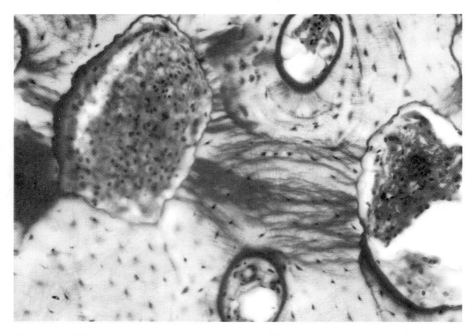

Figure 5　c. Diffuse microdamage (white arrow) lies between two active osteons with both resorption and formation. Note both resorption cavities spread into the direction of the microdamage.

SUMMARY

In an open biopsy on a 12 year old boy to rule out tumor, bulk stained histological examination revealed microdamage accumulation and initiation of microdamage repair by remodeling at the stress fracture site. This report is the first histological demonstration of a clinical stress fracture, also showing a repair reaction. Our histological observations suggest that remodeling repairs microdamage, which implies that remodeling is an important physiological function of bone to maintain mechanical integrity against fatigue.

REFERENCES

1. Martin, R.B. and Burr, D.B., Fatigue in bone, in *Structure, Function, and Adaptation of Compact Bone*, Raven Press, New York, 1989, chap. 7.
2. Agarwal, B.D. and Brountman, L.J., *Analysis and Performance of Fiber Composite*, John Wiley & Sons, New York, 1980.
3. Reifsnider, K.L., Shulta, K., and Dyke, J.C., Long-term fatigue characteristics of composite materials. In *Long Term Behavior of Composite Materials STP813,* American Society for Testing and Materials, Philadelphia, 1983.
4. Curry, J.D., Stress concentrations in bone, *Q. J. Microsc. Sci.,* 103, 111, 1962.

5. Carter, D.R., et al., Fatigue behavior of adult cortical bone. The influence of mean strain and stress range, *Acta Orthop. Scand.,* 52, 481, 1981.
6. Burr, D.B., et al., Experimental stress fractures of the tibia. Biological and mechanical aetiology in rabbits. *J. Bone J. Surg.,* 72B, 370, 1990.
7. Mori, S., Bone microdamage and its repair: pathophysiology of bone fatigue, in *Mechanical Loading of Bone and Joints,* Takahashi E., Ed., Springer Verlag, Tokyo, 1999, 139.
8. Frost, H.M., *Orthopedic Biomechanics,* Charles C. Thomas, Springfield, IL, 1973.
9. Freeman M.A., Todd, R.C., and Pirie, C.J., The role of fatigue in the pathogenesis of senile femoral fractures, *J. Bone J. Surg.,* 56B, 698, 1974.
10. Frost, H.M., The pathomechanics of osteoporosis, *Clin. Orthop.,* 200, 198, 1985.
11. Johnston, C.C. and Slemenda, C.W., Pathogenesis of osteoporosis, *Bone,* 17, 19S, 1995.
12. Cooper, C., Epidemiology of fragility fractures: a role of bone quality? *Calcif. Tissue Int.,* 53, S381, 1993.
13. Burr, D.B. and Schaffler, M.B., The involvement of subchondral mineralized tissues in osteoarthrosis: quantitative microscopic evidence, *Microsc. Res. Tech.,* 15, 343, 1997.
14. Frost, H.M., Presence of microscopic cracks *in vivo* in bone, *Bull. Henry Ford Hosp.,* 8, 25, 1960.
15. Burr, D.B. and Stafford, T., Validity of the bulk-staining technique to separate artifactual from *in vivo* bone microdamage, *Clin. Orthop.,* 260, 305, 1990.
16. Burr, D.B. and Hooser, M., Alteration to the en bloc basic fuchsin staining protocol for the demonstration of microdamage produced *in vivo*, *Bone,* 17, 431, 1995.
17. Mori, S., Harruff, R., Ambrousius, W., and Burr, D.B., Trabecular bone volume and microdamage accumulation in the femoral heads with and without femoral neck fractures, *Bone,* 12, 521, 1997.
18. Wenzel, T.E., Schaffler, M.B., and Fyhrie, D.P., *In vivo* trabecular microcracks in human vertebral bone, *Bone,* 19, 89, 1996.
19. Fazzalari, N.L., Forwood, B.A., et al., Three-dimensional confocal images of microdamage in cancellous bone, *Bone,* 23, 373, 1998.
20. Boyce, T.M., et.al., Damage types and strain mode associations in human compact bone bending fatigue, *J .Orthop. Res.,* 16, 322, 1998.
21. Trafton, P.G., Fatigue fracture in *Skeletal Trauma,* Vol. 2, Browner, B.D., Ed., Saunders, Philadelphia, 1992, 1860.
22. Forwood, M.R. and Parker, A.W., Microdamage in response to repetitive torsional loading in the rat, *Calcif. Tissue Int.,* 45, 47, 1989.
23. Mori, S. and Burr, D.B. Increased intracortical remodeling following fatigue damage, *Bone,* 14, 103, 1993.
24. Schaffler, M.B., Choi, K., and Milgrom, C., Aging and matrix microdamage accumulation in human compact bone, *Bone,* 17, 521, 1995.
25. Norman, T.L. and Wang, Z., Microdamage of human cortical bone: incidence and morphology in long bone, *Bone,* 20, 375, 1997.
26. Bogumill, G.P. and Schwamm, H.A., Stress fracture, in *Orthopedic Pathology,* W.B. Saunders, Philadelphia, 1984, 87.
27. Martin, B., Mathematical model for repair of fatigue damage and stress fracture in osteonal bone. *J .Orthop. Res.,* 13, 309, 1994.

CHAPTER **11**

Bone Fatigue and Remodeling in the Development of Stress Fractures

Mitchell B. Schaffler

CONTENTS

Introduction...161
Does Bone Fatigue Within the Normal Range of Physiological Strains and
    Cycles?...162
How Does Bone Behave When Fatigue-Loaded At Lower, More Physiological
    Strains?..162
Fatigue Microdamage in Compact Bone 164
Remodeling and Repair of Microdamage in Bone..167
How Does Stress Fracture Occur? 170
How Can Increased Remodeling Drive Microdamage Accumulation in Bone?....174
References..177

INTRODUCTION

Stress fractures result from repetitive loading and occur commonly among physically active individuals. Stress fractures are not associated with a specific history of trauma. Rather, they are frequently reported in soldiers, ballet dancers, joggers, and other individuals who have increased their levels of repetitive-type physical activities.[4,28,30,52,55,74-76,78,81] As such, they have been often regarded as a mechanical fatigue-driven process. Stress fractures are ranked between the second and eighth most common running injury, with incidences reported between 4 and 14%.[48,59] Rates of occurrence of stress fracture in the U.S. military were reported by Jones et al.[59] to be in the range of less than 4%. However, recent studies by Hise et al.[52] found that stress fracture incidence among female soldiers in basic training was considerably higher, at nearly 8%. In other military training environments, such as the Israeli army, the incidence of stress fracture among soldiers has been reported as high as 31 percent.[74,75]

Clinically, stress fractures present as bone tenderness, often with radiographic evidence of a periosteal callus; less frequently observed is occurrence of an actual fracture line.[30,81,109] Typically, stress fractures occur after four to six weeks of increased activity. This is estimated to correspond to about 100,000 load use cycles.[24,30] In recent years, diagnosis of stress fracture has shifted from radiology to bone scintigraphy using ^{99m}technetium (^{99m}Tc).[46,74-76,91,109,114,115]

There are two hypotheses regarding the cause of stress fractures. One hypothesis holds that stress fractures are the result of development, accumulation, and growth of microcracks within the bone.[20-25,29,35,80] In this view, stress fractures are considered a purely mechanical damage occurrence, i.e., fatigue failure of the skeleton. An alternative hypothesis models stress fracture as a positive feedback mechanism: increased mechanical usage stimulates bone turnover, which results in focally increased bone remodeling space (porosity) and decreased bone mass. With continued loading of this focally, transiently osteopenic bone, local stresses are markedly elevated, leading to accelerated damage and failure. Fracture is the result of continued repetitive loading superimposed on the decreased bone mass caused by more and larger resorption spaces.[30,58,68,97,98]

DOES BONE FATIGUE WITHIN THE NORMAL RANGE OF PHYSIOLOGICAL STRAINS AND CYCLES?

Bone can fracture with relatively few loading cycles when cyclic stresses or strains are large. Carter and Caler[20,21] showed that bone can fail in fatigue in as few as 1000 to 100,000 loading cycles at strain ranges of 5000 to 10,000 microstrain (0.5 to 1 percent deformation). However, *in vivo* bone strain studies indicate that habitual peak physiological strain ranges in living animals are considerably lower, typically less than 1500 microstrain in tension and 2500 microstrain in compression.[62,92,93] Very high bone strains (in the range of 4000 to 5000 microstrain) in muscularly fatigued, growing racehorses have been reported by Nunamaker et al.[80] However, other studies have not observed comparably high strain levels in race horses.[93,94] Recently, Burr and co-workers[18,44,53] applied strain gages to the tibial shafts in Israeli soldiers during intensive training regimes and found that repetitive strains did not exceed 2000 microstrain for any voluntary activity, no matter how extreme the regimen. They also observed that after extreme muscular fatigue, strain magnitudes did not change but strain rates increased significantly.[44] In summary, these data indicate that maximum bone strains *in vivo* during vigorous activities, in humans and in animals, are in the range of about 2000-2500 microstrain.

HOW DOES BONE BEHAVE WHEN FATIGUE-LOADED AT LOWER, MORE PHYSIOLOGICAL STRAINS?

At physiological strains in the range of 1500 to 2500 microstrain, the *predicted fatigue life to failure* of compact bone (defined as fracture) is extremely long — up to 10 million load cycles. However, Schaffler et al.[97,98] showed that during cyclic loading at such low strains as encountered in habitual loading, bone sustains a significant amount of fatigue damage. This fatigue is evidenced by up to 10% stiffness (modulus) loss in bone test specimens over the first few hundred thousand cycles of loading. A number of other studies have since reported similar observations for fatigue in bovine, canine, equine, and human bone.[17,47,85,100] The mechanical loss of material stiffness, or modulus reduction, during fatigue is correlated to the accumulation of microdamage. All of these studies found that the fatigue process begins early in the loading history, with most of the modulus degradation occurring within several hundred thousand cycles of loading. Stiffness loss then stabilizes for the duration of the experimental loading period and does not progress to failure for up to several million load cycles (Figure 1). Thus, at the levels of stress and strain which are habitually developed *in vivo*, the fatigue life to failure for compact bone is extremely long — 1 to 10 million load cycles, which corresponds to approximately five to ten years of use in life. However, significant amounts of fatigue damage occur throughout the loading history. This damage must be repaired in order to avoid failure of skeletal elements. It should also be noted that strain rate, or the rate at

Fatigue behavior of compact bone at habitual physiological strains

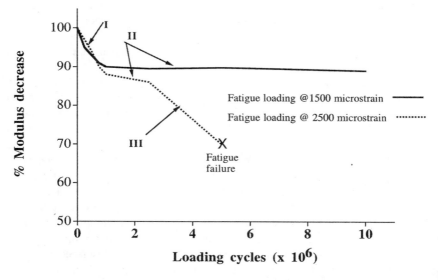

Figure 1   Summary of fatigue behavior of compact bone loaded at two strain levels characteristic of the physiologic loading environment. At the lower strain, characteristic of rapid walking, bone sustains damage and loses stiffness (shown as percentage decrease from the initial elastic modulus) early in its loading history (phase I). Stiffness loss then slows and remains stable (phase II) for up to 10 million cycles. At 2500 microstrain, the strain level characteristic of normal running, bone shows a similar early degradation of modulus (I). Damage accumulation then slows and remains stable for 1 to 2 million cycles (II). At this higher strain, however, modulus degradation will resume and progress to fatigue failure (phase III) after several million cycles of loading.

which peak strains are generated in bone, has a significant effect on damage accumulation. In laboratory fatigue tests, loading at strain rates characteristic of running were more damaging to bone than loading at lower rates, regardless of the magnitude of strain or load.[97]

The key point of these data is that bone readily sustains fatigue damage at modest stresses or strains. An analogous temporal pattern of fatigue behavior occurs in many fiber–reinforced composite materials.[1,89] Under low stress or strain cyclic loading conditions, stiffness loss occurs early in the loading history, corresponding structurally to the initiation of new cracks and voids in the material. Stiffness loss then slows until very late in the loading history, when it again resumes and progresses rapidly to failure. This three-phase failure behavior for low stress/strain cyclic loading failure of composite materials, and apparently compact bone as well, stands in contradistinction to the earlier idea that compact bone can be characterized as a material that has a linear, progressive loss of stiffness leading to failure. Thus, at the low stress/strain levels at which bone is habitually loaded, bone sustains fatigue damage quickly, but that damage does not readily progress to failure.

FATIGUE MICRODAMAGE IN COMPACT BONE

Loss of stiffness with fatigue loading is direct mechanical evidence for the existence of damage within the matrix in composite material such as bone.[1,8,22,85,97,98,100] However, given that bone is a comparatively brittle, inhomogeneous material, it has been problematic to visualize matrix damage and validate that matrix cracking is not an artifact of microscopic preparation techniques.

Frost[40] reported the first observations of microdamage (small, 30 to 100 µm-long cracks) in human rib samples obtained at autopsy. He suggested that such microcracks result from fatigue *in vivo*. Frost's simple and elegant approach for visualizing microscopic damage in bone is still central to bone fatigue and matrix damage research some 40 years after its original description.[11,17,47,101,104] Large blocks of bone tissue were stained in a dye (basic fuchsin) which binds non-specifically to open bone surfaces prior to histological sectioning. Microcracks existing in the bone prior to sectioning were stained; new cracks introduced during sectioning for microscopic observation remained unstained and could therefore be readily distinguished as artifact. This bulk staining approach has been updated to include fluorescent and heavy metal dyes, allowing studies using confocal microscopy and electron microscopy.[64,99,103]

Bone microcracks, of the typical linear morphology first described by Frost (Figure 2), have been produced experimentally by applying physiological levels of stress or strain cyclically to devitalized bone samples[17,19,97,98,100] and *in vivo* as well.[5,15,77,108] Moreover, bone is a hierarchical, inhomogeneous material, and cracks can potentially form at any level in its microstructural organization. Thus, it is clear that there can be other levels of matrix failure in bone which occur early in the fatigue process and strongly influence its fatigue behavior. In experiments from our laboratory,[100] human compact bone samples were fatigued to increasing amounts of damage, as evidenced by modulus degradation. Typical linear-type microcracks (Figure 3a) were observed rarely in specimens at lower fatigue level (15% modulus

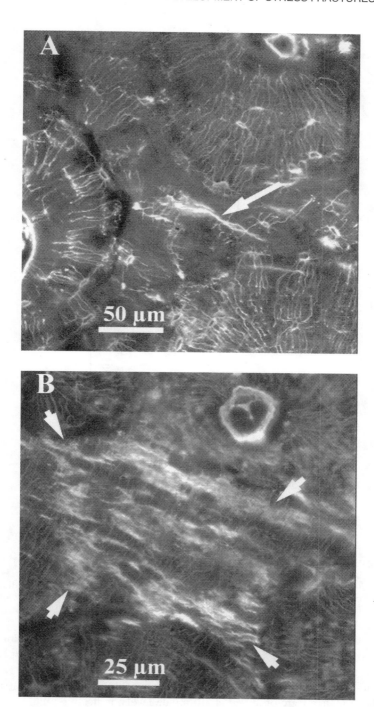

Figure 2   Confocal photomicrographs of microdamage in human bone samples. Upper panel (A) shows a linear microcrack (arrow) typical of that first described by Frost.[40] Lower panel (B) shows a higher magnification view of a region of diffuse matrix damage, comprised of large numbers of very small microcracks.

(a)

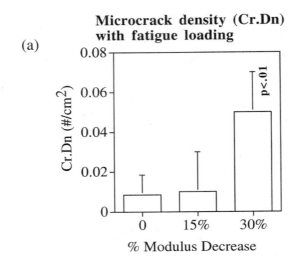

(b)

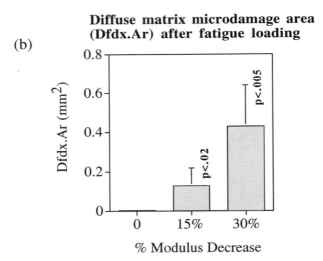

Figure 3 Linear microcrack density (Cr.Dn) and diffuse damage content (Dfdx.Ar) in human bone specimens experimentally loaded to increasing levels of fatigue. a. For linear microcracks, increased Cr.Dn occurs after a 30% modulus decrease. b. In contrast, diffuse damage content increases in direct relation to increasing amounts of fatigue in these samples.

loss) but were observed routinely at higher levels of fatigue (30% modulus degradation). In studies of whole bone fatigue in canine long bones, Burr et al.[9] also reported that linear microcracks were not observed until 15% stiffness loss. However, in fatigue-loaded human bone specimens, patches of diffuse basic fuchsin staining of the bone matrix were observed at all fatigue levels, indicating a fatigue-induced change in bone matrix permeability to the stain. The amount of this diffuse staining increased in direct relation to increasing specimen fatigue levels (Figure 3b).

Confocal microscopy showed these patches of diffuse basic fuchsin staining in fatigued bone to be comprised of very fine matrix cracking at the sub-lamellar level (<5 μm) size order in bone. (Figure 2). Occasional foci of dye uptake were observed within regions of identifiable matrix microcracking, for which no cracks could be resolved using confocal microscopy. As the maximum lateral resolution of confocal microscopy is ~200 nanometers, these foci indicate that some damage occurs at even finer levels of bone matrix structure. Zioupos and Currey,[113] in their recent studies of fracture toughening mechanisms in bone, reported similar early mechanisms of matrix failure. The principal bone matrix structures at the level of organization of these very small cracks in bone are hydroxyapatite crystals and their aggregates, suggesting that early matrix failure in bone might occur principally at the level of these structures.

In summary, compact bone undergoes fatigue and sustains matrix-level damage as a result of cyclic loading at the magnitudes of stress or strain that can be generated with habitual physiological activities. However, at these same stresses/strains, fatigue does not progress to failure within a time frame consistent with the development of stress fractures *in vivo*. These data suggest that other mechanisms must be involved in the development of so-called fatigue or stress fractures *in vivo*.

Studies show that different amounts of fatigue in compact bone lead to different amounts of microdamage, but also to different qualities of the damage present (i.e., diffuse matrix microdamage early in fatigue; typical microcracking later in fatigue). It is well established in materials science that microdamage content (quality and quantity) compromises the residual (remaining) mechanical properties of a material. Diminished residual properties in bone after fatigue were first demonstrated by Carter and Hayes.[22] In order to assess how different amounts and types of damage with different levels of bone fatigue alter functional-mechanical properties, Boyce et al.[8] examined the residual properties of human compact bone after fatigue, using matched contralateral femurs to those used in fatigue experiments described in the preceding section. After completion of fatigue loading, specimens were tested mono-tonically to failure. Residual properties of ultimate stress (strength), ultimate strain, and work to fracture were measured from stress-strain curves. Among specimens loaded to the lower level of fatigue (15% modulus decrease), residual stress, strain, and work to fracture were reduced in general proportion to the amount of modulus degradation. In contrast, bone specimens fatigued to greater levels (30% modulus decrease) showed losses of ultimate strength and work to fracture far greater than expected based on the stiffness changes in these specimens (67 and 76% reductions, respectively). Most striking, however, is that bone specimens fatigued to the higher level of fatigue showed effectively no post-yield deformation (Figure 4). In other words, the accumulation of fatigue damage caused a disproportionate loss of the ability of bone to withstand a catastrophic fracture.

REMODELING AND REPAIR OF MICRODAMAGE IN BONE

Unlike synthetic engineering materials, bone is capable of detecting and repairing fatigue damage at the microscopic level. Numerous investigators have suggested that

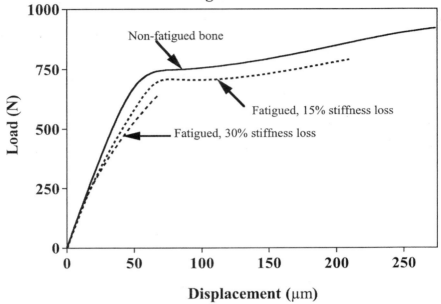

Load-displacement characteristics for human compact bone at different fatigue levels

Figure 4 Residual mechanical properties for bone specimens after different amounts of fatigue. Non-fatigued bone shows well-defined elastic, yield, and plastic regions of the loading curve. At a modest level of fatigue (15% modulus decrease), the bone mechanical properties are reduced in close proportion to the induced fatigue level. At the higher fatigue level (30% modulus loss), bone stiffness and strength are reduced proportionally. However, the load-displacement curve no longer shows a yield point or any post-yield region. These data show that higher levels of fatigue cause a disproportionate loss of bone's fracture toughness, or the ability of bone to withstand fracture.

a primary function of osteonal remodeling in the adult skeleton is reparative: remodeling serves to remove and replace fatigue-damaged regions of compact bone.[5,15,19,40-42,68,69,77,84,97,98,101] Specifically, repair of matrix microdamage occurs through a microscopic "drill and fill" process, in which osteoclasts tunnel into bone and remove damaged regions. Osteoblasts then concentrically fill in the resorption space, forming a completed osteon. The remodeling repair response is summarized schematically in Figure 5. How bone remodeling units (tunneling osteoclast followed by osteoblasts) target damaged areas of bone is not understood. Osteocytes, the resident cells buried within the mineralized matrix of bone, appear to play a critical role in this process. Indeed, despite the widely held concept that bone remodeling functions in the repair of microdamage, empirical data demonstrating this basic physiological mechanism are scant, owing to the difficulty and complexity of performing such studies.

Burr, Martin, Schaffler, and Radin,[15] and Mori and Burr[77] showed experimentally that bone resorption spaces are associated with remodeling of linear microcracks in experimentally loaded canine compact bone. Recently, Bentolila et al.[5] reported an

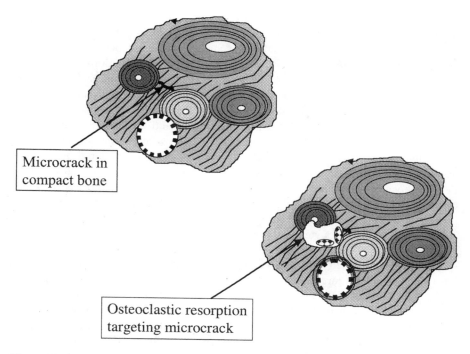

Microcrack in
compact bone

Osteoclastic resorption
targeting microcrack

Figure 5 Schematic diagram showing microdamage in compact bone and targeted removal of the damage by osteoclastic resorption.

in vivo fatigue model based on end-load ulnar bending in adult rats, in which bone fatigue levels can be monitored as changes in whole bone stiffness. After fatigue loading, bone remodeling was activated and was observed in association with both linear microcracks and areas of diffuse matrix damage. Remodeling was effective in removing both damage types from the bone. Recent studies by Mashiba and co-workers[70] have taken a different approach to examining the relationship between microdamage and remodeling in normal bone physiology. They found that inhibiting bone remodeling in normally active dogs, using two types of bisphosphonate,[2,3] leads to a significant increase in bone microdamage content in the axial skeleton (ribs and vertebral bodies) as well as in long bones (femurs). These experiments show very convincingly that without an active remodeling-repair system, microdamage will accumulate in skeletal tissues as a result of normal, mechanically nominal levels of mechanical usage.

The cellular mechanisms by which groups of osteoclasts target regions of bone for resorption are unknown. However, it is reasonable to presume that osteocytes, the only cells embedded in the bone matrix, would be involved. Osteocytes and their elongated cell processes (in their lacunae and canaliculi, respectively) are widely and extensively distributed throughout the bone matrix. These cells are attached to their surrounding bone matrix with numerous attachment molecules, and to their neighboring cells through electrical connections known as gap junctions.[31,32] Osteocytes are highly responsive to mechanical loading.[63,103] Matrix disruption from microdamage can be expected to directly injure osteocytes, disrupt their attachments to bone matrix, interrupt their communication through canalicular cellular and fluid flow processes, or alter their metabolic exchange. When osteocytes are lost from bone, complete fatigue fracture occurs. Examples include radiation-induced death of osteocytes,[72] allograft bone[6] and avascular necrosis.[60] Dunstan et al.[33] showed that the absence of osteocytes is associated with hip fracture. Osteocytes are focally lost in areas of microcrack accumulation in aging human bone.[86]

The involvement of osteocytes in bone fatigue and remodeling was recently demonstrated by Verborgt et al.[108] using the rat *in vivo* fatigue model. They found that with fatigue *in vivo*, osteocytes surrounding microcracks are injured and undergo an ordered cell disintegration process following a genetically regulated program, i.e., apoptosis. Regulated cell death is the ubiquitous biological process by which cells break down at the end of their functional life,[10,61,106] with the resulting cell breakdown products targeted by phagocytic cells. Osteoclasts belong to the phagocytic cell lineage. Osteocyte apoptosis has been observed in other metabolic situations associated with bone resorption.[9,79,106] Thus, osteocytes, and in particular the events surrounding their death, appear to provide a key part of the signaling process by which osteoclasts target microdamaged bone for removal and focal repair.

Left undetected and unrepaired, the accumulation of microdamage in bone leads to compromised mechanical properties and bone fragility. Damaged bone has significantly reduced mechanical properties in terms of strength and stiffness, and especially fracture toughness. Even small amounts of ultrastructurally based microdamage associated with early fatigue will compromise the functional-mechanical properties of bone. Fatigue damage has both mechanical and biological consequences. Stress fractures are the obvious application of the damage and repair concept in bone. However, bone microdamage, repair, and fragility are also implicated in bone aging, bone implant failure, and fractures associated with long-term usage of drugs that suppress bone remodeling physiology.[19,37,54,101] Suppressing remodeling may allow damage accumulation that will have deleterious mechanical consequences.

HOW DOES STRESS FRACTURE OCCUR?

There are two hypotheses regarding the causes of stress fractures. One hypothesis holds that stress fractures are the result of the accumulation and growth of microcracks within the bone. In this view, stress fractures are considered a purely mechanical damage occurrence, i.e., fatigue failure of the skeleton. However, fatigue to fracture as the primary mechanical causation for stress fractures is not supported by the experimental data (reviewed above). Alternatively, stress fracture has also been variously described as being primarily a biological process in which bone remodeling processes and periosteal reaction constitute the key features. However, there is little direct data on the pathophysiology of stress fractures. Attempts to understand the stress fracture process from human clinical studies have met with only limited success because of the inability to study bone tissue mechanisms directly. Mechanistic studies have not been performed in animals because of lack of a suitable experimental system until recently.

Of the few studies of human stress fracture tissues, those of Johnson and co–workers,[58] from the Armed Forces Institute of Pathology, stand out as the most critical in gaining insight into the physiology of stress fracture processes (also see Morris and Blickenstaff[78] for detailed discussion of Johnson's work). They obtained biopsies of stress fracture lesions from military recruits. Johnson observed woven bone reactions in numerous samples. Perhaps most significantly, however, focally increased intracortical remodeling was observed at stress fracture sites even in the absence of any woven bone response. Johnson's studies were based on histopathological biopsies of the lesions, taken at single time points, and therefore did not systematically examine the underlying development or physiology of the stress fracture lesions. Nevertheless, these data indicate that increased intracortical remodeling is one of the earliest and most prominent features in human stress fracture.

The association of remodeling and damage is supported by the stress fracture biopsy study presented by Mori in Chapter 10. Photomicrographs of the biopsy show accumulation of both diffuse damage and multiple linear microcracks in the region where the stress fracture occurred. Moreover, the bone surrounding the damaged regions is highly porous because of the presence of numerous active resorption cavities which are actively removing the damaged bone. These observations show that extensive microdamage is associated with the stress fracture and that bone mounts a repair reaction that will ultimately remove this damage.

Milgrom and co-workers in Israel[74,75] examined the time course of development of stress fractures among military recruits using serial ^{99m}Tc bone scans. They found that scintigraphic activity in bones destined for stress fracture increased significantly well before the existence of any increase in observable periosteal reaction. Early increased ^{99m}Tc uptake provides intriguing, albeit indirect evidence that increased bone turnover processes may be a significant early component in the development of stress fractures.

Recently, Stover and colleagues[104] reported histopathological data from racehorses with stress fracture that suggests that increased remodeling precedes the occurrence of microdamage in stress fracture. They obtained paired long bones from horses that had suffered complete (catastrophic) stress fractures of one limb. Cortical bones adjacent to the fracture sites showed elevated intracortical porosity. Most remarkable, however, is that comparable increases of intracortical porosity were also present at the same locations of the contralateral non-fractured long bones. Based on these findings, the authors suggested that increased intracortical porosity might be a necessary prerequisite to the development of stress fracture. As these were single time point studies, questions about the exact role of this increased bone turnover in the pathogenesis of stress fracture were not addressed.

Li et al.[66] reported experimental serial histological observations on the development of stress fractures in an animal model (Chapter 14). They produced stress fracture in rabbits by a chronic repetitive activity model. Animals were forced to jump and run in their cages for several hours per day for two months. Li et al. found that initial intracortical remodeling of the tibial diaphysis was the earliest observable change in the stress fracture sequence, with increased vascularity and osteoclastic resorption evident within the first week of repetitive loading. Periosteal reaction was not evident until the onset of intracortical resorption.

In our laboratory, we have developed an experimental animal model for stress fractures in rabbits, using repetitive impulsive loading of hindlimbs (Chapter 14).[12,16,102] Microfractures of trabecular bone and remodeling of the subchondral bone are a well established consequence of the repetitive impulsive loading model.[36,87,88] Adapted for use in diaphyseal bone, this model reproduces the scintigraphic and radiographic changes typically observed with stress fractures, including progressive increase in [99mTc] uptake in bone, periosteal callus formation, and presence of microscopic cracks within the bone.[12,102] In this model, hindlimbs of skeletally mature rabbits were loaded to produce tibial diaphyseal stress fractures. Briefly, right hindlimbs were subjected to repetitive impulsive loading, using a cam-driven loading device. Loading is at 1.5 time body weight for a 50 millisecond cycle duration at 1 Hz. Animals receive 2400 load cycles daily. This regime causes stress fracture in the distal tibial diaphysis after five to six weeks of loading.

In the first series of experiments using this model, Burr et al.[12] showed that stress fractures in rabbits result from repetitive cyclic loading at low stresses. The lesions, which occurred in the distal third of the tibial diaphysis, were characterized at the organ level by progressive increases in bone [99mTc] activity, followed later and variably by a periosteal reaction (Figure 6). In subsequent studies,[16] we measured tibial diaphyseal strains at the stress fracture site in the range of 500 to 1000 microstrain, which is within the normal physiological strain range (see above discussion). Strain rates, though increased somewhat over normal, were also within the range reported for normal locomotor activities.[93]

Recently, Schaffler and Boyd[102] examined bone tissue-level responses in the development of stress fracture in the rabbit stress fracture model. They showed that increases in intracortical porosity precede the accumulation of bone microdamage in experimentally induced stress fracture in this model. Intracortical remodeling at the stress fracture site was markedly increased by three weeks of loading, with the number of resorbing sites increased almost sixfold over control levels (Figure 7a). Intracortical remodeling activity was further increased by six weeks of loading, with resorption number increased more than tenfold over control levels). Resorption

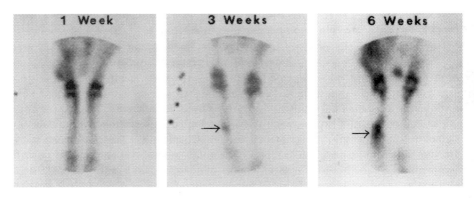

Figure 6   [99mTc] bone scans of rabbit tibiae during development of experimental stress fracture. Arrows indicate increased isotope uptake in distal diaphyses of loaded limbs after 3 and 6 weeks of loading. Lesion severity progresses from 3 to 6 weeks.

Intracortical resorption activity in rabbit tibiae during development of stress fracture

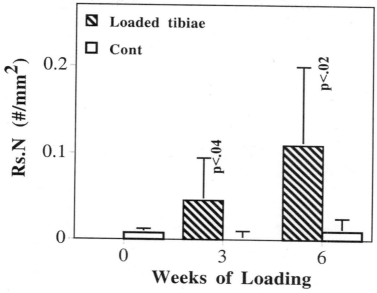

Figure 7a   Intracortical resorption activity, as measured from resorption space number, at stress fracture site in rabbit distal tibial diaphyses after 3 and 6 weeks of repetitive loading. Significance values are shown relative to internal, nonloaded control limbs.

occurred primarily in the anterior and posterior tibial cortices, corresponding to the location of stress fracture and highest strain rate in this model. Bone microdamage was not observed in control bones or experimentally after three weeks of loading. By six weeks of loading, there was a significant increase in the number of microcracks observed in diaphyses Figure 7b. Typically, these were small cracks (mean length = 24 ± 7 μm). In addition, microcracks were observed only in those areas of the cortex that were undergoing intracortical remodeling (Figure 7c). Acute fatigue loading experiments, in which the equivalent of six weeks of loading was performed in one day, showed little microdamage induced by the loading alone (Figure 7b), confirming that rapid microdamage accumulation occurred only in the presence of increased bone remodeling.

The stimulus for activation of new remodeling sites in these experiments is not clear, as the experimental stress fracture site experiences a complicated series of changes relative to baseline in normal rabbit tibiae. These changes include altered strain distribution, increased loading rate with concomitant high frequency signal, and small amounts of microdamage, all of which have been shown to activate intracortical remodeling. Otter and co-workers[82] recently put forth the intriguing hypothesis that inadequate bone perfusion and reperfusion type injury in bone under chronic loading also might be a stimulus to activate bone remodeling in stress fracture. Thus, several lines of clinical, histopathological, and experimental data

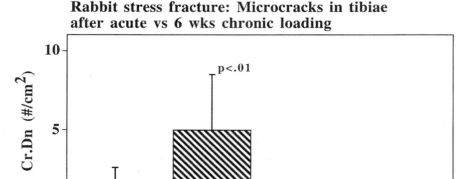

Figure 7b   Microcrack content at stress fracture site in rabbit distal tibial diaphyses after 6 weeks of daily (chronic) loading versus acute loading (continuous loading for 20 hours to produce equivalent number of cycles to 6 weeks of daily loading). Acute loading, which occurs without increases in intracortical remodeling, results in a slight increase in bone microdamage content. Chronic loading, which occurs in the presence of significant increases in bone remodeling, causes a dramatic increase in microdamage.

show that increased bone remodeling occurs early in the stress fracture process. Activation of local remodeling activity results in focally increased bone porosity. Accordingly, increased intracortical porosity may be necessary for the later rapid accumulation of bone microdamage and development of stress fracture.

HOW CAN INCREASED REMODELING DRIVE MICRODAMAGE ACCUMULATION IN BONE?

A number of studies demonstrate that increased intracortical remodeling results from increased cyclic loading,[7,14,50,77] with direct mechanical effects (strain distribution, strain rate, frequency), matrix microdamage, and local cytokines among the possible stimuli for activating turnover. While the specific stimulus for activation of increased intracortical remodeling remains unclear, these studies all support the idea that early remodeling occurs with increased mechanical usage. In 1990, Schaffler, Radin, and Burr proposed a hypothesis for how elevated intracortical remodeling might drive the stress fracture process. They argued that increases in intracortical porosity, resulting from activation of intracortical remodeling, will have a dramatic effect on decreasing the stiffness of cortical bone. Continued loading of this focally osteoporotic bone will increase local stresses and strains, accelerate bone microdamage accumulation, cause periosteal hypertrophy and, ultimately, result in stress fracture. In essence, stress fracture would result when mechanical loading is sustained on a region of high turnover bone, creating a positive feedback loop leading to fracture, as summarized in Figure 8 (see Chapter 12).

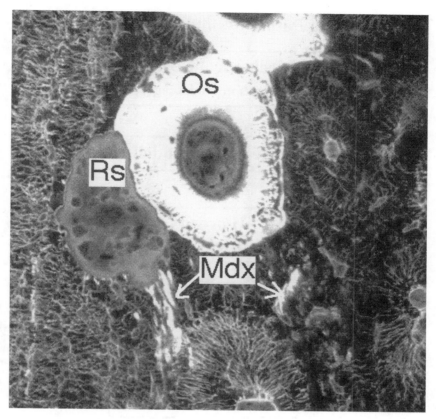

Figure 7c   Confocal photomicrograph of rabbit tibial compact bone at 6 weeks of loading, showing intracortical resorption (Rs) and new osteon (Os) in association with bone microdamage (Mdx arrows) (Field width = 400 µm).

Intracortical remodeling begins by activation of new remodeling sites and recruitment of bone cells to the active surface. In the first phase of remodeling, osteoclasts resorb pre-existing bone, resulting in more and larger porosity within the cortex. In humans, the resorption phase is estimated to last for about six to seven weeks.[34,57] Thus, increased intracortical remodeling results in increased bone porosity, which lasts several months after onset. As a consequence of the increase in remodeling space, void (i.e., porosity) volume in bone expands at the expense of bone tissue volume (total tissue volume = bone volume + porosity). Numerous investigations have shown that stiffness of bone decreases with decreasing bone volume (or increasing porosity), following a power-law type relationship. In trabecular bone, stiffness is proportional to the cube of bone volume.[23] Compact bone stiffness is even more highly dependent on mass. Schaffler and Burr found that stiffness in compact bone decreases to the seventh power of decreasing bone volume, indicating that the stiffness of compact bone is profoundly sensitive to its porosity or bone volume.[95] Similar exponential relationships for compact bone stiffness and density/porosity

Hypothesis: Pathophysiology of Stress Fracture

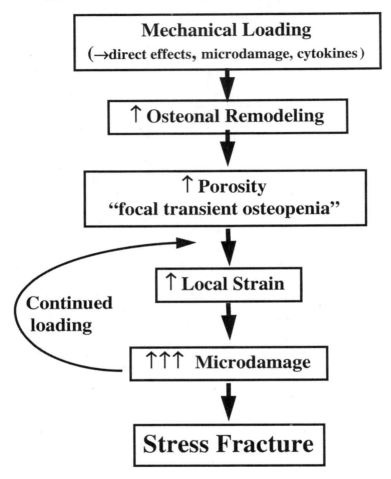

Figure 8   Schematic diagram summarizing the mechanism hypothesized for development of stress fracture, wherein increased bone remodeling and porosity (resulting from increased mechanical usage) are a prerequisite for the development of stress fractures. Increased local strains during continued loading would accelerate the accumulation of bone microdamage and the development of stress fracture in a positive feedback type manner.

were reported recently by Les et al.,[65] confirming that compact bone stiffness changes dramatically in response to small changes in intracortical porosity or bone volume.

The recent mathematical model for stress fracture development by Martin[68] is of particular interest in this regard (Chapter 12). Using a feedback model to examine the effects of increasing porosity on the mechanical properties of compact bone and development of stress fracture, Martin showed that there is a critical porosity — load interaction threshold. Once this point is reached, through increased bone porosity and/or through increased local loading, Martin demonstrates that the system becomes unstable (i.e., positive feedback), and bone fails rapidly and catastrophically.

In summary, experimental data and several lines of clinical, histopathological data support the idea of a complex interplay between mechanical loading and bone remodeling in the etiology of stress fractures. While bone readily sustains fatigue microdamage during the course of repeated loading at the stresses or strains encountered in normal activities, it does not lead to fracture in the time course seen for the development of stress fracture. The model that best explains the development of stress fracture is that of a biologically (remodeling) driven damage accumulation system. In this model, stress fracture occurs as a positive feedback mechanism (Figure 8), wherein increased mechanical usage stimulates bone turnover, which results in focally increased bone remodeling space (porosity) and decreased bone mass. There is a wide range of factors (low level fatigue, altered mechanical loading, injury, cytokines, vascular) that can potentially activate local bone remodeling. All of these can occur in the development of stress fracture. With continued loading of this focally, transiently osteopenic bone, local stresses would be markedly elevated, leading to accelerated matrix damage and failure. Fracture is the result of continued repetitive loading superimposed on the decreased bone mass caused by more and larger resorption spaces

REFERENCES

1. Agarwal, B.D. and Broutman, L.J. *Analysis and Performance of Fiber Composites*, John Wiley & Sons, New York, 1980.
2. Antic, V.N., Fleisch, H., and Mulbauer, R.C., Effect of bisphosphonates on the increase in bone resorption induced by a low calcium diet, *Calcif. Tissue Int.*, 58, 443, 1996.
3. Balena, R., et al., The effects of 2-year treatment with the aminobisphosphonate alendronate on bone metabolism, bone histomorphometry and bone strength in ovariectomized nonhuman primates, *J. Clin. Invest.*, 92, 2577, 1993.
4. Beck, T.J., et al., Dual-energy x-ray absorptiometry derived structural geometry for stress fracture prediction in male U.S. Marine Corps recruits, *J. Bone Miner. Res.*, 11, 645, 1996.
5. Bentolila, V., et al., Intracortical remodeling in adult rat long bones after fatigue loading, *Bone*, 23, 275, 1998.
6. Berry, B.H., et al., Fractures of allografts: frequency, treatment and end results, *J. Bone Jt. Surg.*, 72A, 825, 1990.
7. Bouvier, M. and Hylander, W.L., Effect of bone strain on cortical bone structure in macaques (*Macaca mulatta*), *J. Morphol.*, 167, 1, 1981.
8. Boyce, T.M., et al., Residual mechanical properties of human cortical bone following fatigue loading, *Am. Soc. Biomech.*, 20, 23, 1996.
9. Bronckers, A.L.J.J., et al., DNA fragmentation during bone formation in neonatal rodent assessed by transferase mediated end labeling, *J. Bone Miner. Res.*, 11, 1281, 1996.
10. Buja, L.M., Eigenbrodt, M.L., and Eigenbrodt, E.H., Apoptosis and necrosis — basic types and mechanisms of cell death, *Arch. Pathol. Lab. Med.*, 117, 1208, 1993.
11. Burr, D.B. and Stafford, T., Validation of the bulk-staining technique to separate artifactual from *in vivo* bone microdamage, *Clin. Orthop.*, 260, 305, 1991.

12. Burr, D.B., et al., Experimental stress fractures of the tibia, *J. Bone Jt. Surg.*, 72B, 370, 1990.

13. Burr, D.B., et al., Skeletal change in response to altered strain environments: Is woven bone a response to elevated strain, *Bone*, 10, 223, 1989.

14. Burr, D.B., et al., The effects of altered strain environments on bone tissue kinetics, *Bone*, 10, 215, 1989.

15. Burr, D.B., et al., Bone remodeling in response to *in vivo* fatigue microdamage, *J. Biomechan.*, 18, 189, 1985.

16. Burr, D.B., et al., High strain rates are associated with stress fractures, *Trans. Orthop. Res. Soc.*, 20, 526, 1995.

17. Burr, D.B., et al., Does bone microdamage accumulation affect the normal mechanical properties of bone, *J. Biomech.*, 31, 337, 1998.

18. Burr, D.B., et al., *In vivo* measurement of human tibial strains recorded during dynamic loading, *Bone*, 19, 405, 1996.

19. Burr, D.B., et al., Bone microdamage and skeletal fragility in osteoporotic and stress fractures, *J. Bone Miner. Res.*, 12, 6, 1997.

20. Caler, W.E. and Carter, D.R., Bone creep-fatigue damage accumulation, *J. Biomechan.*, 22, 625, 1990.

21. Carter, D.R. and Caler, W.E., Cumulative damage model for bone fracture, *J. Orthop. Res.*, 3, 84, 1985.

22. Carter, D.R. and Hayes, W.C., Compact bone fatigue damage: a microscopic examination, *Clin. Orthop.*, 127, 265, 1977.

23. Carter, D.R. and Hayes, W.C., The compressive behavior of bone as a two phase porous structure, *J. Bone Jt. Surg.*, 59A, 954, 1977.

24. Carter, D.R., et al., Fatigue behavior of adult cortical bone: the influence of mean strain and strain range, *Acta Orthop. Scand.*, 52, 481, 1981.

25. Carter, D.R., et al., Uniaxial fatigue of human cortical bone: the influence of tissue physical characteristics, *J. Biomechan.*, 14, 461, 1981.

26. Chamay, A. and Tschantz, P., Mechanical influences in bone remodeling: experimental research on Wolff's law, *J. Biomechan.*, 5, 173, 1972.

27. Chestnut, C.H., Drug Therapy: Calcitonin, bisphosphonates, anabolic steroids, and hPTH, in *Osteoporosis: Etiology, Diagnosis, and Management*, Riggs, R.L. and Melton, L.J., Eds., Raven Press, New York, 1988, 1.

28. Clement, D.B., A survey of overuse running injuries, *Phys. Sportsmed.*, 9, 47, 1981.

29. Currey, J.D., *The Mechanical Adaptation of Bones,* University Press, Princeton, 1984.

30. Devas, M., *Stress Fractures,* Charles Blackstone, London, 1975.

31. Doty, S.B., Morphological evidence of gap junctions between bone cells, *Calcif. Tissue Int.*, 33, 509, 1981.

32. Doty, S.B., Robinson R.A., and Schofield B., Morphological and histochemical staining characteristics of bone cells, in *Handbook of Physiology*, Auerbach, G.D., Ed., American Society of Physiology, Washington, 1976, 3.

33. Dunstan, C.R., Somers, N.M., Evans, R.A., Osteocyte death and hip fracture, *Calcif. Tiss. Int.*, Suppl. 53, 113, 1993.

34. Eriksen, E.F., Axelrod, D.W., and Melsen, F., *Bone Histomorphometry,* official publication of the American Society of Bone and Mineral Research, Raven Press, New York, 1995.

35. Evans, F.G. and Riolo, M.L., Relations between the fatigue life and histology of adult human cortical bone, *J. Bone Jt. Surg.*, 52A, 1579, 1970.

36. Farkas, T.A., et al., Early vascular changes in rabbit subchondral bone after repetitive impulsive loading, *Clin. Orthop.*, 219, 259, 1987.

37. Flora, L., et al., The long-term skeletal effects of EHDP in dogs, *Metab. Bone Dis. Rel. Res.*, 3, 289, 1981.

38. Forwood, M.R. and Parker, A.W., Microdamage in response to repetitive torsional loading in the rat tibia, *Calcif. Tissue Int.*, 45, 47, 1989.

39. Fraser, W.D., Paget's disease of bone, *Curr. Opin. Rheumatol.*, 9, 347, 1997.

40. Frost, H.M., Presence of microscopic cracks *in vivo* in bone, *Henry Ford Hosp. Med. Bull.*, 8, 27, 1960.

41. Frost, H.M., *Bone Dynamics in Osteoporosis and Osteomalacia,* Charles C. Thomas, Springfield, IL, 1966.

42. Frost, H.M. Bone microdamage: factors that impair its repair, in *Current Concepts in Bone Fragility,* Uhthoff, H.K., Ed., Springer-Verlag, Berlin, 1985.

43. Frost, H.M., *Intermediary Organization in the Skeleton,* CRC Press, Boca Raton, 1985.

44. Fyhrie, D.P., Effect of fatiguing exercise on longitudinal bone strain as related to stress fracture, *Ann. Biomed. Eng.*, 26, 660, 1998.

45. Genant, H.K., Bone-seeking radionuclides: an *in vivo* study of factors affecting skeletal uptake, *Radiology,* 113, 373, 1984.

46. Geslien, G.E., et al., Early detection of stress fractures using ^{99m}Tc polyphosphonate, *Radiology,* 121, 683, 1976.

47. Gibson, V.A., et al., Fatigue behavior of the equine third metacarpus, *J. Orthop. Res.*, 13, 861, 1995.

48. Grazier, K.L., et al., *The Frequency of Occurrence, Impact and Cost of Musculoskeletal Conditions in the United States,* American Academy of Orthopedic Surgeons, Chicago, 1984.

49. Griffiths, W.E.G., Swanson S.A.V., and Freeman M.A.R., Experimental fatigue fracture of the human cadaveric femoral neck, *J. Bone Jt. Surg.*, 53B, 136, 1971.

50. Hert, J., Liskova, M., and Landgrot, B., Influence of long-term continuous bending on bone, *Folia Morphol.*, 17, 389, 1969.

51. Hert, J., Pribylova, E., and Liskova, M., Reaction of bone to mechanical stimuli: microstructure of compact bone after intermittent loading, *Acta Anat.*, 82, 218, 1971.

52. Hise, L., et al., Quantitative ultrasound predicts stress fracture risk during basic training in female soldiers, *Trans. Orthop. Res. Soc.*, 22, 186, 1997.

53. Hoshaw, S.J., et al., A method for *in vivo* measurement of bone strains in humans, *J. Biomech.*, 30, 521, 1997.

54. Hoshaw, S.J., Fyhrie, D.P., and Schaffler, M.B., The effect of implant insertion and design on bone microdamage, in *The Biological Mechanisms of Tooth Eruption, Resorption and Replacement by Implants*, Davidovitch, Z., Ed., Harvard Society for the Advancement of Orthodontics, Boston, 1994, 735.

55. Hulkko, A. and Orava, S., Stress fractures in athletes, *Int. J. Sports Med.*, 8, 221, 1987.

56. Igarashi, K., et al., Anchorage and retentive effects of a bisphophonate (AHBuBP) on tooth movements in rats, *Am. J. Orthod. Dentofacial Orthopaed.*, 106, 279, 1994.

57. Jee, W.S.S., The skeletal tissues, in *Cells and Tissues*, Weiss, L.J., Ed., Elsevier Press, Amsterdam, 1989.

58. Johnson L.C., et al., Histogenesis of stress fractures, *J. Bone Jt. Surg.*, 45A, 1542, 1963.

59. Jones B.H., et al., Exercise-induced stress fractures and stress reactions in bone: epidemiology, etiology, and classification, *Exerc. Sport Sci. Rev.*, 17, 379, 1993.

60. Kenzora, J.E., et al., Experimental osteonecrosis of the femoral head in adult rabbits, *Clin. Orthop.*, 130, 8, 1978.

61. Kerr, J.F.R., Wyllie, A.H., and Currie, A.R., Apoptosis: a basic phenomenon with wide-ranging implications for tissue kinetics, *Br. J. Cancer*, 26, 239, 1972.

62. Lanyon, L.E., et al., Bone deformation recorded in vivo from strain gages attached to the human tibial shaft, *Acta Orthop. Scand.*, 46, 256, 1975.

63. Lanyon, L.E., Osteocytes, strain detection and bone modeling and remodeling *Calcif. Tiss. Int.,* Suppl. 53, 102, 1993.

64. Lee, T.C., Myers, E.R., and Hayes, W.C., Fluorescence-aided detection of microdamage in compact bone, *J. Anat.*, 193, 179, 1998.

65. Les, C.M., et al., Estimation of material properties in the equine metacarpus with use of quantitative computed tomography, *J. Orthop. Res.*, 12, 822, 1994.

66. Li, G., et al., Radiologic and histological analysis of stress fracture in rabbit tibias, *Am. J. Sports Med.*, 13, 285, 1985.

67. Martin R.B., Porosity and specific surface of bone, *CRC Crit. Rev. Biomed. Eng.,* 10, 3, 179.

68. Martin, R.B., Mathematical model for repair of fatigue damage and stress fracture in osteonal bone, *J. Orthop. Res.*, 13, 309, 1995

69. Martin, R.B. and Burr, D.B., A hypothetical mechanism for the stimulation of osteonal remodeling by fatigue damage, *J. Biomechan.,* 15, 137, 1982.

70. Mashiba, T., et al., Suppressed bone turnover by bisphosphonates increases microdamage accumulation and reduces some biomechanical properties in dog rib, *J. Bone Miner. Res.*, 15, 613, 2000.

71. Matheson, G.O., et al., Stress fractures in athletes: a study of 320 cases, *Am. J. Sports Med.*, 15, 46, 1987.

72. Mellanotte, P.L. and Follis, R.H., Early effects of x-radiation on cartilage and bone, *Am. J. Pathol.*, 39, 1, 1961.

73. Meunier, P.J. and Vignot, E., Therapeutic strategy in Paget's disease of bone, *Bone*, 17, 489S, 1995.

74. Milgrom, C., et al., Multiple stress fractures: a longitudinal study of a soldier with 13 lesions, *Clin. Orthop.*, 192, 174, 1985.

75. Milgrom, C., et al., Stress fractures in military recruits: a prospective study showing an unusually high incidence, *J. Bone Jt. Surg.*, 67B, 732, 1985.

76. Mills, G.Q., Marymount, J.H., and Murphy, D.A., Bone scan utilization in the differential diagnosis of exercise-induced lower extremity pain, *Clin. Orthop.*, 149, 207, 1980.

77. Mori, S. and Burr, D.B., Increased intracortical remodeling following fatigue damage, *Bone*, 14, 103, 1993.

78. Morris, J.M. and Blickenstaff, L.D., *Fatigue Fractures,* Charles C. Thomas, Springfield, IL, 1967.

79. Noble, B.S., et al., Identification of apoptotic changes in osteocytes in normal and pathological human bone, *Bone*, 20, 273, 1997.

80. Nunamaker, D.M., Butterweck, D.M., and Provost, T.M., Fatigue fractures in thoroughbred racehorses: relationship with age, peak bone strain and training, *J. Orthop. Res.*, 8, 604, 1990.

81. Orava, S. and Hulkko, A., Stress fractures of the mid-tibial shaft, *Acta Orthop. Scand.*, 55, 35, 1984.

82. Otter, M.W., et al., Does bone perfusion/reperfusion initiate bone remodeling and the stress fracture syndrome, *Med. Hypotheses*, 53, 363, 1999.

83. Parfitt, A.M., Stereologic basis of bone histomorphometry: theory of quantitative microscopy and reconstruction of the third dimension, in *Bone Histomorphometry: Techniques and Interpretation*, Recker, R.R., Ed., CRC Press, Boca Raton, 1983.

84. Parfitt, A.M., A new model for the regulation of bone resorption with particular reference to the effect of bisphosphonates, *J. Bone Miner. Res.*, 11, 150, 1996.

85. Pattin, C.A., Caler, W.E., and Carter, D.R., Cyclical mechanical property degradation during fatigue loading of compact bone, *J. Biomechan.*, 29, 69, 1996.

86. Qiu S.J., Boyce, T.M., and Schaffler, M.B., Osteocyte loss and microdamage in aging human compact bone, *Trans. Orthop. Res. Soc.*, 22, 88, 1997.

87. Radin, E.L., et al., Response of joints to impact loading. 3. Relationship between trabecular microfractures and cartilage degeneration, *J. Biomechan.*, 6, 51, 1973.

88. Radin, E.L., et al., Effects of mechanical loading on the tissues of the rabbit knee, *J. Orthop. Res.*, 2, 221, 1984.

89. Reifsnider, K.L., Schultz, K., and Duke J.C., Long-term fatigue behavior of composite materials, in *Long Term Behavior of Composites,* ASTM STP, Philadelphia, 1983, 813, 136.

90. Rice, J.C., Cowin, S.C., and Bowman, J.A., On the dependence of the elasticity and strength of cancellous bone on apparent density, *J. Biomechan.*, 21, 155, 1988.

91. Roub, L.W., et al., Bone stress: a radionuclide imaging perspective, *Radiology*, 132, 431, 1979.

92. Rubin, C.T., Skeletal strain and the functional significance of bone architecture, *Calcif. Tissue Int.*, Suppl. 36; 11, 1984.

93. Rubin, C.T. and Lanyon, L.E., Limb mechanics as a function of speed and gait: a study of functional strains in the radius and tibia of horse and dog, *J. Exp. Biol.*, 101, 187, 1982.

94. Rubin, C.T., et al., The correlation of metabolic fatigue to changes in the skeleton's milieu, *13th Annu. Am. Soc. Biomech.*, 246, 1989.

95. Schaffler, M.B. and Burr, D.B., Stiffness of compact bone: effects of porosity and density, *J. Biomechan.*, 21, 13, 1988.

96. Schaffler, M.B., et al., Skeletal tissue responses to thermal injury: an experimental model, *Bone*, 9, 397, 1988.

97. Schaffler, M.B., Burr, D.B., and Radin, E.L., Mechanical and morphological effects of strain rate on fatigue in compact bone, *Bone*, 10, 207, 1989

98. Schaffler, M.B., Radin, E.L., and Burr, D.B., Long-term fatigue behavior of compact bone at low strain magnitude and rate, *Bone*, 11, 321, 1990

99. Schaffler, M., Examination of compact bone microdamage using back-scattered electron microscopy, *Bone*, 15, 483, 1994.

100. Schaffler, M.B., Boyce, T.M., and Fyhrie, D.P., Tissue and matrix failure modes in human compact bone during tensile fatigue, *Trans. Orthop. Res. Soc.*, 21, 57, 1996.

101. Schaffler, M.B., Choi, K., and Milgrom, C., Aging and microdamage accumulation in human compact bone, *Bone*, 17, 521, 1995.

102. Schaffler, M.B. and Boyd, R.D., Bone remodeling and microdamage accumulation in experimental stress fracture, *Trans. Orthop. Res. Soc.*, 22, 113, 1997.

103. Skerry, T.M., et al., Early strain related changes in enzyme activity in osteocytes following bone loading *in vivo*, *J. Bone Miner. Res.*, 4, 783, 1989.

104. Stover, S., Spontaneous fractures in equine long bone, First International Workshop on Overuse in the Equine and Human Athletes, Tufts University, 1996.

105. Sullivan, D., et al., Stress fractures in 51 runners, *Clin. Orthop.*, 187, 188, 1984.

106. Tomkinson, A., et al., The role of estrogen in the control of rat osteocyte apoptosis, *J. Bone Miner. Res.*, 13, 1243, 1998.

107. Tschantz, P. and Rutishauser, E., La surcharge mechanique de l'os vivant, *Ann. Anat. Pathol.*, 12, 223, 1967.

108. Verborgt, O., Gibson, G.J., and Schaffler, M.B., Loss of osteocyte integrity in association with microdamage and bone remodeling after fatigue *in vivo*, *J. Bone Miner. Res.*, 15, 60, 2000.

109. Wang, D.C., Kottamasu, S.R., and Karvelis, K., Scintigraphy in metabolic bone disease, in *Primer on Metabolic Bone Disease and Disorders of Mineral Metabolism,* Fauvas, M.J., Ed., American Society of Bone and Mineral Research, Kelseyville, CA, 1990.

110. Weibel, E.R., *Stereological Methods,* Academic Press, New York, 1980.

111. Weinreb, M., et al., Histomorphometrical analysis of the effects of the bisphosphonate alendronate on bone loss caused by experimental periodontitis in monkeys, *J. Periodontal Res.,* 29, 35, 1994.

112. Wyllie, A.H., Cell death: the significance of apoptosis. *Int. Rev. Cytol.,* 68, 251, 1980.

113. Zioupos, P. and Currey, J.D., The extent of microcracking and the morphology of microcracks in damaged bone, *J. Mater. Sci.,* 29, 978, 1994.

114. Zwas, S.T., et al., Early diagnosis of stress fractures in soldiers by ^{99m}Tc-MDP bone scan: evaluation of efficiency and scintigraphic patterns of appearance and resolution, in *Fifth Congress of Nuclear Medicine in Israel,* 4, Czerniak, P. and Noam, N., Eds., Ramat Aviv: Baruk Institute for Radioclinical Research and Publication Sale Division, Tel Aviv University, 1980, 52.

115. Zwas, S.T., Elkanovitch, R., and Frank, G., Interpretation and classification of bone scintigraphic findings in stress fracture, *J. Nucl. Med.,* 28, 452, 1987.

Figure 4 C r o s s - s e c t i o n a l photomicrograph of stress fracture (H&E stained, ×15.6). New woven bone was formed on the periosteal envelope, and cortical bone was highly porous with a number of cutting cones. No inflammatory changes such as infiltration of neutrophils were observed.

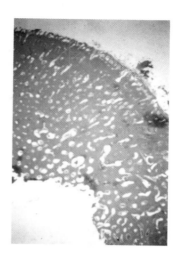

Figure 5-a, b, c
Photomicrographs of microdamage in the bulk stained sections (x62.5).

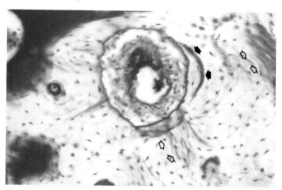

a) Debonding microdamage on the cement line (black arrow), and diffuse microdamage in interstitial bone (white arrow) are associated with resorption cavity.

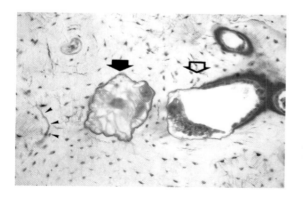

b) An osteon in active resorption phase (black arrow) and another osteon showing both resorption and formation (white arrow) in association with a linear microcrack (black triangle).

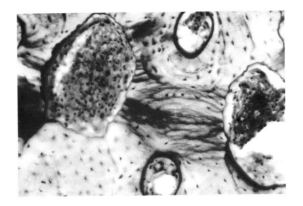

c) Diffuse microdamage (white arrow) lies between two active osteons with both resorption and formation. Note both resorption cavities spread into the direction of the microdamage.

CHAPTER 14

Figure 5 Contour plot of compressive (left) and Tresca (shear, right) stresses on the anterior aspect of the rabbit tibia. The scale is given in Mpa. "X" denotes lateral. High stress concentrations are located on the anterior and anterolateral aspect of the distal tibia, coincident with the region where rabbits present with stress fractures.

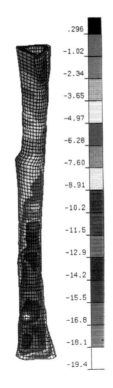

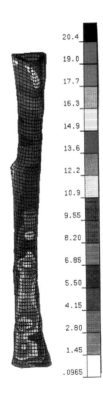

CHAPTER 12

The Role of Bone Remodeling in Preventing or Promoting Stress Fractures

R. Bruce Martin

CONTENTS

Introduction 184
Theory 185
    Mathematical Model 168
    Model Results 192
        Equilibrium State 192
        Responses to Additional Loading 192
        Adding a Periosteal Response 195
        Discontinued Loading 197
Discussion 198
    Remodeling and Homeostatic Damage Control 198
    Failure of Homeostatic Damage Control 199
Summary 200
References 200

GLOSSARY OF MATHEMATICAL NOTATION

Symbol	Definition
F	force, N
A_C	cortical area, mm^2
σ	stress, Pascals, or N/mm^2
E	elastic modulus, Pascals, or N/mm^2

Symbol	Definition
ε	strain, or strain range, $\mu\varepsilon$ (microstrain, 10^{-6} m/m)
q	exponent on strain range, dimensionless
R_L	loading rate, load cycles/day
k_D	damage formation rate coefficient, day cycle^{-1} mm^{-1} $\mu\varepsilon^{-q}$
D	microdamage, crack length/unit section area, mm^{-1}
$\dot{D}_F$	damage formation rate, mm^{-1} day^{-1}
R_C	osteon or resorption cavity radius, mm
A_O	osteon or resorption cavity area, mm^2
A_S	section area, mm^2
ΔD	damage expected to be removed by a BMU, mm^{-1}
Δt	time interval, days
ΔD_T	damage removed in a time interval Δt, mm^{-1}
f_a	remodeling activation frequency, BMUs mm^{-2} day
$\dot{D}_R$	damage removal rate, mm^{-1} day^{-1}
D_E	equilibrium damage, mm^{-1}
D_0	equilibrium value of damage
f_{amax}, f_{amin}	maximum and minimum activation frequency values, respectively, BMUs mm^{-2} day^{-1}
k_R	coefficient for f_a versus D dose-response curve, mm^2 day BMU^{-1}
N_R, N_I, N_F	numbers of resorbing, reversing, and refilling BMUs per mm^2 of section, respectively
T_R, T_I, T_F	resorbing, reversing, and refilling periods, respectively, days
Q_C, Q_B	mean rates of resorption and formation in individual BMUs, respectively, mm^2 day^{-1}
P	porosity, dimensionless area or volume fraction

INTRODUCTION

Other chapters of this book have covered in detail the elements of mechanical loading and biological responses that are thought to contribute to stress fractures. The mechanical elements include application of repetitive loading over periods of days, weeks, or months; mode of loading; magnitude and number of cycles per day of this loading; type and magnitude of strains the loading produces in the bone; and resulting fatigue damage to bone tissue. The biological elements include muscle fatigue, hypothesized to increase bone strain and strain rate through diminished shock absorption, and bone responses engendered by strain or damage, including modeling of periosteal or endosteal surfaces and intracortical remodeling of the bone material.

Several studies have suggested that the occurrence of stress fractures cannot be entirely explained on the basis of fatigue failure (i.e., mechanical elements). One of the most significant of these studies was the experiment of Schaffler and co-workers,[1] which showed that human bone specimens loaded at physiologic strain rates to physiologic strain levels consistently sustain tens of millions of cycles without fracturing and without substantial loss of stiffness. Assuming that a cycle of loading is equivalent to a stride covering 1.5 meters, 10 million cycles corresponds to 1500 kilometers of running or walking. This is 4 to 5 times greater than the 320 kilometers that military recruits who experience stress fractures are estimated to run and walk during 12 weeks of basic training.[2] Furthermore, most stress fractures occur well before the end of basic training, and only a minority of recruits experience such fractures. Thus, the mechanical test data do not support fatigue failure as the sole cause of stress fractures. Also, there are inadequate explanations for why such failures happen to some individuals and not to others under similar loading conditions.

The observed and surmised biological responses to fatigue damage have also been described in other chapters. These include two principal responses: increased internal remodeling and the production of woven bone on adjacent periosteal surfaces. These are noninvasively observed with bone scans and plane film radiographs, respectively, and have occasionally been directly observed in histologic sections. The purpose of this chapter is to present a theory to explain the occurrence of stress fractures under loading conditions that would not produce fatigue failure in an *ex vivo* laboratory experiment. It may also explain why such fractures are so difficult to predict, given similar loading conditions.

THEORY

The theory begins with the long held premise that bone remodeling serves to remove fatigue damage from bone. This idea, perhaps first suggested by Frost,[3-5] has become a basic tenet of orthopedic science. The hypothesis has been strengthened by abundant circumstantial evidence that fatigue microdamage serves as a stimulus that, within a few days, activates a remodeling basic multicellular unit (BMU) in spatial proximity to the damage.[6-9] The details of the biological pathway for this response are not fully elucidated,[10] but there is little doubt that a feedback mechanism exists for activating BMU-based remodeling in close proximity to fatigue damage. This hypothesis is consistent with several clinical and experimental observations of abundant remodeling and associated porosity (remodeling space) in the vicinity of stress fractures, including those in Chapter 10 and References 6 and 11–14.

The theory described here predicts that while remodeling normally removes fatigue damage approximately as fast as it occurs, excessive rates of fatigue damage formation can overload this homeostatic system and cause it to become unstable. The mechanism for this instability derives from the fact that resorption precedes formation in the remodeling process, so that increased remodeling is always associated with increased porosity. This "remodeling space" reduces the bone's elastic modulus, which in turn increases strain. This in turn increases the rate of damage formation, and creates a positive feedback loop that exacerbates rather than controls the amount of damage. Thus, there are two feedback loops relating damage and remodeling rate, a "good loop" that leads to *reduced* damage, remodeling, and porosity, and a "bad loop" that *increases* them. The question is, which of these loops prevails when the system is challenged by increased loading? In this chapter, a mathematical model is used to analyze this problem. The purpose of this model is not to predict the outcome of any specific case, but to explore the behavior of the system. Specifically, the model will be used to examine the hypotheses that (1) remodeling can homeostatically control fatigue damage under varying loading conditions, and (2) remodeling space contributes to stress fractures through the "bad loop" of the block diagram.

Mathematical Model

The model described here is similar to that of Martin[15] and incorporates concepts developed in Martin et al.[16] Formulation of the model begins at the top of the block diagram in Figure 1. The model is intended to provide a credible demonstration of the system's general behavior without going into unnecessary detail. Therefore, for the sake of simplicity, we assume a cylindrical cortex of cross-sectional area A_C

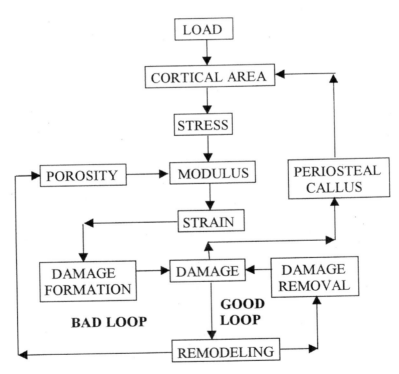

Figure 1 A block diagram organizing the mechanical and biological factors of interest in stress fractures. In the case of a bone diaphysis loaded in compression, the load acts through the cortical area to produce stress, which in turn produces bone strain in inverse proportion to the elastic modulus. High strains cause damage formation, and damage activates remodeling, which removes damage. Remodeling also increases bone porosity, which diminishes the modulus and increases strain and damage formation. Thus, remodeling has "good" and "bad" feedback loops. The effects of the bad loop can be alleviated if damage also activates the production of a periosteal callus, which increases cortical area and reduces stress and strain.

bearing an axial compressive load that cycles between zero and some peak value F. The exact temporal waveform of this force is assumed to be unimportant. The stress throughout the bone is assumed to be homogeneous with a waveform similar to the load and a peak value equal to:

$$\sigma = F/A_C \tag{1}$$

The bone is assumed to have a linear stress-strain relationship, so the strain range, ε, is likewise homogeneous and time-varying with a peak value:

$$\varepsilon = \sigma/E \tag{2}$$

where E is the elastic modulus. (E will be related to porosity below.)

Pattin et al.[17] and others have found that the fatigue life of bone is inversely related to the strain range raised to a power. It is reasonable to assume that the damage formation rate, $\dot{D}_F$, is similarly proportional to the strain range raised to a power. If the damage formation rate is also linearly proportional to the loading rate, R_L (i.e., the number of applied load cycles/day), we have:

$$\dot{D}_F = k_D \, R_L \, \varepsilon^q \tag{3}$$

where k_D is a damage formation coefficient. This equation could represent the production of damage from one particular kind of strain-producing activity — walking, for example. Other kinds of activity could involve different values of R_L and ε. If we assume that the damage produced by each of a variety of different activities can be summed, and identify these activities by the subscript $_i$, we have:

$$\dot{D}_F = \sum k_D \, R_{Li} \, \varepsilon_i^q \tag{4}$$

where the summation is over i = 1, 2, 3, etc. In this demonstration of the model, we will simplify matters by assuming there are only two activities: sedentary and an optional exercise regimen.

We now address the question of the rate at which remodeling can be expected to remove fatigue damage from bone. We initially assume that both damage and BMU activation are randomly distributed within the bone volume. It is easier to formulate this problem in the context of a two-dimensional histologic cross-section than volumetrically, and this can be done because stereology shows that representative area and volume fractions are equivalent.

Let a representative section from the volume contain total area A_S. Suppose the section also contains D damage per mm², as shown in Figure 2. Damage could be defined in various ways, such as total crack length per unit section area or the area of diffuse damage per unit section area. Because all forms of fatigue damage would be removed when a moiety of bone is resorbed by remodeling, the definition of damage is not important at this stage. If a single new BMU enters this section at a

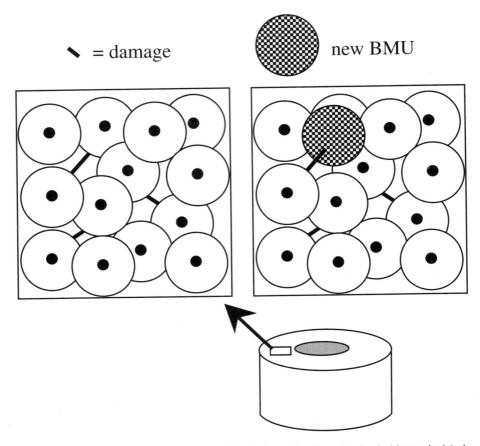

Figure 2 At upper left is a representative histologic section from the loaded bone depicted below. This section contains osteonal bone and damage in the form of three microcracks. Damage could be defined as D = total microcrack length per unit cross-sectional area. Assume that a new BMU arrives at this section, opening a resorption cavity at a random location, as shown at upper right. The expected amount of damage, ΔD, "overlapped" or actually obliterated by this new BMU, is proportional to D and the area of the resorption cavity.

random location, excavating a resorption cavity of radius R_C and area $A_O = \pi R_C^2$, how much of D can this BMU be expected to remove? If the damage is randomly distributed throughout the specimen, the fraction of the damage removed (ΔD/D) is expected to equal the fraction of the area removed (A_O/A_S). Therefore,

$$\Delta D = D\, A_O/A_S \tag{5}$$

Now suppose that as time goes by more BMUs pass through the section. If the BMU activation frequency is f_a BMUs/mm^2/day, then over a time increment Δt, the number of BMUs added is $f_a A_S \Delta t$ and the amount of bone (temporarily) removed from the section is $f_a A_S A_O \Delta t$. The total damage removed is:

$$\Delta D_T = D\, f_a\, A_S\, A_O\, \Delta t / A_S = D\, f_a\, A_O\, \Delta t \tag{6}$$

In the limit as $\Delta t \to 0$, the rate of damage removal is:

$$\dot{D}_R = D\, f_a\, A_O \tag{7}$$

The work of Burr and co-workers[7,8,18] provides evidence that the origination of new BMUs is not spatially random, but tends to occur in the vicinity of damage. It is also possible that BMUs "steer" toward damage as they tunnel through the bone far from their site of origin, but there is no evidence for this. In any event, the location of BMUs in a section seems not to be random with respect to the locations of damage, but preferentially aimed at damage. We may account for this in Equation 8 by adding a "remodeling specificity factor," F_S:

$$\dot{D}_R = D\, f_a\, A_O\, F_S \tag{8}$$

with $F_S > 1$ when "aiming" occurs.

If the damage removal rate equals the damage formation rate, the system is in equilibrium; in this state the equilibrium damage (i.e., damage waiting to be removed) is found by equating Equations 3 and 8 and solving for D. The result is:

$$D_E = k_D\, R_L\, \varepsilon^q / f_a\, A_O\, F_S \tag{9}$$

When the system is not in equilibrium, the daily change in damage may be calculated from the difference between $\dot{D}_F$ and $\dot{D}_R$. Thus, if $\Delta t = 1$ day,

$$D_{TODAY} = D_{YESTERDAY} + \left[\dot{D}_F - \dot{D}_R \right] \Delta t \tag{10}$$

We now need a "dose-response" relationship between damage, D, and remodeling activation frequency, f_a. Here the definition of damage presumably is important, but no explicit data are available for the numerical relationship between f_a and any form of damage. Therefore, a reasonable approach is to assume a sigmoidal function relating the range of possible activation frequency values to a range of damage values. Such a function is shown in Figure 3, and can be represented by the equation:

$$f_a = \frac{f_{amax} f_{amin}}{f_{amin} + \left(f_{amax} - f_{amin} \right) \exp\left[-k_R\, f_{amax}\, (D - D_0)/D_0 \right]} \tag{11}$$

Here, k_R is a coefficient that governs the slope of the curve, f_{amax} and f_{amin} are the maximum and minimum values of f_a, and D_0 is the value of damage at which $f_a = f_{amin}$. It was assumed that the sedentary loading condition is associated with the left end of the curve, so that $f = f_{amin}$ and $D = D_0$ in the sedentary state. (It is assumed

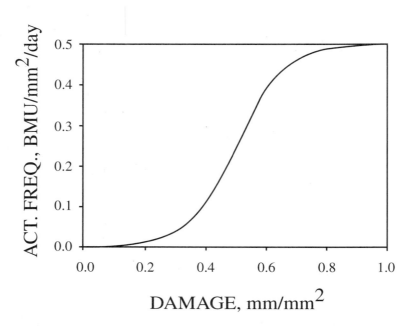

Figure 3 Assumed sigmoidal dose-response relationship between activation frequency (ACT. FREQ.) and fatigue damage (DAMAGE).

that remodeling is activated by other factors as well, but these components of activation are assumed to be constant at a low basal level f_{amin} in this model.)

The following f_a and damage data and their original sources may be found in Tables 3.1, 3.6, and 5.20 in Reference 16. f_{amin} and f_{amax} were chosen with reference to experimental measurements of cortical bone remodeling at relatively slow and rapid rates. For cortical bone in ribs, mean values of f_a range from 0.003 to 0.05 BMU/mm²/day in humans, depending on age. However, ribs remodel at a higher rate than limb long bones. Based on the rate of osteon accumulation with age in human femurs and tibias, f_{amin} was taken to be 0.001 BMU/mm²/day. The upper limit of activation frequency was based on data for young rhesus monkeys (0.076 ± 0.04 BMU/mm²/day). Assuming that activation could exceed this by several fold in a stress fracture, $f_{amax} = 0.5$ BMU/mm²/day was used.

The limits of the damage axis in Figure 3 were set using the microcrack density data of Schaffler et al.[19] for human femoral cortical bone. Averaging together the male and female mean crack density at age 20 years predicted by Schaffler's age regression equations yields 0.065 microcracks/mm². Multiplying by an assumed mean crack length of 0.088 mm,[18] crack density was converted to 0.0057 mm/mm², which was rounded to define $D_0 = 0.006$ mm/mm². The highest femoral crack densities approached 6 mm⁻², or $D = 6 \times 0.088 = 0.53$ mm/mm². It was assumed that this value would be well below that associated with f_{amax}, so k_R was chosen to make f_a reach its maximum value when $D = 1.0$ mm/mm². While the numerical values used to construct this dose–response curve are somewhat arbitrary, the exact shape of the curve and the specific values on the axes are not critical to the general behavior of the model.

Active BMUs can be divided into three populations: resorbing, intermediate (resorption concluded but formation not yet initiated), and refilling. The number of BMUs/mm^2 in these three populations can be designated N_R, N_I, and N_F, respectively. These populations depend on the time required for each remodeling phase to occur. Let T_R, T_I, and T_F represent these periods. By keeping track of the f_a history, the current values of N_R, N_I, and N_F can be calculated each day. Because resorption occurs first, all the resorbing BMUs were initiated (born) during the last T_R days, and N_R may be found by integrating the activation frequency over this period:

$$N_R = \int_{-T_R}^{0} f_a \, dt \tag{12}$$

The intermediate BMUs were born during the period between T_R and $(T_R + T_I)$ days ago, so:

$$N_1 = \int_{-(T_R+T_1)}^{-T_R} f_a \, dt \tag{13}$$

The refilling BMUs were born between $(T_R + T_I)$ and $(T_R + T_I + T_F)$ days ago, so:

$$N_F = \int_{-(T_R+T_I+T_F)}^{-(T_R+T_I)} f_a \, dt \tag{14}$$

Changes in bone porosity due to remodeling are calculated as follows. During the resorption phase, each BMU removes πR_C^2 mm^2 of bone from the cross-section in T_R days. The mean rate of bone resorption at the BMU level is then:

$$Q_C = \pi R_C^2 / T_R \tag{15}$$

Each refilling BMU adds $\pi (R_C^2 - R_H^2)$ mm^2 of bone in T_F days, R_H being the completed Haversian canal radius. Thus, the mean rate of bone formation at the BMU level is:

$$Q_B = \pi \left(R_C^2 - R_H^2 \right) / T_F \tag{16}$$

The daily change in porosity can then be found from the relationship:

$$P_{TODAY} = P_{YESTERDAY} + \left(N_R Q_R - N_F Q_F \right) \Delta t \tag{17}$$

where $\Delta t = 1$ day. The elastic modulus of the bone, in GPa, is assumed to vary with porosity as

$$E = 20.0 \, (1 - P)^3 \qquad\qquad (18)$$

a modification of other empirical E–P relationships.[20] This sequence of computations can be repeated using a computer program or spread sheet to track the response of the system to changes occurring over many days.

Model Results

Equilibrium State

Suppose the model represents a diaphyseal segment having a cross-sectional area of 500 mm² that is loaded 2000 cycles/day (cpd) by a force cycling between 0 and 2614 N. This load produces a peak stress of 5.23 MPa, and if the initial porosity (due to Haversian canals and active BMUs) is 0.0448, then the elastic modulus is 17.4 GPa and the strain range is 300 microstrain ($\mu\varepsilon$). Using the parameters shown in Table 1, the system will remain in equilibrium under this loading regimen, with damage formation and removal rates equal, if the activation frequency is f_{amin} = 0.001 BMU/mm²/day. The equilibrium damage is D_0 = 0.006 mm⁻². This is considered to be the model's "sedentary" state.

Responses to Additional Loading

Now consider the behavior of this model when additional loading is imposed. Suppose the above equilibrium state represents a sedentary young person, and we are interested in the effects of suddenly adding a new exercise regimen to the person's normal activities. This regimen could represent (in a greatly simplified way) athletic or military training. To simulate this, *in addition to* the sedentary 300 $\mu\varepsilon$, 2000 cpd loading (i = 1 in Equation 4), the bone model is loaded so as to cycle between 0 and 2000 $\mu\varepsilon$ for 1000 cpd (i = 2 in Equation 4). In both cases, the magnitude of the applied

Table 1   Values Assigned to Model Parameters

Variable	Value	Units
R_H	20	μm
R_C	95	μm
T_R	23	days
T_I	3	days
T_F	62	days
F_S	5	dimensionless
q	4	dimensionless
k_D	52505	mm/mm²
f_{amax}	0.5	BMU/mm²/yr
f_{amin}	0.001	BMU/mm²/yr
k_R	0.151	mm² day/BMU
k_P	10	μm/day/mm/mm²
D_C	0.001	mm/mm²
$k_P{}^*$	2.0	μm/day/mm/mm²
$D_C{}^*$	0.057	mm/mm²

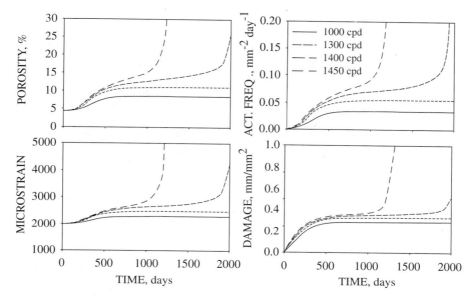

Figure 4 Changes in damage, activation frequency, porosity, and strain are plotted for the responses of the initial model (no periosteal response) to an exercise regimen that initially produces 2000 µε. The solid line refers to an additional 1000 cpd of this exercise regimen superimposed on the usual baseline daily activity. Dashed lines show the effects of 1300, 1400, and 1450 cpd, respectively, of this additional activity. In this and subsequent plots, the strain graph shows the strain produced by the exercise load.

load remains constant and the reference strain is that *initially* produced by the load. As the bone responds to the loading, strain may change. It is assumed that each of these two activities adds damage independently, the damage is homogeneous, and the daily remodeling response in the bone depends on the current total damage.

The lowest curve in each of the graphs in Figure 4 shows the effect of this additional loading. Damage, activation frequency, porosity, and strain all increase over a period of about two years, then plateau at new equilibrium values. The figure also shows the responses when the number of cycles of 2000 µε loading is increased to 1300 cpd: the increases in each variable are greater, but a new equilibrium state is still reached. However, when 1400 cpd of 2000 µε loading are applied, the model's variables start to plateau, but then begin to increase again after about four years, and these increases accelerate over time. At 1450 cpd this phenomenon occurs more quickly. This response may be thought of as a stress fracture because damage and strain values rapidly become very large. Consequently, this behavior will be called "fracture" in the context of this model.

To give a more graphic appreciation of the porosity changes in the bone, Figure 5 simulates the appearance of the active BMUs in histologic sections after 500 days of remodeling for the 1000 and 1450 cpd exercise regimens. These active BMUs contain the remodeling space that increases strain. Note that the 1450 cpd illustration shows porosity very early in the stress fracture response.

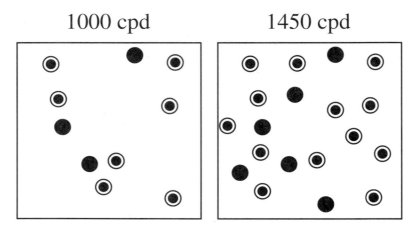

Figure 5 Schematic illustrations of the numbers of active BMUs in a 4 mm² region of the model after 500 days of remodeling with an exercise regimen initially producing 2000 με. The daily number of cycles is shown above each illustration. Resorption cavities are the larger black rings; refilling BMUs are the rings with black centers. For simplicity, all the BMUs are shown as the same size, and completed Haversian canals are not shown. The model only tracks numbers of active BMUs; their positions in these figures were arbitrarily chosen.

Figure 4 suggests that the four variables grow without limit in a fracture response, but this is not the case if there is an upper limit to f_a, as in Figure 3. Figure 6 shows, with expanded scales, the results for 1450 cpd of 2000 με loading. In the model each variable plateaus when f_a reaches its upper limit. However, at more than 43,000 με the maximum strain substantially exceeds cortical bone's failure strain, implying failure before the plateau is reached. This further supports the interpretation that this response is tantamount to stress fracture of the model. When f_{amax} is reduced to 0.1 BMU/mm²/day, remodeling space is limited to the point that fracture of the model does not occur. Thus, the fracture phenomenon depends critically on the upper limit of f_a, because this governs the magnitude of the "bad loop" effect (Figure 1). (Of course, other variables, such as osteonal diameter, affect this criticality, too.) These results suggest that a drug that inhibits remodeling could lower f_{amax} and prevent stress fracture, but the bone would then be liable to "fatigue failure" as damage accumulated.

These results show that this model system is able to adjust to significantly increased loading (e.g., 1300 cpd at 2000 με) by increasing the rate of remodeling so that the damage removal rate increases to match the damage formation rate. Two aspects of this response are of particular interest. First, the time to reach a new equilibrium is several times greater than the remodeling period (sigma) as it is observed in histologic sections. That is, the remodeling period for the model is 88 days, but the time required for equilibrium to be reached is about 2 years. It takes several remodeling cycles for the four interrelated variables shown in Figure 4 to reach a common equilibrium state. The second interesting thing about the response is that its capacity to deal with increased loading is limited. That is, exercise initially resulting in a high but physiologic strain of 2000 με produced model fracture at

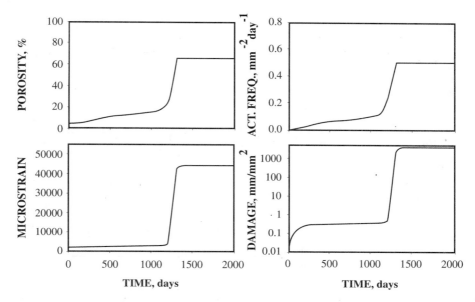

Figure 6   Similar to Figure 4 but with expanded ordinate scales to show how the upper limit of f_a limits the other variables in the 2000 με, 1450 cpd overload case. However, strain values reach failure magnitudes before f_a reaches its upper limit. Note the logrithmic damage scale; one would also expect failure long before the upper damage values shown here were reached.

1450 cpd; if the exercise were running, this would be less than 2 miles/day for a large mammal. Thus, strains that are physiologic in animals lead to fracture in the model after relatively modest numbers of cycles. However, the model described so far omits an essential element of the stress fracture response: the production of a periosteal callus. Adding this component to the model substantially improves its ability to cope with additional loading.

Adding a Periosteal Response

To facilitate the addition of a periosteal response to the model, assume that the endosteal diameter of the diaphysis is half the periosteal diameter; consequently, for a 500 mm² cortex, the endosteal radius is 7.28 mm and the periosteal radius is 14.56 mm. Next, assume periosteal modeling in the formation mode is provoked by fatigue damage, and that the apposition rate (in μm/day) is linearly proportional to the amount by which damage exceeds a critical level, D_C. Thus,

$$M_P = k_P \left(D - D_C \right) \tag{19}$$

where k_P is a coefficient and $M_P = 0$ when $D \le D_C$. The apposition rate is not allowed to exceed 30 μm/day, assumed to be the maximum rate at which woven bone can be formed, based on periosteal data for rats.[21] Also, elastic modulus differences

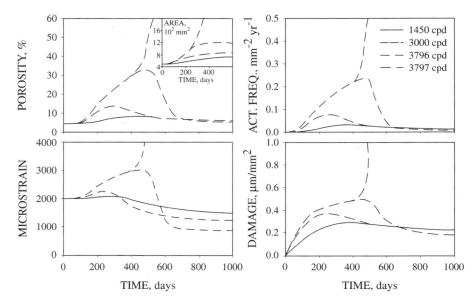

Figure 7   Changes in damage, activation frequency, porosity, and strain are plotted for the model with a periosteal callus response simulated. The exercise regimen again initially produced 2000 µε, with the daily number of cycles as shown. Up to 3796 cpd, the porosity, activation frequency, and damage responses are all characterized by an initial increase, followed by a decline as the periosteal new bone increases cortical area (inset). Then, at 3797 cpd, each of these variables fails to decline, and instead rapidly increases as the model fractures. The strain plots start at the imposed 2000 µε and diminish as cortical area increases and bone stress is reduced. However, at fracture, strain rapidly increases to values above bone's yield strain.

between woven and lamellar bone are ignored for simplicity's sake. As damage increases in the model, periosteal modeling will accompany increased internal remodeling.

When the exercise regimen that produced fracture in the previous model (2000 µε, 1450 cpd) is applied to the revised model (with $k_P = 0.05$ µm/day/mm/mm^2 and $D_C = 0.2$ mm/mm^2), it behaves as indicated by the solid curves in Figure 7. Periosteal new bone increases the cortical area (inset) by 42% over 33 months, compensating for increased remodeling space, and fracture does not occur. Furthermore, the loading that initially produced 2000 µε produces less than 1500 µε in the enlarged cortex.

As the daily number of cycles is further increased to 3000 and 3796 cpd, the remodeling responses increase, but within a year damage, activation frequency, porosity, and strain have all peaked and are declining. However, at 3796 cpd the model has reached a critical point. When one more cycle per day is added, the model fractures. Activation frequency increases to its limit, and the resulting porosity rapidly elevates peak strain above 16,000 µε, which is greater than cortical bone's compressive yield strain (about 10,000 µε for human and cow bone).[22] At this strain, catastrophic fracture would presumably occur in a few cycles.

The critical nature of the model's "fracture" or failure behavior when the periosteal response is present is striking; one additional cycle per day spells the difference between recovery and failure. This suggests that small individual differences could govern the occurrence of stress fractures. For example, in the context of military training, slight differences in a recruit's activities, or in the recruit's bone biology or initial bone structure, could determine whether or not a stress fracture occurs. The model's failure is similar to the bucking of a column in that the transition is sudden and unpredictable by direct observation: as the loading is gradually increased, there is no indication that failure is going to occur. This criticality could help explain the apparently capricious nature of stress fractures.

Discontinued Loading

While the model's variables do not reveal signs of failure beforehand, real bones are often painful when a stress fracture is imminent. Clearly, a more realistic scenario than unabated loading is one in which pain causes the exercise regimen to be stopped before a stress fracture occurs, or after a partial fracture. To simulate this, a 2500 µε, 4000 cpd exercise regimen that would have fractured the model in less than 4 months was applied for only 50 days. As shown by the solid curves in Figure 8, the model

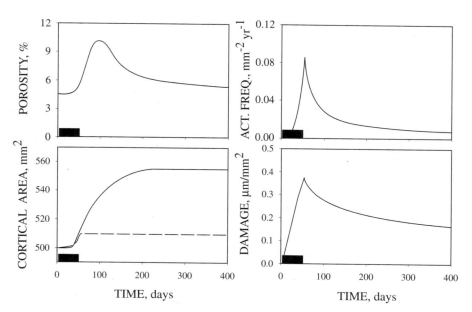

Figure 8 Plot of results for a stress fracture simulation in which a 500 cpd exercise regimen initially producing 2500 µε, is stopped after 50 days, as indicated by the black bars. Note that the strain plot is replaced by one for cortical area. The solid curves show responses when periosteal response is proportional to all damage existing in the bone. Dashed curves show results for the revised model in which the periosteal apposition rate is proportional to only the damage created during the past week. In this case fracture is prevented without adding as much cortical area to the bone. (Except for the area plot, dashed curves underlie solid curves.)

begins to recover as soon as the exercise regimen stops, but the return to normal takes several months. Note also that the periosteal response has continued to add bone long after the exercise loading was stopped. This is because the periosteal apposition rate was assumed to depend on the accumulated damage in the bone, and considerable time is required to bring that below D_C, the critical level at which periosteal apposition was assumed to occur.

An alternative system would have the periosteal response depend only on the most recently occurring damage, that is, if Equation 19 is changed to:

$$M_P = k_P* \left(D* - D_C*\right) \tag{20}$$

where the * notation refers to damage that has occurred within a specified time. If this period is the last 7 days, and the values $k_P* = 2.0$ μm/day/mm/mm^2 and $D_C* = 0.057$ mm/mm^{-2} are used, the model's response to an exercise regimen that does not stop is similar to that previously shown. However, when the 2500 με, 4000 cpd exercise regimen is applied for 50 days and stopped, the cortical area stops increasing within a few weeks, and the model recovers without adding unnecessary bone mass (dashed curve, Figure 8).

DISCUSSION

Prior to drawing conclusions from this model, it is important to review its purpose and limitations. At this point, the model is not intended to be predictive; instead, it is a tool for testing hypotheses about stress fracture etiology and visualizing the implications of various assumptions. It is one thing to discuss a multifaceted concept such as the role that remodeling space plays in stress fracture etiology; it is quite another to quantitatively show that it is plausible, and discern its secondary and tertiary ramifications. That is the present function of this model. Ultimately, when the missing dose-response data and other shortcomings are resolved, the model may become predictive, but in the meanwhile it serves to demonstrate several important phenomena and raise some important questions.

Remodeling and Homeostatic Damage Control

First, the model supports the hypothesis that remodeling can control fatigue damage by removing it in a homeostatic manner. While data on the specific relationships between damage and BMU activation are lacking, the model shows that, given histomorphometrically measured BMU characteristics, reasonable increases in activation frequency could accommodate significant increases in damage formation rates. However, the model also indicates that the time required for such accommodation may be longer than has been imagined. Investigators usually assert that the time required for bone remodeling to reach a new equilibrium following a disturbance is on the order of one remodeling period, as observed in a histologic section; i.e., about three months. The model predicts that when mechanical and biological processes interact, the time required for all the interacting variables to equilibrate is much longer than the remodeling period itself.

It is interesting to compare the model's responses with data from an experiment by Burr and co-workers.[23] In dogs, an exercise regimen (running 45 minutes/day, 5 days/week for 1 year) superimposed on normal ("sedentary") kennel activities significantly increased BMU activation by 272% in the diaphysis of the humerus. If the dogs ran at 2 hz, the average loading rate would have been 3857 cpd. When an exercise regimen defined by 3857 cpd at 1100 $\mu\varepsilon$ was applied to the present model, activation frequency increased 262% after 1 year. The model also tracks the time course of changes in damage, porosity, strain, the numbers of BMUs in each remodeling phase, the numbers of single and double-labeled BMUs, and periosteal apposition rate. Fitting the model to the results of a similar but more elaborate experiment in which these variables were measured at several time points could go a long way toward producing a model with predictive capability.

Failure of Homeostatic Damage Control

The model also illustrates how the capacity of remodeling to control fatigue damage must be limited by the effects of remodeling space. Certainly, many of the model's parameters need to be more precisely determined, and the model needs to be experimentally verified. However, the basic phenomenon of ever-increasing porosity and damage, rather than attainment of equilibrium, when loading reaches a critical level is not a fluke associated with certain parameter choices. As long as loading produces damage, damage activates sufficient remodeling, and observed BMU geometry and remodeling periods are approximated, the model will behave in this way when the loading is sufficiently increased, either in terms of strain magnitude or load cycles per day.

It is probably not feasible to produce this effect experimentally by exercising an experimental animal, but an experimental model which seems capable of doing so is described by Rubin and co-workers.[24] Using the isolated turkey ulna model, they applied 30,000 cpd at 2000 to 3000 $\mu\varepsilon$ for up to 54 days. They observed both numerous large intracortical resorption spaces and periosteal woven bone formation. They did not stain and examine their specimens for microcracks, and did not attribute the increase in remodeling activity to microdamage. However, they concluded that their specimens looked like bones experiencing stress fracture, and stated that weakening of the bone was caused by the remodeling porosity rather than fatigue damage. However, their observations are also consistent with the present model. If damage was present and responsible for the increased remodeling, the isolated avian ulna might be used to obtain data on the mathematical model's parameters in the range of actual stress fractures by sampling the bone at various times and assessing microdamage as well as activation frequency, porosity, elastic modulus, and the periosteal response.

The model suggests that the periosteal response would be more efficient if it were based on recent rather than total accumulated damage. The isolated avian ulna could also be used to test this hypothesis, as well as the equivalent hypothesis with respect to internal remodeling activation. It is conceivable that the periosteal modeling and internal remodeling responses are different in this respect. In adults, periosteal modeling responses are usually acute and associated with trauma, while remodeling is ongoing and activated by a variety of stimuli. The periosteum contains different cells and a different environment than the Haversian canals where remodeling is activated. Experimental data are required to clarify these issues.

SUMMARY

This chapter has argued that bone remodeling plays an essential role in both preventing and promoting stress fractures. Remodeling normally prevents fatigue fracture but can promote stress fracture. That is, remodeling removes fatigue damage in a homeostatic way, and this normally prevents fatigue failure during an individual's lifetime. However, there are limits to the rate at which this damage removal process can be effective because of the remodeling space. The theory views the periosteal expansion of the cortex as an essential adjunct to remodeling in that it counteracts increased remodeling space so that greater loading challenges can be surmounted. However, when loading and damage formation reach a critical point and failure occurs, it can be attributed as much to the increased bone porosity as to fatigue damage. That is the sense in which remodeling promotes stress fracture.

REFERENCES

1. Schaffler, M. B., Radin, E. L., and Burr, D. B., Long-term fatigue behavior of compact bone at low strain magnitude and rate, *Bone*, 11, 321, 1990.
2. Jones, B. H., Harris, J. M., Vinh, T. N., and Rubin, C., Exercise-induced stress fractures and stress reactions in bone: epidemiology, etiology, and classification, *Exerc. Sport Sci. Rev.*, 17, 379, 1989.
3. Frost, H. M., Presence of microscopic cracks *in vivo* in bone, *Henry Ford Hosp. Med. Bull.*, 8, 25, 1960.
4. Frost, H. M., *Bone Remodeling and Its Relationship to Metabolic Bone Diseases*, Charles C. Thomas, Springfield, IL, 1973.
5. Frost, H. M., Mechanical microdamage, bone remodeling, and osteoporosis: a review, in *Osteoporosis*, DeLuca, H. F., Frost, H. M., Jee, W.S.S., and Johnston, C. C., Eds., University Park Press, Baltimore, 1980.
6. Rahn, B. A., Gallinaro, P., and Schenck, R. K., Compression interfragmentaire et surcharge locale de l'os, In Interarthrite de l'epaule, in *Osteogenese et Compression*, Boitzy, A., Ed., Huber, Bern, 1972.
7. Burr, D. B., Martin, R. B., Schaffler, M. B., Radin, E. L., Bone remodeling in response to *in vivo* fatigue microdamage, *J. Biomech.*, 18, 189, 1985.
8. Mori, S. and Burr, D. B., Increased intracortical remodeling following fatigue damage, *Bone*, 14, 103, 1993.
9. Bentolila, V., Boyce, T. M., Fyhrie, D. P., Drumb, R., Skerry, T. M., and Schaffler, M. B., Intracortical remodeling in adult rat long bones after fatigue loading, *Bone*, 23, 275, 1998.

10. Verborgt, O., Gibson, G.J., and Schaffler, M.B., Loss of osteocyte integrity in association with microdamage and bone remodeling after fatigue *in vivo, J. Bone Miner. Res.*, 15, 60, 2000.

11. Tschantz, P. and Rutishauser, E., La surcharge mechanique de l'os vivant, *Ann. Anat. Path.*, 12, 223, 1967.

12. Chamay, A. and Tschantz, P., Mechanical influences in bone remodeling. Experimental research on Wolff's Law, *J. Biomech.*, 5, 173, 1972.

13. Scully, T. J. and Besterman, G., Stress fracture — a preventable training injury, *Mil. Med.*, 147, 285, 1982.

14. Stover, S. M., Stress fractures, in *Current Techniques in Equine Surgery and Lameness,* White, N. A. and Moore, J. N., Eds., W.B. Saunders, Philadelphia, 1998, 451.

15. Martin, R. B., A mathematical model for fatigue damage repair and stress fracture in osteonal bone, *J. Orthop. Res.*, 13, 309, 1995.

16. Martin, R. B., Burr, D. B., and Sharkey, N. S., *Skeletal Tissue Mechanics*, Springer-Verlag, New York, 1998.

17. Pattin, C. A., Caler, W. E., and Carter, D. R., Cyclic mechanical property degradation during fatigue loading of cortical bone, *J. Biomech.*, 29, 69, 1996.

18. Burr, D. B. and Martin, R. B., Calculating the probability that microcracks initiate resorption spaces, *J. Biomech.*, 26, 613, 1993.

19. Schaffler, M. B., Choi, K., and Milgrom, C., Aging and matrix microdamage accumulation in human compact bone, *Bone*, 17, 521, 1995.

20. Martin, R. B., Determinants of the mechanical properties of bones, *J. Biomech.*, 24 (Suppl. 1), 79, 1991, (see also erratum, 25, 1251, 1992).

21. Turner, C. H., Forwood, M., Rho, J.-Y., and Yoshikawa, T., Mechanical loading thresholds for lamellar and woven bone formation, *J. Bone Miner. Res.*, 9, 87, 1994.

22. Cowin, S. C., *Bone Mechanics*, CRC Press, Boca Raton, FL, 1989.

23. Burr, D. B., Yoshikawa, T., and Ruff, C. B., Moderate exercise increases intracortical activation frequency in old dogs, *Trans.Orthop. Res. Soc.*, 20, 204, 1995.

24. Rubin, C. T., Harris, J. M., Jones, B. H., Ernst, H. B., and Lanyon, L. E., Stress fractures: the remodeling response to excessive repetitive loading, *Trans. Orthop. Res. Soc.*, 9, 303, 1984.

CHAPTER **13**

Bucked Shins in Horses

David Nunamaker

CONTENTS

Natural History 203
Classical Etiology/Pathogenesis 204
Experimental Studies to Determine Etiology/Pathogenesis 207
Prevention 213
Synthesis 216
References 219

NATURAL HISTORY

The young North American Thoroughbred racehorse represents an excellent example of a naturally occurring model of fatigue failure in bone.

It has been reported that 70% of young Thoroughbred racehorses in training develop a repetitive loading injury (bucked shins) in their third metacarpal bone (MCIII).[1] This injury occurs most commonly in 2 year-old animals during the first six months of their training and may occur bilaterally. If the condition does occur bilaterally, the left limb is usually involved before the right. This seems to be associated with the fact that horses train and race in a counter–clockwise direction and are on the left lead of their gait when in the turns. Clinically, the condition is diagnosed by palpation of MCIII, revealing heat, pain, tenderness, and swelling over the dorsal surface of the third metacarpal bone. The animals tend to be short strided, uncomfortable at exercise, or lame. Radiographic diagnosis may be delayed from the clinical onset of signs but is evidenced by periosteal new bone formation over the dorsal or dorsomedial aspect of this bone.[1] This proliferation of periosteal new bone may be extreme in some cases (Figure 1). With few exceptions, once the condition occurs and subsequently resolves, the animals do not experience this problem again. This "vaccination", or adaptation phenomenon, is important in distinguishing animals at risk from those that are not. It is interesting to note that the condition of bucked shins occurs in young horses entering training. These animals are typically 2 year-olds and are equivalent to human adolescents. They are still growing and will have open physes (growth plates). If by chance older adult animals are entered into training as 3 or 4 year–olds, they may develop bucked shins as well. Racehorses that have trained and raced successfully in Europe may develop bucked shins when they race in North America. The interesting thing to note is that these horses are running on a harder surface in North America than in Europe, where they usually run on turf courses as opposed to dirt tracks in North America.

Some animals (~12%) that "buck their shins" will develop a radiographically visible "stress fracture" on the *dorsolateral* surface of MCIII up to one year after the original injury (Figure 2).[2] Clinically, this injury is usually seen as a fracture line first, with periosteal callus formation and cortical remodeling during the healing phase. Cortical remodeling can precede the occult fracture line seen radiographically. Horses that develop these stress fractures will have a previous history of bucked shins, usually with significant evidence of periosteal new bone formation at that time. Catastrophic complete fractures of MCIII can occur when horses with these stress fractures are exercised at speed or raced.

It is particularly interesting that this injury, while occurring commonly in Thoroughbred racehorses, is uncommon in Standardbred racehorses. These two breeds train and race in different gaits at different speeds, with the Thoroughbred training in several different gaits and racing in a galloping or running gait, while the Standardbred trains and races at a trot or pace, only varying the speed of travel. The Thoroughbred has a faster racing gait (64 km/h) than the Standardbred (48 km/h). These observations of the naturally occurring injury to bone suggest that understanding the details of mechanical loading may play an important role in determining how and why bone fatigue occurs *in vivo*.

CLASSICAL ETIOLOGY/PATHOGENESIS

Bucked shins as a disease/condition of racehorses has been described for years. The classical description of its etiology and pathogenesis was associated with other fractures of bone. Basically the story told was that of small, multiple fractures on the surface of MCIII as a result of high-speed exercise. The healing pattern was presumed to be secondary fracture healing with callus formation. Little observation or experimentation was performed to study the etiology or pathogenesis. Micro fractures had not been demonstrated histologically. Classical treatments of MCIII involved pin firing (the use of a pointed hot branding iron to create a pattern of thermal necrosis points through the skin and soft tissue to bone over the injured area) and rest.

This classical description appeared to show no association with the described pathogenesis and treatment. In addition, secondary fracture healing with callus

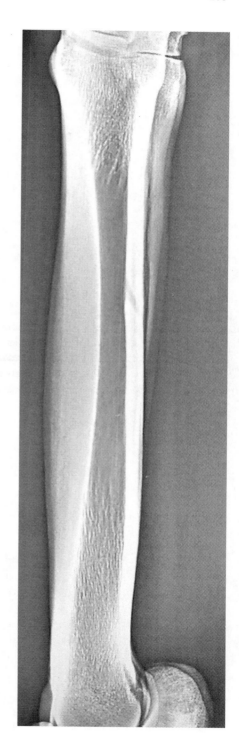

Figure 1 This xeroradiograph shows a clinical example of bucked shins. The periosteal reaction can be seen as an elevation of the dorsal cortical surface with the original cortex still defined.

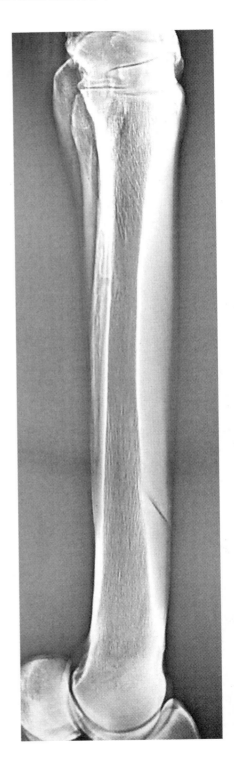

Figure 2 A stress fracture is seen in the distal third of the dorsolateral cortex of MCIII in this xeroradiograph.

formation occurs when there is motion associated with the ends of the fracture. Primary healing or direct remodeling would be expected in stress fracture, as the bone was intact. A repetitive motion injury associated with high strain cyclic fatigue seemed probable.

EXPERIMENTAL STUDIES TO DETERMINE ETIOLOGY/PATHOGENESIS

To elucidate a more realistic hypothesis for the etiology and pathomechanics/pathogenesis of this condition, a number of *in vitro* and *in vivo* experimental studies will be presented to demonstrate how this model relates to fatigue failure of bone.

Because Thoroughbred racehorses have such a high incidence of bucked shins, while Standardbred racehorses do not, a starting point was to determine if the *in vitro* fatigue properties of Thoroughbred MCIII were different from those of the Standardbred.

In this study, 26 dumbbell–shaped specimens machined from MCIIIs of 5 adult Thoroughbreds, and 25 specimens machined from MCIIIs of 5 adult Standardbred horses were tested in fully reversed cyclic bending experiments, using a constant strain rotating cantilever model that measured load decrement.[3] All specimens were tested fresh, and tests were completed within three hours after the death of the horse. All tests were performed at 40 Hz, following a pilot study examining the differences between 10, 20, and 40 Hz that showed no significant differences in fresh bone. Testing of all specimens continued until the specimen broke or had a 30% loss of stiffness. Three different offsets were used to establish nominal strains of 7500, 6000, or 4500 microstrain in the specimens.

Data were analyzed using a power regression model for each horse and each breed. Differences were not found in the curves for individual horses of the same breed, or for the curves between the two breeds. Pooling the data resulted in a data set that described the *in vitro* fatigue characteristics of cortical MCIIIs from Thoroughbreds and Standardbreds, greater than four years of age, subjected to fully reversed cyclic loading (Figure 3).

In vitro fatigue studies of equine MCIII have been the subject of several papers. Gibson et al. described the fatigue behavior of equine MCIII using rectangular beams of cortical bone ($10 \times 4 \times 100$ mm) tested monotonically and in fatigue in 4–point bending.[4] Deformations reaching 10,000 $\mu\varepsilon$ were used for the fatigue tests. The beams were machined from the four quadrants of the bone in the mid diaphysis. The animals were between two and five years old. Two were in race training and the other four had raced numerous times. The authors reported a loss of modulus in the medial and lateral regions but not in the dorsal regions as the fatigue tests approached failure. The standard deviations of their fatigue data in the dorsal regions were consistently higher than the means of the fatigue data in this region, which may have been related to the histories of the specimens that included two horses in race training and the others having raced. The authors provided a good discussion of problems associated with *in vitro* fatigue testing, i.e., temperature variation, cyclic

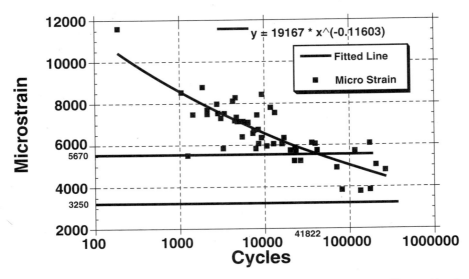

Figure 3 Fatigue data are presented using strain versus number of cycles. The Thoroughbred and Standardbred data are combined, as they were not different (r^2 = 0.486). Superimposed on this data set is the average *in vivo* strain recorded for the young Thoroughbred horses in training (5670 με) and the older horse (3250 με). The strain levels for young horses intersect the *in vitro* fatigue regression line at 41,822 cycles, while the older horse does not intersect this data set. (From Nunamaker, D.M., Butterweck, D.M., and Black, J., *Am. J. Vet. Res.*, 52, 97, 1991. With permission.)

rate, and loading methodologies. They concluded that "*in vitro* laboratory fatigue testing does not account for the *in vivo* biological responses to fatigue damage."

The same group evaluated the residual strength of equine MCIII following *in vitro* fatigue loading.[5] Using the same methodology, they cycled bone specimens from 0 to 5000 με for 100,000 cycles and then compared their strength in bending with matched monotonically loaded specimens from the same individual. They showed that the modulus of the specimens did not degrade over the 100,000 cycles tested. The residual strength was only 3% lower in the cycled specimens versus the monotonically loaded ones.

Using the same model once more, this group looked at remodeling and microcrack damage created *in vitro* in monotonically loaded specimens and those subjected to cyclic fatigue at 10,000 με.[6] Following failure, they bulk stained the specimens in basic fuchsin, and 100 μm cross–sections were cut and examined microscopically. Two types of cracks were seen. The unstained cracks seen in woven bone were thought to be damaged Sharpey's fibers, with their length increasing after failure. The stained cracks were larger, and were seen near the fracture surface and on compressed surfaces. They were more numerous in specimens with a higher modulus and shorter fatigue life. Prior remodeling of bone did not appear to influence the presence of microdamage in these studies.

Because *in vitro* fatigue data of equine MCIIIs showed no difference by breed, it appeared that other factors were important in the pathogenesis of fatigue failure of bone in the Thoroughbred racehorse. Since fatigue of structures can be associated with material properties or sectional geometric properties, these sectional properties of the two breed's MCIIIs were examined. To see if the bone's inertial properties were different we examined 30 pairs of second, third, and fourth metacarpal bones of the racehorse (10 Standardbred and 20 Thoroughbred horses).[7] Data on the Thoroughbred bones were grouped by age into 5 groups: yearlings, 2 year olds, 3 year olds, 4 year olds and "aged" horses (older than 5 years of age). The Standardbred data were divided into two groups, five pairs in each group: yearlings and "aged" horses. Comparisons were made between breeds of a particular age group and between the age groups of a particular breed. Mean sectional properties were then plotted against percent of bone length in order to observe patterns, proximal to distal, for each property measured.

Results of this study showed that age and breed were the only factors affecting sectional properties, i.e., there were no left–right differences. In the Thoroughbred group, all sectional properties were much lower for yearlings than for any other age group. Minimal differences were seen in cross-sectional areas in horses over two years of age. Changes in the second moments of area that relate to bending stiffness in a particular direction did show significant differences by age. These second moments related to bending of the bone in the dorsopalmar direction, and bending in the medial to lateral direction were used to determine the principal moments I_{min} and I_{max}. The most significant changes in the bone occurred at the mid-diaphysis between the ages of one and two, but continued change occurred until age four. No observable changes took place after four years of age. I_{min} was smaller in the yearling Thoroughbred than the yearling Standardbred, but was larger in the adult Thoroughbred than in the adult Standardbred (Figure 4); therefore, the Thoroughbred changes

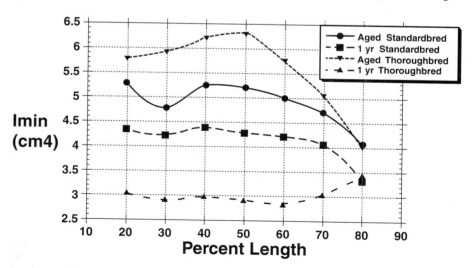

Figure 4 Graphical representation of MCIII inertial properties related to dorsopalmar bending of the MCIII is demonstrated by breed and age. The Thoroughbred racehorse increases its Imin with age to a much greater extent than does the Standardbred racehorse. (From Nunamaker, D.M., Butterweck, D.M., and Provost, M.T., *J. Biomech.*, 22, 129, 1989. With permission.)

this property to a greater extent than the Standardbred during the first two to four years of life, just when the animal is at risk for bucked shins. One could hypothesize that the inertial property I_{min} changes as the horse undergoes training and must enlarge to reduce strain or deformation in the bone. As the animal gets older and increases its inertial properties because of training, deformation of the bone would decrease with the same applied loads.

In a classic publication in 1979 Goodship et al. showed that the strains in the forelimb of the pig would double by resecting the ulna and allowing the pig to run around on its radius.[8] By the time the radius and healing ulna regenerated the same area of bone in the cross–section, the strains would return to normal. The authors did not look at inertial properties, but used a cross-sectional area. This same phenomenon may be at work in the horse with young, small diameter bones that are being asked to carry a larger load during high speed training. The inertial properties must increase to handle that load.

The next step was to record bone strain on the MCIIIs of horses training for racing at or near racing speed. To determine if differences existed between young (2 year-olds) and older established racehorses, four 2 year-old horses were purchased and trained for approximately six months.[9] A veteran 12 year-old Thoroughbred racehorse that had raced more than 40 times was also used in this study. All the horses were trained by professional trainers and were exercised with rosette strain gages mounted on their MCIIIs on a dirt racetrack, and all but one horse raced prior to strain gage measurement. All animals were exercised at work, i.e., their racing gait at racing speed (breeze). Speed was monitored with a stopwatch using furlong poles as distance markers. An onboard tape recorder captured the data, and strain measurements were made continuously throughout the workout. One channel of the tape was used to record a voice overlay of the jockey during the workout to fit the gait patterns to the bone strain. All horses were urged to their maximum effort for one quarter of a mile, which included the stretch run.

In vivo strains measured during these experiments using the rosette gages were resolved using Mohr circle analysis and reported as principal strains and directions when possible. The four 2 year-olds recorded peak compressive strains: horse 1, –4,761 microstrain; horse 2, –4,533 microstrain; horse 3, –5,670 microstrain; and horse 4, –4,400 microstrain (mean = –4841 ± 572 {SD} microstrain). The 12 year-old racehorse recorded strains of –3,317 microstrain. Horse 3 developed clinical signs compatible with the diagnosis of bucked shins. His strain gage measurements were approximately six standard deviations above the average maximal strains of horses 1, 2, and 4 (mean = –4,565 ± 182.6 microstrain).

Changes in speed from a trot to the racing gallop (breeze) changed the principal strain direction by more than 40 degrees on the dorsolateral surface of MCIII at the site of strain gage placement in all horses studied. Animals that were trotting showed tensile strains in the long axis of the bone on the dorsal/dorsolateral surface of MCIII. At racing speeds this same surface of the bone showed compressive strains.

Following the acquisition of *in vivo* strain data from these young horses, an attempt was made to correlate this data with the *in vitro* fatigue data previously generated by determining the average number of cycles that a young Thoroughbred racehorse would gallop in training prior to the onset of bucked shins. To accomplish this, the records of six 2 year-old Thoroughbred racehorses in training that had developed bucked shins were examined to establish the distances the animals trained prior to the onset of fatigue failure of bone.[3] To determine the number of cycles galloped over these distances, six 3 year-old racehorses were exercised at a canter, gallop, and at work (racing speed) to evaluate the length of stride in each of these gaits. The stride length was then divided into a mile to determine the number of strides (cycles) per mile. The total number of gait cycles of the six animals under study was estimated based on the distances covered in a canter, gallop, and at work. These horses were trained in these gaits between 10,000 and 12,000 cycles per month. The six horses were diagnosed with bucked shins between 35,284 and 53,299 training cycles.

Superimposition of the *in vivo* strain gage data from the four young Thoroughbred horses (5670 με) on the *in vitro* fatigue data previously compiled, along with the *in vivo* numbers of cycles data for the incidence of bucked shins in the six commercially trained Thoroughbred racehorses, showed a remarkable overlap (Figure 3). Furthermore, superimposition of the 12 year-old horse (3250 με) on this data showed that older horses would not reach the critical strain-number of cycles line of the fatigue curve for more than 200,000 cycles (16 to 20 months). This should give the bone adequate time to remodel without being at risk. Older horses do not train as much as younger horses as they continue to race.

To evaluate changes in whole bone stiffness and changes in local surface strains over time with superimposed training, twelve yearling Thoroughbred racehorses were purchased at auction and divided into four groups.[10] Three horses were kept as controls and allowed free exercise at pasture. The other nine horses were trained in groups of three per year by a professional trainer using a classical training regimen. Complete training records were kept, and each horse's MCIII was strain gaged at two different times. The right MCIII was strain gaged after each horse was broken to saddle and able to gallop a mile (1.5 km) at 11.2 m/sec. The left MCIII was strain gaged several months after the right side, well into the training process. Use of a radar gun and radar detector marking the tape recordings allowed comparisons of the two different strain gage sessions at the same speed. Maximum principal strains were compared between the first and second strain gage sessions where possible, to determine the effect of training on measured bone strain.

One horse developed bucked shins after the first strain gage session and was too lame to be instrumented a second time. Another horse had equipment problems and was only measured once. Seven horses had both sessions recorded, and four of these horses increased their bone strains from the first to the second session (mean increase = 1384 ± SD 819 με). Two horses showed a decrease in bone strain from the first session to the second, and two horses were essentially unchanged. It is interesting to note increased strains in some individuals when one might expect decreasing strains based on increasing inertial properties (sectional properties) of the bone. If the change in inertial properties did not occur, then strains would be expected to remain the same; conversely, if material properties degrade (modulus) then the strains would be expected to rise.

Measurements of whole bone stiffness and/or bone material properties from animals in the normal population and animals trained for racing might delineate the

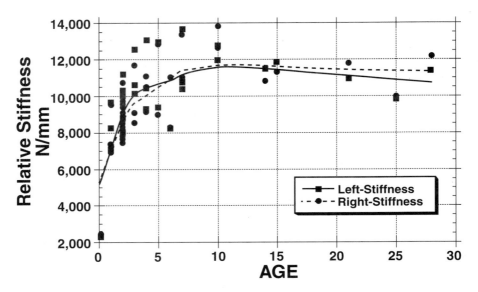

Figure 5 Paired whole bone *in vitro* stiffness measurements show increasing bone stiffness for the first 5 to 6 years. Animals in different stages of training make up the group between 2 and 5 years, where large differences are seen. The stiffness of each bone is shown in this figure relative to the 160 cm bone span used for the 3–point bending measurements (i.e., a shorter unsupported length would have resulted in a higher stiffness).

changes associated with increasing strain measurements in the face of continued training. Whole bone stiffness was measured in 40 pairs of MCIIIs from animals 2 months to 28 years of age, using non-destructive 3–point dorsopalmar bending tests *in vitro*.[10] Bone stiffness measurements were calculated from load displacement values obtained using a jig and clip gage assembly mounted on each bone coupled to the load cell of an Instron 1331 testing machine. The bones showed general increases in stiffness until they reached a plateau at about 6 years of age (Figure 5).

The intact MCIIIs of twelve experimental 2 year-old Thoroughbred racehorses were included in these tests using nondestructive 3–point bending *in vitro*, following the *in vivo* portion· of another experiment. Paired bone stiffness measurements showed dramatic changes in three of the trained horses, with differences between right and left MCIIIs of 16, 27, and 23%. One of these horses bucked its shin between strain gage sessions and was not strain gaged the second time (see above). The other two horses had clinical evidence of bucked shins. Three other trained horses showed differences in bone stiffness in the 6 to 8% range, and three trained and three control horses showed no difference between their right and left limbs.[10]

These studies showed that paired limbs from young Thoroughbred racehorses in training may not have the same mechanical properties. The dramatic change in stiffness noted in three of the horses versus no change in the controls was presumed to be related to the training on an oval track. The animals train in a counter–clockwise direction making the animal use his left lead in the turns. Thus, changes in the bone are graded so that they occur first in the left forelimb and then the right. The natural history of bucked shins shows that the left is usually involved, and precedes the right when both are affected. The enigma presented by the data was that the left leg in two of the three horses was stiffer than the right, while the right leg of the third horse was stiffer than the left.

Besides being a model for fatigue failure in bone, bucked shins in the North American Thoroughbred racehorse represents a significant clinical problem for the horse racing industry. Therefore, understanding the etiology and pathogenesis of this condition should help point to a method of treatment or prevention. Experimental studies showed that the inertial properties of Thoroughbred racehorses increase dramatically at the same time when growth and superimposed training leads to bucked shins. This would seem reasonable, since horses that do not train for racing do not develop the same inertial properties. To prevent bucked shins, it would seem necessary to change the inertial properties early in the training period. In addition, it was shown that the dorsal surface of MCIII is under tension when the animal is training in a slow gait and changes to compression when the animal races. Classical training methods for Thoroughbred racehorses consist of long, slow gallops, with racing speed and gait used sparingly. Therefore, horses that train in a classical manner with a lot of tensile forces across the dorsal surface of the MCIII would be well suited for training but may not be so for racing. Horses that mimic racing in their training may be more suited for racing, since the dorsal surface of the MCIII will be loaded in compression. It seems obvious that bone that models and remodels for tensile forces on the dorsal aspect of MCIII will be poorly adapted for the large compressive strains that are seen during racing. High strain cyclic fatigue (bucked shins) occurs quickly in the young training Thoroughbred racehorse, usually at about the time of the first start, when the animal is running in its racing gait.

PREVENTION

Because exercise is the problem, a change in the pattern of exercise may also be the solution. Our hypothesis was that training that mimics racing should produce a bone structure that decreases the incidence of bucked shins by changing the inertial properties.

With the understanding that slow speed gaits produce tensile strains on the dorsal surface of MCIII while high speed exercise induces compressive strains in this region, a study was undertaken to determine the effects of different training regimens and track surfaces on the modeling and remodeling of MCIII in the Thoroughbred racehorse.[11]

Eight 2 year-old Thoroughbred horses were purchased at auction prior to any training and divided into four groups of two horses each. Classical training methods were used for the horses in Groups I and II. Group I horses trained on a dirt track only, while Group II horses trained on a wood chip track only. Group III horses (control group) were not trained but were allowed free exercise in a five acre pasture. Group IV horses were trained using a modified classical training program on a dirt track only.

The classical training program comprised daily gallops (~18 second furlongs, ~11.2 m/sec) of one to two miles per day (1.6 to 3.2 km) followed by shorter "works" or "breezes" at racing speed (~14 second furlongs, ~14.4 m/sec) once every seven to ten days and increasing in distance from two to six furlongs (0.4 to 1.2 km) progressively over the course of the study. The modified classical training method used daily gallops of one mile but the frequency of the high-speed "works" increased to three times a week, while distances increased progressively from one to four furlongs (0.2 to 0.8 km.). The study was completed over a five month period.

Following five months of training or pasture turnout, the animals were killed, and the MCIIIs of all horses collected and cross-sectional inertial property measurements made using methods described previously.

Examination of the inertial properties of the mid-diaphyseal sections of MCIIIs from the different groups showed that the minimum principal moments of inertia (I_{min}) of Groups I and II (classically trained) were similar to Group III horses that did not train at all. The principal moment, I_{min}, of Group IV (modified classical) horses was greater than the other groups and was similar to the I_{min} moments previously reported for mature, successful racehorses (Figure 6).

Gross evaluation of the microradiographic cross-sections from the mid-diaphysis of MCIIIs from these horses showed that bone remodeling occurred only medially and laterally in Groups I and II. The filling of secondary Haversian systems with new bone was more complete in Group I specimens, indicating that the remodeling process was further advanced in the group that was exercised on the harder dirt track surface. There seemed to be a distinct lack of remodeling activity in the dorsal and

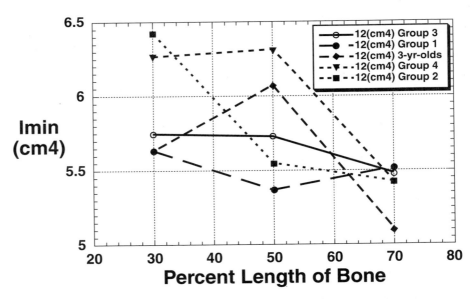

Figure 6 MCIII inertial properties at the mid-diaphysis (50%) of horses trained using different regimens show that classical training (bottom two lines, Groups 1 and 2) has no effect when compared to horses that don't train (middle line, Group 3). Modified training that includes short distance fast exercise (high strain cycles) provides changes (top line, Group 4) that equal or surpass adult trained horses (second line, 3 year-olds). Note the large difference between groups at the 30% (proximal third) level, indicating fusion of the second metacarpal, with the third in Groups 2 and 4.

dorsolateral regions of these sections in Groups I and II. Group III and IV horses showed extensive remodeling throughout the cortex. Groups III and IV specimens revealed remodeling in the dorsal and dorsolateral aspects of the bone which was not seen in Groups I and II.

Interpretation of the data from this experiment suggested that horses that train on a harder track surface seemed to remodel their bone at a faster rate than horses that exercised on a more compliant surface. Previous studies have shown that classically trained horses that exercise on a hard surface seem to have a higher incidence of bucked shins than horses training or racing on a more compliant surface.[12] One horse in Group I in this study bucked its shins during the training period. Classical training methods applied to horses training on a hard or soft track did not effectively change the inertial properties (I_{min}) that influence bending of MCIII in a dorsopalmar direction. In contrast, exercise regimens (Group IV) that stressed MCIII in compression on its dorsal surface did change I_{min} in a significant manner, consistent with adult racehorses evaluated previously that were no longer at risk for bucked shins.

The results of this study supported the concept that exercise could be designed to optimize the shape of MCIII. This, in turn, should influence (decrease) the incidence of bucked shins in this Thoroughbred racehorse model, and hence the problem within the industry.

To prove the efficacy of such an hypothesis it was necessary to design and carry out a large scale study of young Thoroughbred racehorses in training, using different training modalities. Based on these previous experiments, a training program was designed around the modified classical regimen.[13] To determine the efficacy of this adaptive training program to decrease the incidence of bucked shins, a prospective study was started using five commercial training stables. A retrospective review was also made based on logs of the horses' training. Two of the stables (2 and 5) were aware of our modified classical training program and were using it as a basis for their training regimen. The other stables (1,3, and 4) were thought to be training in the classical manner. Stables 1 and 2 used the same racetrack for training. Stable 4 trained on a race track as well, while stables 3 and 5 trained on their own farm training tracks.

To be part of this study, trainers kept complete daily records of each horse's training with accurate accounts of distances the animal jogged, galloped, and breezed. These distances were collected and used in the data analysis as rates (miles/week). In addition, physical exams and indications of events not related to bucked shins were recorded. Horses entered into the study had to be 2 year-old Thoroughbreds being entered into race training for the first time. The animals were followed for 365 days after training began. Data collection stopped when the horses bucked their shins, were sold, or stopped training because of another event not related to bucked shins. The study included 11 years of training data from 226 two year-old Thoroughbred racehorses, but all years were not represented by all stables. Fifty-six of the 226 horses bucked their shins, and the other 170 either completed the 365-day observation period or were sold while in training.

Using STATA statistical software,[14] regression analysis and survival analysis techniques were used to explore the data. Survival in this analysis indicates horses that did not buck their shins. Using the log rank test, we found a significant difference

(P < 0.05) in survivability of the two-year olds at the five stables. Since stable 2 had the best survival and stable 1 and 4 the worst, evaluation of the relationships between jogging, galloping, and breezing among these stables was carried out. Stable 2, with the highest breezing rate, had the lowest incidence of bucked shins, while stables 1 and 4 had the highest galloping rates and the highest incidence of bucked shins.

The next step was to explore the significance of dependence of survivability on each of the three training activities. This was accomplished using a Cox regression stratifying on stable. Since jog rate was not a statistically significant predictor (P = 0.113), the Cox regression was repeated without the jog rate data and showed that gallop rate (P = 0.005) and breeze rate (P = 0.007) were significant predictors of survivability. The hazard ratio for this data set showed that galloping increased the likelihood of bucked shins by 33%/mile galloped/wk, while breezing was protective, reducing the likelihood of bucked shins by 98% mile breezed/wk.

SYNTHESIS

Seventeen years of evolutionary experiments, based on an initial observation of a marked difference in the incidence of fatigue fractures between two different breeds of racehorses, have led to a more complete understanding of a natural model for fatigue failure of bone. We now can compare *in vitro* and *in vivo* fatigue behavior and observe bone adaptation to different exercise regimes. Adaptive exercise has been shown to change the geometric properties of MCIII, to influence bone modeling and remodeling, and to reduce the incidence of fatigue failure of MCIII.

Comparisons of the Thoroughbred with the Standardbred racehorse show major changes in inertial properties of MCIII as a result of growth and superimposed training. Comparisons of young Thoroughbreds that are susceptible to fatigue failure (bucked shins) with older resistant animals suggest that changes in bone inertial properties are an important factor affecting the incidence of this injury. Large MCIII I_{min} values reflect probable increases in MCIII stiffness in the dorsopalmar direction and, thus, reduced peak strain during high speed exercise. The inertial properties of the proximal tibia have been shown to be predictive for the development of fatigue fractures in military recruits,[15,16] just as the inertial property measurement of the 5 year-old Thoroughbred MCIII shows that the animal is no longer at risk for bucked shins.

In vivo strain measurements of Thoroughbred MCIIIs demonstrated higher peak strains under physiological loading than previously reported in any animal species. Although all *in vitro* test conditions differ from the *in vivo* loading, most involve significant bending components that can be expected to produce accumulated fatigue failure in composites such as bone. Therefore, while the *in vitro* data may not produce the *in vivo* intrinsic fatigue mechanism, the superimposition of the *in vivo* strains reported for the young and older horses at racing speed produce a striking predictive relationship for risk of developing this fatigue injury (Figure 2).

Large surface strains, measured *in vivo* at high speeds on the dorsolateral aspect of MCIIIs in young 2 year-old Thoroughbred racehorses in training, contrast dramatically with the smaller strains measured in adult racehorses that have raced successfully. Strains measured on the surface of bone under a given load regimen relate to both the bone's modulus and its inertial properties. Since inertial properties have been shown to increase with age, and bone strains during high speed exercise have been shown to decrease in older horses, it was hypothesized that changes in bone inertial properties and/or modulus lower the peak bone strains as the young racehorse matures. However, it is possible that training regimens can outpace adaptive response. In fact, we observed that a certain percentage of young animals actually increased MCIII surface strains after several months of training. Whole bone stiffness measurements showed right to left differences of up to 27% in horses in training, while there was never a right to left difference in the non-trained control animals. Since bucked shin occurs bilaterally but sequentially in young Thoroughbreds, usually on the left side before the right, it is possible that the developmental stiffness changes in limbs are not synchronized, but may respond to the predominance of the left lead used by the horse in its racing gait as the horse travels in a counterclockwise direction around the racetrack. Maximal strains at exercise and bone stiffness parameters probably both change with time, and may be declining on one side while increasing on the other. Increasing bone strain measured at high speed during training, as seen in four of the seven Thoroughbreds reported, is suggestive of rapid bone stiffness change *in vivo* due to exercise.[10] There are three possible related explanations for this:

1. Bone stiffness <u>decreases</u> *in vivo*, much as it does *in vitro*, when the bone undergoes cyclic fatigue.
2. Bone stiffness *increases* due to inertial property changes in MCIII and may or may not be overwhelmed by *decreasing* intrinsic material stiffness.
3. Increasing racing speeds continue to increase bone strains prior to sufficient inertial property changes in MCIII.

If Wolff's law is strictly applied, it follows that a bone that adapts to a particular peak tensile strain may not be adequately prepared to resist far larger peak compressive strains in the same location.

A recent *in vitro* fatigue study of equine MCIIIs showed a difference in fatigue resistance to bending loads in different anatomical quadrants.[4] Bone that was loaded in bending around the physiologic bending axis had greater fatigue resistance than bone bent at 90 degrees to this axis.

We hypothesized that, to adequately adapt for racing, the MCIII should be exposed during training to strains of the actual magnitude and direction experienced during racing. Furthermore, the high incidence of bucked shins in Thoroughbreds suggested that loading to produce such peak strains and concomitant adaptive remodeling did not occur in a large number of Thoroughbreds in classical training programs prior to racing.

Previous *in vivo* studies, using the functionally isolated rooster ulna, have shown that low numbers of loading cycles (four per day) were adequate to maintain bone mass.[17] Thirty-six cycles were enough to stimulate bone formation in this model, but again, the loads, although still physiologic, were such that the bone was loaded in a different direction. The resulting periosteal new bone formation that was seen in this model is the same type of bone reaction observed in the Thoroughbred racehorse MCIII with a compensating fatigue injury.

Taking these observations into account, an exercise (training) regimen was developed that modestly increased the small numbers of high load cycles using peak load magnitudes and directions that are seen during racing. Increasing the number of short distance works (breezes) from once every seven to ten days, as occurs with classical training programs, to three times a week, produced large changes in the modeling, remodeling, and inertial property measurements of MCIII. Classical training produced little progressive change in the inertial properties of MCIII, seemingly no better than no training at all, while the new, modified training program showed inertial property development that equaled or surpassed that observed in established older Thoroughbreds, horses apparently no longer susceptible to bucked shins.

To prove efficacy that adaptive exercise could be used to reduce the incidence of fatigue injuries of bone, an 11 year longitudinal study of 226 commercially trained Thoroughbred racehorses in 5 stables was undertaken. Two of the stables (2 and 5) were aware of the modified training program and carried it out to some extent. Survival analysis of the data showed the influence of weekly jogging, galloping, and breezing rates (miles/week) on the incidence of bucked shins. The hazard ratios for this data set indicated that galloping (1.365) was a training risk for bucked shins, while breezing (0.014) was protective at the distances used. The winter of 1994 brought severe ice storms to the northeast. Stable 2 could not train their horses using the modified program because of the weather conditions, and they reverted to the standard classical program. This then became an unintentional crossover design experiment, and 62% of the horses trained that year from Stable 2 bucked their shins. Without using the 1994 year, only 9.3% of the horses trained by Stable 2 bucked their shins in the five year training period when the modified training program was implemented. Interestingly, stable 1 had 50% of the horses in training buck their shins in 1994, compared to their average not including the 1994 year of 41.3%. These two stables are easily compared, as they both used the same training facility and would have the fewest confounding variables.

When evaluating the hazard ratios, it is necessary to point out that the breezing rate was much lower than the galloping rate (miles/week). Arbitrarily increasing the breezing rate because it is protective would also change the hazard ratios. Certainly, long distance breeze rates would be detrimental, and have been described.[18]

Adaptive exercise has been shown to change the geometric parameters of a specific bone in a way that would be expected to reduce fatigue damage while, at the same time, would significantly reduce the clinical incidence of apparent fatigue injury of this bone. This correlation, although not explicit proof of the interrelationship between the factors measured, is convincing and has already been incorporated into the racing industry on a limited scale to improve the health of this working animal, the North American Thoroughbred racehorse.

Although many questions regarding fatigue failure of bone remain, the ability to use a naturally occurring model to search for answers helps make the connection to large amounts of *in vitro* data in the literature. The problem of relating *in vitro* to *in vivo* data is dependent on a good model, and the Thoroughbred racehorse seems to be a productive one.

REFERENCES

1. Norwood, G.L., The bucked shin complex in Thoroughbreds, in *Proceedings 24th Annual Convention of AAEP*, 1978, 319.
2. Nunamaker, D.M. and Provost, M.T., The bucked shin complex revisited, in *Proceedings of the 37th Annual Convention of AAEP*, 1992, 549.
3. Nunamaker, D.M., Butterweck, D.M., and Black, J., *In vitro* comparison of Thoroughbred and Standardbred racehorses with regard to local fatigue failure of the third metacarpal bone, *Am. J. Vet. Res.*, 52, 97, 1991.
4. Gibson, V.A., Stover, S.M., Martin, R.B., Gibeling, J.C., Willits, N.H., Gustafson, M.B., and Griffin, L.V., Fatigue behavior of the equine third metacarpus: mechanical property analysis, *J. Orthop. Res.*, 13, 861, 1995.
5. Martin, R.B., Gibson, V.A., Stover, S.M., Gibeling, J.C., and Griffin, L.V., Residual strength of equine bone is not reduced by intense fatigue loading: implications for stress fracture, *J. Biomech.*, 30, 109, 1997.
6. Martin, R.B., Lau, S.T., Mathews, P.V., Gibson, V.A., and Stover, S.M., *In vitro* fatigue behavior of the equine third metacarpus: remodeling and microcrack damage analysis, *J. Orthop. Res.*, 14, 794, 1996.
7. Nunamaker, D.M., Butterweck, D.M., and Provost, M.T., Some geometric properties of the third metacarpal bone: a comparison between the Standardbred and Thoroughbred racehorse, *J. Biomech.*, 22, 129, 1989.
8. Goodship, A.E., Lanyon, L.E., and McFie, H., Functional adaptation of bone to increased stress, *J. Bone Jt. Surg.*, 61A, 539, 1979.
9. Nunamaker, D.M., Butterweck, D.M., and Provost, M.T., Fatigue fractures in Thoroughbred racehorses: relationship with age, peak bone strain and training, *J. Orthop. Res.*, 8, 604, 1990.
10. Nunamaker, D.M., Provost, M.T., and Bartel, D.L., Third metacarpal bone strain and stiffness measurements of Thoroughbred racehorses in training, in *Transactions of the 2nd Combined Meeting of the Orthopedic Research Society, USA*, 1995, 11.
11. Nunamaker, D.M. and Butterweck, D.M., Bone modeling and remodeling in the Thoroughbred racehorse: relationships of exercise to bone morphometry, in *Transactions of the 35th Annual Meeting of the Orthopedic Research Society*, 1989, 99.
12. Moyer, W. and Fisher, J.R.S., Bucked shins: effects of differing track surfaces and proposed training regimens, *Proceedings of the 37th Annual Convention of AAEP*, 1992, 541.
13. Boston, R.C. and Nunamaker, D.M., Gait and speed as exercise components of risk factors associated with onset of fatigue injury of the third metacarpal bone in 2-year-old Thoroughbred racehorses, *Amer. J. Vet. Res.*, 61, 602, 2000.
14. STATA Statistical Software, Release 5, *STATA Reference Manual*, 3, 1997.
15. Giladi, M., Milgrom, C., Simkin, A., Stein, M., Kashtan, H., Margulies, J., Rand, N., Chisin, R., Steinberg, R., and Aharonson, Z., Stress fractures and tibial bone width. A risk factor, *J. Bone Jt. Surg.*, 69, 326, 1987.
16. Milgrom, C., Giladi, J., Simkin, A., Rank, N., Kedem, R., Kashtan, H., Stein, M., and Gomori, M., The area moment of inertia of the tibia: a risk factor for stress fractures, *J. Biomech.*, 22, 1243, 1989.
17. Rubin, C.T. and Lanyon, L.E., Regulation of bone formation by applied dynamic loads, *J. Bone Jt. Surg.*, 66A, 397, 1984.
18. Estberg, L., Stover, S.M., Gardner, I.A., et al., Case-control study of a cluster estimate of cumulative exercise distance as a risk factor for fatal musculoskeletal injury in Thoroughbred racehorses, in *Proceeding of the AAEP*, 1994, 171.

CHAPTER 14

Rabbits As An Animal Model for Stress Fractures

David B. Burr

CONTENTS

Introduction 221
Rabbit Models 222
    The Impulsive Loading Model 222
        Advantages of the Impulsive Loading Model 226
        Limitations of the Impulsive Loading Model 228
    The Excessive Jumping Model 229
        Advantages of the Excessive Jumping Model 229
        Limitations of the Excessive Jumping Model 230
Conclusion 230
References 231

INTRODUCTION

Few animal models are well characterized to study stress fractures. In models such as horses and greyhounds, stress fractures occur naturally, making it difficult to control relevant loading variables or to study the pathogenesis of development of the stress fracture over time prior to its occurrence. Consequently, study of the pathophysiology of stress fractures has been delayed because of the difficulty of finding a suitable experimental animal model.

0-8493-0317-6/01/$0.00+$.50

RABBIT MODELS

The Impulsive Loading Model

Several investigators have used the rabbit as an animal model for stress fracture. In the rabbit impulsive loading model,[1] stress fractures can be induced in the tibial diaphysis of rabbits by the repeated application of non-traumatic loads. In this model, the right hindlimb of a rabbit is placed in a splint that prevents the contraction of the gastrocnemius, and impairs its ability to attenuate tensile loads caused by bending. Loads 1.5 x body weight are applied over a period of 25 msec to the heel (Figure 1). Because of soft tissue attenuation, loads on the distal tibia only achieve magnitudes of about 1 x body weight.[2] Skeletally mature rabbits are loaded at 1 Hz for 40 min/day, 5 days/week for up to 9 weeks to create the stress fracture. The loading protocol applies about 12,000 cycles/week at a load equivalent to loads placed on the lower limbs during walking.

Within one week of loading (i.e., <12,000 cycles), nearly 50% of the rabbits show some evidence of a positive ^{99m}Tc bone scan. Following three weeks of loading

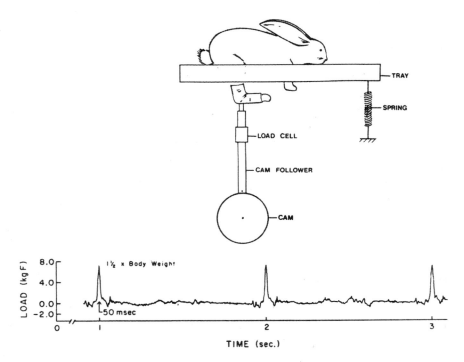

Figure 1   (a) Schematic diagram of the apparatus used to mechanically load the rabbit hindlimb. The device is cam-driven, with the cam follower connected to a splint on the rabbit's leg. The tray that supports the rabbit is counterbalanced by a spring. (b) A typical load-time record from the load cell on the cam-follower. The rise time for the application of the load is about 25 ms. (From Radin, E.L., Martin, R.B., Burr, D.B., Caterson, B., Boyd, R.D., and Goodwin, C., *J. Orthop. Res.*, 2, 221, 1984. With permission.)

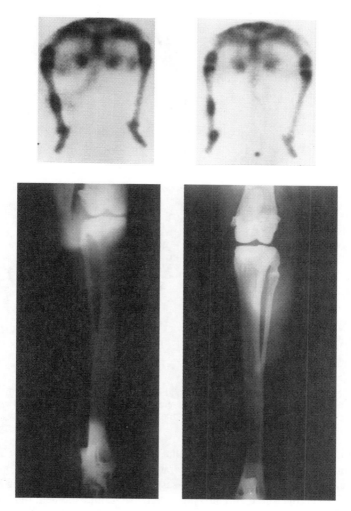

Figure 2 Scintigraphic and radiographic images showing changes indicative of a stress fracture, and progression between three and six weeks in the rabbit impulsive loading model. (a) Increased uptake of ^{99m}Tc in the distal tibia in a rabbit loaded for three weeks. (b) Increased uptake of ^{99m}Tc in the distal tibia in the same rabbit loaded for six weeks. (c) Slight periosteal callus formation can be seen radiographically in the loaded tibia (shown on left), corresponding to the region of increased ^{99m}Tc uptake. The tibia shown on the right is the contralateral control limb.

(~36,000 cycles), 48% of the rabbits demonstrate severe lesions (Figure 2). This increases to 68% following six weeks of loading. Scintigraphic evidence of stress fracture is positively associated with radiologic evidence of periosteal callus, indicative of a stress-induced reaction. More than 90% of the rabbits show radiographic or scintigraphic evidence of a stress fracture after six weeks of loading.

Even with continued loading, some healing occurs between six and nine weeks. All rabbits loaded for nine weeks present with some lesion, even though they typically demonstrate more severe lesions at three or six weeks. Scintigraphic images for rabbits

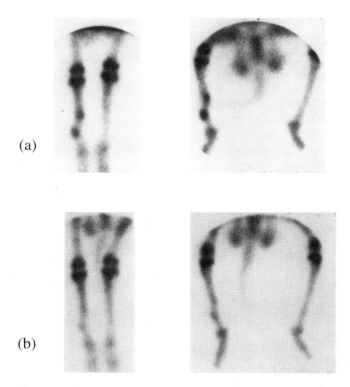

(a)

(b)

Figure 3 Scintigraphic images showing healing between six (a) and nine weeks (b) of loading in the same rabbit. The edges of the stress fracture appear less distinct in the image from nine weeks, and the uptake of the 99mTc is more diffuse.

following nine weeks of loading show that the edges of the lesion are no longer clearly demarcated, and the uptake of the radioactive tracer is diffuse (Figure 3).

The local mechanical strains and stresses that occur in the tibia during impulsive loading have been measured and also predicted, using finite element representations of tibial morphology subjected to the application of a load.[3,4] Local strains at the site of the stress fracture, and at the tibial midshaft, were measured using rosette strain gages during the loading procedure. This analysis showed that strains at the stress fracture site on the cranio-medial cortex of the tibia in rabbits loaded impulsively average about −733 με, while those on the lateral cortex average 822 με (Table 1). These strains are significantly higher than strains on the medial and lateral cortex at midshaft. Strain rates were also highest on the cranio-medial cortex at the stress fracture site ($p < 0.01$), 55% higher than on the analogous cortex at midshaft. These strain magnitudes, and the strain rates that are generated, are very consistent with strains in the human tibia during walking and running,[5] but are very low to create a stress fracture (see Chapter 8), suggesting that the cause of the stress fractures may not be solely the impulsive loading, but may require initiation of a biological reaction to the load that weakens the bone (see Chapters 10 and 12 for

Table 1   Experimentally Measured Strains and Strain Rates in the Rabbit Impulsive Loading Model

Gage Location	Principal Strain (microstrain)	Shear Strain (microstrain)	Strain Rate (Shear) (microstrain/sec)
Stress Fracture Site			
Cranio-medial	−733 (233)[a]	−426 (358)	6083 (1941)[b]
Cranio-lateral	822 (428)[a]	−459 (383)	5076 (2592)
Posterior	677 (345)[c]	−478 (285)[a]	5862 (3625)[a]
Tibial Midshaft			
Medial	−521 (293)	−345 (374)	3933 (1904)
Lateral	490 (280)	−258 (188)	3338 (2356)
Posterior	270 (66)	−253 (118)	3039 (845)

Strains at stress fracture site larger than strains at tibial midshaft, one-tailed t-test:

[a] $p < 0.05$
[b] $p < 0.01$
[c] $p < 0.005$

discussion of this concept). Nevertheless, stress fractures in the rabbit model most frequently involve the cranial cortex of the distal tibia, which is where the highest strains and strain rates in the tibia were found. Perhaps a combination of higher strain magnitudes and strain rates that are 50 to 100% higher than those normally generated during running may contribute to the development of stress fracture.

An isotropic finite element model of the rabbit hindlimb at the moment of peak application of strain shows that the circumferential distribution of the calculated (predicted) principal and shear (Tresca) stresses on the periosteal surface of the tibia at the stress fracture location occur anteriorly, consistent with observations of stress fractures at this location (Figure 4). Tresca stresses along the anterior tibial cortex at the stress fracture site are nearly twice those found at midshaft. Pockets of locally high shear and compressive stress are found on the anterior and anterolateral cortices in the distal third of the femur in the region where stress fractures occur (color Figure 5*).

The correspondence between the location of the stress fractures in this model and the finite element prediction of local shear stress concentrations suggests that high shear stresses may be a significant underlying cause for the stress fractures observed in this model. Tensile stresses cannot be the primary cause because fracture lesions are found on the anterolateral tibial cortex and tensile stresses are calculated to be highest on the posterior cortex. Although compressive stresses are also high on the anterior cortex in the rabbit model, the longitudinal compressive strength of bone is three times greater than its shear strength,[6] and compressive stresses developed on the anterior cortex are not sufficient to cause fracture.

Although there is good correspondence between regions of high shear stress and the locations of stress fractures in the tibia, the strains are much too low to be the sole cause for the stress fractures. Schaffler and his co-workers[7] have examined the

* See color insert following page 182.

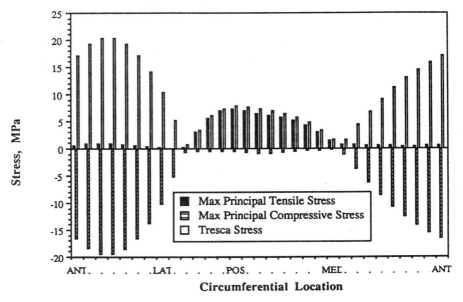

Figure 4   Peak principal compressive, tensile and Tresca (shear) stresses at the tibial stress fracture site in impulsively loaded rabbits, calculated using a finite element model. The highest stresses are located anteriorly, coincident with the location of the stress fracture.

biological response to the application of the load, which they feel may be part of the etiology for the fracture in this model. Rabbits loaded for 32,400 cycles over the course of one day showed no biological evidence of skeletal damage. Rabbits loaded for 37,500 cycles over three weeks also fail to present any histological evidence of skeletal damage, even though 80% of them show evidence of a stress fracture by scintigraphy.[1] The increased [99mTc] uptake in the tibia reflects a sixfold increase in resorption sites. After six weeks of loading there was a significant increase in microcrack density, and cracks were observed only in areas undergoing intracortical remodeling. This may implicate increased bone turnover as a precondition for stress fracture in this model, and suggests a biological remodeling response via positive feedback with loading in the pathogenesis of the stress fracture in this model.

Advantages of the Impulsive Loading Model

The impulsively loaded rabbit model mimics the development of human stress fractures in several respects. Onset of the stress fractures is entirely consistent with the development of stress fractures in military recruits. Stress fracture incidence is generally observed to increase between the second and fourth weeks of training,[8-15] although incidence remains high between five and eight weeks.[11,16,17] Greaney et al.[18] reported that in U.S. Marines 64% of stress fractures occurred in the first two weeks

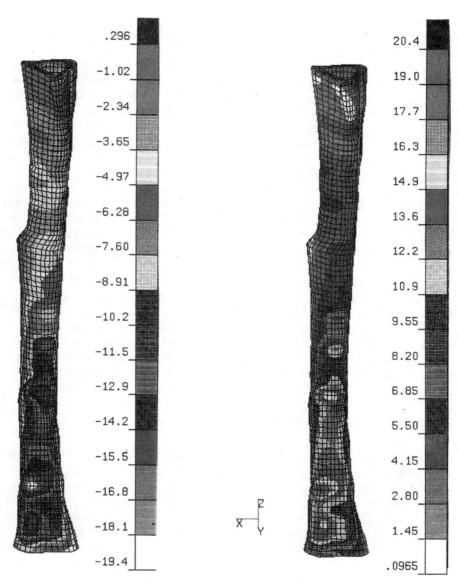

Figure 5 Contour plot of compressive (left) and Tresca (shear, right) stresses on the anterior aspect of the rabbit tibia. The scale is given in MPa. "X" denotes lateral. High stress concentrations are located on the anterior and anterolateral aspect of the distal tibia, coincident with the region where rabbits present with stress fractures. See color insert following page 182.

of training, while Milgrom et al.[19] found that 33% of tibial stress fractures occurred during the first two weeks of training in the Israeli military, with an increased incidence to more than 50% within the first four weeks.

Stress fracture lesions in this model become progressively more severe with loading up to six weeks, although some regression and healing is observed between six and nine weeks of loading. Positive scintigraphic findings are correlated with radiologic evidence of periosteal callus formation. The model demonstrates penetrance in that not all rabbits demonstrated severe stress fractures even under similar loading conditions. The observation of severe lesions in 48% of rabbits by three weeks and 68% of rabbits by six weeks compares favorably with the reported incidence of stress fractures in physically active humans.[19-21] In this rabbit model, 89% of the stress fractures are found in the middle or distal tibia, and 74% of them involve the anterior or the anteromedial cortex. This is similar to sites reported to be most common in human tibial stress fractures.[16,22-34]

Another advantage of the model is that it can be used to predict the risk of future stress fracture under controlled loading conditions. The uptake of ^{99m}Tc at the end of week one of loading predicted the increased ^{99m}Tc uptake at three weeks ($r^2 = 0.67$, $p < 0.01$). Uptake at three weeks predicted the rate of change in uptake between six and nine weeks ($r^2 = 0.96$, $p < 0.02$). Thus, the model shows that quantitative analysis of technetium uptake prior to radiologic signs of overt stress fracture can predict the progression of the condition that eventually leads to the stress fracture. Early quantitative analysis of ^{99m}Tc can, therefore, provide a reasonable screening assessment for the risk of future fracture.

Finally, for econonic reasons, it is important to find a small animal model for stress fractures. The larger animals (greyhounds, horses) that develop stress fractures "naturally" can be very expensive for long term studies. Rabbits represent a feasible model for doing studies in which larger sample sizes or longer experimental periods are necessary.

Limitations of the Impulsive Loading Model

The rabbit impulsive loading model has several limitations as well. First, it relies on a cumbersome mechanical loading apparatus that is not available to most investigators. This apparatus has several flaws. Although the load magnitude and rate can be controlled fairly tightly, the large displacement of the leg during loading (6 to 8 cm) makes it difficult to control out of plane loading. This causes motion in several planes, making the local stress distribution difficult to analyze and understand. This off-axis displacement may result in rubbing between the splint and lower leg, causing periosteal inflammatory reactions that could be unrelated to the development of stress fracture. This inflammatory reaction would create a positive scintigraphic image and could cause the formation of a periosteal callus, both symptomatic of stress fracture. Reducing of off-axis displacements to minimize reactions that may not be related to the pathogenesis of stress fractures requires a very experienced animal handler.

In the model, the only radiographic evidence of a fracture was the formation of callus. No definite fractures were observed on radiographic or post-mortem inspection. There was microscopic damage at some sites of positive bone scans, but these were not always in anatomical association with the periosteal callus, and were not observed in every rabbit with a stress fracture. Therefore, the model would benefit by additional characterization, and by demonstring that friction on the leg by the splint does not contribute to the development of what appears to be a stress fracture.

The Excessive Jumping Model

Li et al.[35] reported a model in which stress fractures could be produced by causing rabbits to run or jump excessively. An electric cage with high voltage but low current was used to induce the rabbits to jump to a height of about 15 cm, and then run. The voltage and current are controlled for intensity (15,000 V and 100 to 200 microamps), duration (0.2 to 0.4 sec), and interval of stimulation (3/min). This stimulation is given for 2 hours each day with a 10 minute break at the halfway mark, 6 days/week over a 60 day period. Over the two month period, rabbits receive 21,600 jolts, and presumably would load the limb from the jump an equal number of times. To characterize the model, rabbits were sacrificed at various times during the 60 day period.

Periosteal callus in the tibia formed within 12 days, consistent with the signs of a stress fracture. Most of the periosteal callus is formed on the anteromedial side of the cortex, in locations adjacent to areas of active bone remodeling in the pre-existing tibial cortex. By 21 days (~6,480 jumps), an incomplete fracture of the tibial cortex occurred in 20% (2 of 10) of the rabbits, and 25% of the rabbits (1 of 4) presented with complete fracture of one cortex of the tibia by day 50.

As with the impulsive loading model, both microcracks and bone remodeling increase in the cortex of loaded rabbits. Microcracks are observed by the 10th day, especially on the anterior and medial aspects of the tibial cortex. Increased remodeling is observed after only 14 days of loading (<4,500 jumps).

Advantages of the Excessive Jumping Model

The advantages of this model are similar to those of the impulsive loading model. The lesions that develop in the tibia are progressive. The lesion begins with a periostitis, as in the human condition, with the ultimate formation of periosteal callus. Unlike the impulsive loading model, these lesions may progress to frank fracture of a single cortex, which is atypical of stress fracture but can occur in cases of continued loading. Stress fractures tend to be located anteromedially, again consistent with the human condition. The model employs no external splinting or loading and avoids the potential complicating factor of periosteal reactions occurring as a response to irritation to the periosteum. Finally, the onset of stress fractures is consistent with onset of human stress fractures, with the initial periosteal stress reaction detected by two weeks, followed at three to eight weeks by the formation of periosteal callus, and frank fracture at seven weeks in a subset of rabbits.

One attractive feature of the model is the use of immature rabbits (2.5 to 2.8 kg). The incidence of stress fractures appears to be higher in younger animals[36] and humans,[37] so the natural history of the stress fracture may be more like that of a naturally occurring stress fracture. It is well known that modeling and remodeling processes are quite different in adolescents and adults, and if biologic feedback is necessary for the pathogenesis of the fracture, this will be duplicated more accurately in a model that uses younger animals.

Limitations of the Excessive Jumping Model

There are several limitations to this model as well, not the least of which is the difficulty of receiving approval from an institutional animal care and use committee to provide such a noxious stimulus to rabbits. Beyond this purely practical and ethical issue, however, the model suffers from several scientific limitations.

Although the intensity, duration, and interval of electrical stimulation can be controlled, the actual load on the rabbit's hindlimb cannot be controlled, nor was it monitored throughout the experiment. This limits the flexibility of the model in that aspects of load and load rate cannot be manipulated to alter the natural progression of stress fracture development.

Some investigators have tried to duplicate this model but have had difficultly getting the rabbits to jump. Most often, once the animals become acclimated, they will simply lift a leg rather than jump. In other cases, the rabbits shorted out the electrical grid by urinating. This model has never been duplicated in another laboratory.

The model would benefit by further validation and characterization. Only one or two animals was observed at each time period, and only two controls were used — one at the beginning of the experiment and one at the end. Varying the intensity and duration of the stimulus in separate groups of rabbits could potenially provide more convincing negative and positive controls for the experiment.

CONCLUSION

These two rabbit models are the only experimental models that have been characterized, although other naturally occurring models exist (see Chapter 13). They produce changes that are consistent with each other, and may provide significant insight into the pathogenesis of stress fractures. Both show evidence of some periosteal reaction by three weeks, with progression and the formation of periosteal callus through about nine weeks. Both involve reactions on the anteromedial aspect of tibia consistent with tibial stress fractures in humans. Interestingly, both involve the formation of microcracks in the bony cortex and subsequent elevation of remodeling rate. This consistency in biological response suggests that microdamage and the remodeling reaction may be part of a positive feedback that underlies the pathogenesis of fracture development. Although similar histological evidence exists for human stress fractures (Chapter 10), these models could help to delineate whether these changes are necessary to development of a stress fracture or are incidental responses that occur in response to the fracture.

REFERENCES

1. Burr, D.B., Milgrom, C., Boyd, R.D., Higgins, W.L., Robin, G., and Radin, E.L., Experimental stress fractures of the tibia. Biological and mechanical aetiology in rabbits, *J. Bone Jt. Surg.*, 72B, 370, 1990.
2. Farkas, T., Boyd, R.D., Schaffler, M.B., Radin, E.L., and Burr, D.B., Early vascular changes in rabbit subchondral bone after repetitive impulsive loading, *Clin. Orthop. Rel. Res.*, 219, 259, 1987.
3. Burr, D.B., Bone, exercise, and stress fractures, *Exerc. Sport Sci. Rev.*, 25, 171, 1997.
4. Burr, D.B., The mechanical behavior of cortical bone *in vivo*, *J. Jpn. Soc. Bone Morphom.*, 8, 1, 1998.
5. Burr, D.B., Milgrom, C., Fyhrie, D., Forwood, M., Nyska, M., Finestone, A., Hoshaw, S., Saiag, E., and Simkin, A., *In vivo* measurements of human tibial strains during vigorous activity, *Bone*, 18, 405, 1996.
6. Reilly, D.T. and Burstein, A.H., The mechanical properties of cortical bone, *J. Bone Jt. Surg.*, 56A, 1001, 1974.
7. Schaffler, M.B. and Boyd, R.D., Bone remodeling and microdamage accumulation in experimental stress fracture, *Trans. Orthop. Res. Soc.*, 22, 113, 1997.
8. Garcia, J.E., Grabhorn, L.L., and Franklin, K.J., Factors associated with stress fractures in military recruits, *Mil. Med.*, 152, 45, 1987.
9. Gilbert, R.S. and Johnson, H.A., Stress fractures in military recruits — a review of twelve years' experience, *Mil. Med.*, 131, 716, 1966.
10. Kowal, D.M., Nature and causes of injuries in women resulting from an endurance training program, *Am. J. Sports Med.*, 8, 265, 1980.
11. Lee, C-H., Tsai, C-S., Lin, L-C., Pai, W-M., and Au, M-K., Stress fractures in military recruits — a report of 518 cases, *J. Orthop. Surg. ROC*, 10, 1, 1993.
12. Pester, S. and Smith, P.C., Stress fractures in the lower extremities of soldiers in basic training, *Orthop. Rev.*, 21, 297, 1992.
13. Reinker, K.A. and Ozburne, S., A comparison of male and female orthopaedic pathology in basic training, *Mil. Med.*, 144, 532, 1979.
14. Scully, T.J. and Besterman, G., Stress fracture — a preventable training injury, *Mil. Med.*, 147, 285, 1982.
15. Wilson, E.S. and Katz, F.N., Stress fractures, *Radiology*, 92, 481, 1969.
16. Giladi, M., Aharonson, Z., Stein, M., Danon, Y.L., and Milgrom, C., Unusual distribution and onset of stress fractures in soldiers, *Clin. Orthop. Rel. Res.*, 192, 142, 1985.
17. Protzman, R.R. and Griffis, C.G., Comparative stress fracture incidence in males and females in an equal training environment, *Athletic Training*, 12, 126, 1977.
18. Greaney, R.B., Gerber, F.H., Laughlin, R.L., Kmet, J.P., Metz, C.D., Kilcheski, T.S., Rao, B.R., and Silverman, E.D., Distribution and natural history of stress fractures in U.S. Marine recruits, *Radiology*, 146, 339, 1983.
19. Milgrom, C., Giladi, M., Stein, M., Kashtan, H., Margulies, J.Y., Chisin, R., Steinberg, R., and Aharonson, Z., Stress fractures in military recruits: a prospective study showing an unusually high incidence, *J. Bone Jt. Surg.*, 67B, 732, 1985.
20. Meurman, K.O. and Elfving, S., Stress fractures in soldiers: a multifocal bone disorder. A comparative radiological and scintigraphic study, *Radiology*, 134, 483, 1980.
21. Rosen, P.R., Micheli, L.J., and Treves, S., Early scintigraphic diagnosis of bone stress and fractures in athletic adolescents, *Pediatrics*, 70, 11, 1982.
22. Armstrong, J.R. and Tucker, W. E., *Injury in Sport: The Physiology, Prevention and Treatment of Injuries Associated with Sport*, Staples Press, London, 1964.

23. Belkin, S.C., Stress fractures in athletes, *Orthop. Clin. North Am.*, 11, 735, 1980.

24. Clement, D.B., Taunton, J., Smart, G.W., and McNicol, K.L., A survey of overuse running injuries, *Phys. Sportsmed.*, 9, 47, 1981.

25. Hulkko, A. and Orava, S., Stress fractures in athletes, *Int. J. Sports Med.*, 8, 221, 1987.

26. Matheson, G.O., Clement, D.B., and McKenzie, D.C., Stress fractures in athletes: a study of 320 cases, *Am. J. Sports Med.*, 15, 46, 1987.

27. McBryde, A.M., Jr., Stress fractures in athletes, *J. Sports Med.*, 3, 212, 1975.

28. McBryde, A.M., Jr., Stress fractures in runners, *Clin. Sports Med.*, 4, 737, 1985.

29. Orava, S., Puranen, J., and Ala-Ketola, L., Stress fractures caused by physical exercise, *Acta Orthop. Scand.*, 49, 19, 1978.

30. Orava, S. and Hulkko, A., Stress fractures of the mid-tibial shaft, *Acta Orthop. Scand.*, 55, 35, 1984.

31. Sullivan, D., Warren, R.F., Pavlov, H., and Kelman, G., Stress fractures in 51 runners, *Clin. Orthop. Rel. Res.*, 187, 188, 1984.

32. Taunton, J.E., Clement, D.B., and Webber, D., Lower extremity stress fractures in athletes, *Phys. Sportsmed.*, 9, 77, 1981.

33. Walter, N.E. and Wolf, M.D., Stress fractures in young athletes, *Am. J. Sports Med.*, 5, 165, 1977.

34. Zwas, S.T., Elkanovitch, R., and Frank, G., Interpretation and classification of bone scintigraphic finds in stress fractures, *J. Nucl. Med.*, 28, 452, 1987.

35. Li, G., Zhang, S., Chen, G., Chen, H., and Wang, A., Radiographic and histologic analyses of stress fracture in rabbit tibias, *Am. J. Sports Med.*, 13, 285, 1985.

36. Nunamaker, D.M., Butterweck, D.M., and Provost, M.T., Fatigue fractures in thoroughbred racehorses: relationships with age, peak bone strain, and training, *J. Orthop. Res.*, 8, 604, 1990.

37. Milgrom C., Finestone, A., Shlamkovitch, N., Rand, N., Lev, B., Simkin, A., and Wiener, M., Youth is a risk factor for stress fracture, *J. Bone Jt. Surg.*, 76B, 20, 1994.

CHAPTER 15

Prevention of Stress Fractures by Modifying Shoe Wear

Aharon S. Finestone

CONTENTS

Introduction..233
Heel Strike Shock Wave and Stress Fractures..234
Shoe Fit and Shoe Last Effects...236
Arch Height and Stress Fractures 237
Custom-Made Orthotics 239
Summary..243
References..243

INTRODUCTION

The idea that the incidence of stress fractures might be reduced by the use of orthotics or by changing shoe parameters is attractive. It promises a solution that does not require modifying or supervising training programs. The only requirement is purchase of the proper product. Manufacturers' frequent recommendations of shock absorbing inserts and soles are easily accepted into a simplistic concept that stress fractures are caused by a shock wave arising from the ground and propagated through the body. This lends itself to the idea that shock absorbers could diminish the stress fracture problem. The truth, as usual, is not so clear. In theory, the effect of footwear on any health parameter can be divided into three categories: a shock absorbing effect, biomechanical effects related to arch height and subtalar joint position manipulation, and effects that can be related to the shoe last.

HEEL STRIKE SHOCK WAVE AND STRESS FRACTURES

The shock wave initiated by the heel strike propagates through the body to the skull,[1] and is attenuated along the way.[2] Wearing inserts or shoes with better shock absorbing properties reduces the incoming shock wave at any particular site.[3,4] This concept has been applied to stress fracture prevention on several occasions in very different research environments.

Gardner et al. conducted a large prospective study among U.S. Army recruits at the Marine Training Center at Parris Island, South Carolina.[5] 3,025 basic training recruits participated in the study. Boots with sorbothane polymer insoles were issued to recruits in even-numbered platoons, and boots with a standard mesh insole were issued to recruits in odd-numbered platoons. Stress fracture incidence proximal to the foot decreased from 95 to 64%, but there was a non-significant increase in stress fractures in the foot from 20 to 71%. Gardner et al.'s negative results might be related to their method of diagnosing stress fractures (a pooling of radiologically positive findings with "clinically significant symptoms"). Another reason for the authors not finding a significant effect might be related to the insoles they used. Cinats et al. published a critical study on the insoles used in Gardner's study (Sorbothane, I.E.M. Orthopaedics, Aurora, Ohio). They found that the insoles had a long relaxation time of 2 seconds, compared with the foot strike, which is approximately 0.1 second while running. They concluded that these insoles might reduce 10% of the stress transmitted, but the claim that 95% of the impact energy is absorbed "is difficult to substantiate".[6]

Schwellnus et al. published results of a prospective, randomized study of recruits in the South African Army. They randomly issued neoprene insoles impregnated with nitrogen bubbles to 237 recruits, and a control group of 1151 recruits was not issued orthotics. They found significantly fewer overuse injuries in the group using the shock absorbing insoles, and fewer stress fractures in that group, but the latter was not statistically significant. Their diagnosis of stress fractures was based on plain film radiography, so some of their recruits with "tibial stress syndrome" and foot pain might have been under-diagnosed. This may explain their overall low incidence of stress fractures: 0% in the insole group, 1.4% in control group.[7] Sherman et al. found no effect of shock absorbing inserts on overuse injuries in U.S. Army basic trainees at Fort Lewis, as reported in post-training questionnaires and medical records.[8]

In a prospective study among elite Israeli infantry recruits, Milgrom et al. randomly assigned 187 recruits to train wearing basketball shoes, with a control group (203 recruits) training in standard military boots. Mechanical durometry tests showed that the basketball shoes had superior shock attenuation to that of the military boots. The maximum decelerations were 75 g at 3.8 ms for the basketball shoes and 128 g at 2.4 ms for the military boots. Proof of the *in vivo* shock attenuation was provided by comparing the shock wave at the tibial tubercle, while each recruit wore his allocated shoes. This was performed towards the end of the basic training at a time when the shoes were already broken in. At this point the shoes may have already lost some of their shock absorbency (running shoes' shock absorbency deteriorates significantly as a function of miles run, with only 45 to 60% of the initial shock

Tibial tubercle accelerations

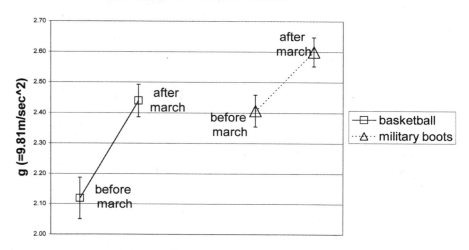

Figure 1 Accelerometry wearing different shoes, before and after a 23 km march.[12]

Table 1   Overuse Injuries in Basic Training, According to Shoe Type[12]

	Basketball Shoe (N = 187)	Standard Infantry Boot (N = 203)	P Value
Femoral stress fx	22 (11.8%)	16 (7.9%)	N. S.
Tibial stress fx	34 (18.2%)	33 (16.3%)	N. S.
Metatarsal stress fx	0	7 (3.4%)	<0.05
Total stress fx	49 (26.2%)	44 (21.7%)	N. S.
Ankle sprains	32 (17.1%)	37 (18.2%)	N. S.
Foot problems*	29 (15.5%)	59 (29.1%)	<0.001
Total injuries	169 (90.4%)	184 (90.6%)	N. S.

fx = fracture

* Not including stress fractures.

absorbency remaining after 500 miles).[9-11] There were significantly lower tibial accelerometry using the basketball shoes compared with the military boots, both before and after a 23 km march (Figure 1).[12] Training with basketball shoes rather than the standard boots resulted in a statistically significant reduction in metatarsal stress fractures and other overuse injuries of the feet, but no decrease in stress fractures of the long bones, overall stress fractures, or overall overuse injury incidence (Table 1). An obvious explanation for the decrease in metatarsal stress fractures when training in basketball shoes is their superior shock attenuation (even though the effect of shoe last factors cannot be ruled out.)[12,13]

The finding that better shoe shock attenuation reduced metatarsal stress fractures but not stress fractures of the femur and tibia clearly depicts a different mechanism for fractures in these locations. Metatarsal stress fractures are related to the vertical forces transferred from the ground to the foot, and these can be attenuated with shoe-wear shock absorbency. This is in agreement with other data, showing that stress fractures of the long bones are probably not related directly to these longitudinal forces, and are almost certainly not related to shock waves. Giladi et al. and Milgrom et al. demonstrated that tibial stress fractures are caused by bending and twisting forces.[14-17]

SHOE FIT AND SHOE LAST EFFECTS

Another parameter that has been examined is the effect of appropriateness of shoe fit on stress fractures. Shoe sizes are based on length. A USA size 10 or a european size 44 are made for a foot of the same length. With a multi-width system, after choosing the length, the width (or mid-foot circumference) is chosen. In a system where there is only one width per length, narrow foot subjects would "wobble" mediolaterally in the shoes to a certain extent (this can be partially compensated for with tighter lacing). Wide foot individuals would have to compensate by choosing larger sizes (lengths). This would probably entail some antero-posterior foot play in the shoe. This assumption regarding the choice of shoe sizes was clearly proved by Finestone et al.[18] Recruits chose military boots and basketball shoes larger than predicted by their foot length (european size = 3/2 foot length in cm). The quartile of recruits with the largest foot width chose larger shoes than those in the other three quartiles. The difference between expected and chosen was significantly different (military boot 3.4 versus 2.9, $P < 0.0001$; basketball shoe 4.7 versus 4.3, $P < 0.05$). There were significantly more overuse injuries in the top and bottom quartiles than in the center ones (94.2 versus 86.7%, $P < 0.02$), but no significant difference was found in stress fracture incidence.[18]

Several studies have been performed in the U.S. Army comparing different types of boots. Bensel found no difference in clinically diagnosed foot stress fractures when comparing tropical and leather combat boots.[19] Bensel and Kish found more sick call and reduced duty in soldiers wearing hot weather boots versus black leather boots. This was probably due to the higher incidence of blisters and lace lesions, but no difference was seen in stress fracture incidence.[20]

Milgrom et al. measured tibial strains while walking and running in different types of shoes.[21] Shoes that reduce strains or strain rates might be expected to reduce the risk for stress fracture.[22] When comparing standard lightweight Israeli infantry boots to boots made with identical soles but on different lasts (Zohar®, Zohar shoe manufacturer, Tel Aviv, Israel), significantly lower strains and strain rates were noted with the Zohar boot on treadmill walking. No difference was found in track running. The Zohar last is characterized by a deep heel cup, and broad midfoot support, and it allows for increased toe motion.

These findings imply that the type of shoe last can affect tibial strains, but the mechanism is not clear. As so little research has been published on any aspect of shoe lasts, there is definitely a need for further investigation. This should probably include the shoe lasts' effect on all measurable parameters in the foot and leg, including metatarsal strains.

ARCH HEIGHT AND STRESS FRACTURES

The relationship between arch height and stress fractures has been studied, with conflicting results.[19,23-26] This is probably due to the fact that there is no clear definition of arch height (bony versus soft tissue, where the height should be measured, and whether the measurement should be performed while weight bearing). An important consequence of this is the high inter-observer variance among health care providers of different disciplines regarding structural pathologies of the foot related to the arch. In some cases, normal healthy young subjects are divided into 40% low arch, 30% high arch, and 30% normal. Even if this were based on objective scientific methods of examination, accepting so much pathology infers some error.

In a subjective evaluation of arch height by informal observation, Giladi et al. found fewer overall femoral and tibial stress fractures in low arch subjects.[27] Simkin et al. measured arch height by performing weight-bearing true lateral radiography of both feet[28] by the method previously described by Clark.[29] They measured three parameters: 1) the calcaneal angle (CA), between the horizontal and inferior surfaces of the calcaneus, 2) the forefoot angle (FOR) between the horizontal and the line between the medial sesamoid and inferior talar surface, and 3) the height–length ratio (H/L), where height is the distance from the platform to the inferior talar surface and length is from the posterior calcaneus to the first metatarsophalangeal joint (MTPJ) (Figure 2). Comparing these three measurements did not yield high correlation coefficients. When calcaneal angle was taken as the measurement of arch height, recruits with low arches had significantly fewer femoral stress fractures than their high-arched counterparts (2.6 versus 15.5%, P < 0.006). There were also fewer tibial stress fractures (9.8 versus 15.7%, NS), but *more* metatarsal stress fractures (6.3% versus 3.2%, NS). This suggests a different pathophysiology for stress fractures of the long bones than for stress fractures of the metatarsals.

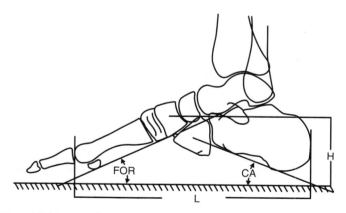

Figure 2   Measurements used to quantitate arch height.[28] CA, calcaneal angle, between the horizontal and inferior surface of the calcaneus. FOR, forefoot angle, between the horizontal and the line between the medial sesamoid and the inferior talar surface. H/L, height–length ratio, where height is the distance from the platform to the inferior talar surface, and the length is from the posterior calcaneus to the first MTPJ. (From Simken et al., Combined effect of foot arch and an orthotic device on stress fractures, *Foot Ankle*, 10, 25, 1989. With permission.)

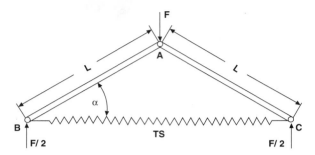

Figure 3 Simkin's simplified model of the foot as an energy absorbing device. A,B,C: Friction-less hinges. L: length of rigid elements; α: inclination angle of rigid elements; TS: tension spring; F: vertical load. (Modified from Simkin et al., Role of the calcaneal inclination in the energy storage capacity of the human foot, *Med. Biol. Eng. Comput.*, 28, 149, 1990. With permission.)

Examining the effect of a non-custom, semi-rigid 3° varus hind foot posted orthotic device dispensed randomly to 113 of 285 elite infantry recruits, Milgrom et al. found fewer femoral, tibial, and metatarsal stress fractures in the group using the orthotics, but the results were only statistically significant for femoral stress fractures.[30]

Simkin et al. analyzed these data according to arch height,[28] and found a different effect in high and low arched subjects. High arched recruits using the orthotic had fewer femoral stress fractures than those not using the device (5.1 versus 15.5%, $P < 0.003$). An opposite effect was noted among low arched subjects: using the orthotic increased femoral stress fracture incidence more than threefold (from 2.6 to 7.9%, NS). In low arched subjects, defined by height/length ratio, using the device was correlated with fewer metatarsal stress fractures (0 versus 6.0%, NS).

Simkin et al. conceptualized the foot as an energy absorbing device (Figure 3). Feet with low arches absorb more energy while training, and therefore the foot is more susceptible to stress fracture. However, the energy that is propagated to the tibia and femur will be less, thereby decreasing the likelihood of stress fracture in these bones. Feet with higher arches will absorb less energy, and therefore be injured less. The energy will be transferred upwards and increase the likelihood of tibial and femoral stress fracture. The authors observed clinically that by using their semi-rigid shock absorbing orthotic device in high arched subjects (with low energy absorbing capacity) it was possible to reduce the energy transferred to the long bones. Using this same device in low arched subjects seemed to interfere with the natural energy absorbing capacity of the foot, and therefore increased femoral stress fractures but lowered the incidence of metatarsal stress fractures. To substantiate their energy absorbing model, they created a biomechanical model of the foot based on spring physics. This model indeed demonstrated that the foot could be looked upon as an energy absorbing device, and more importantly, that more energy would be dissipated with lower arches.[31]

Another study of foot shape performed by a different group of researchers on Israeli soldiers reached similar conclusions. The longitudinal arch was measured by analyzing plantar foot pressures. Significantly more stress fractures were found in high arched subjects than in low arched subjects.[32] The obvious limitations of this study are its retrospective nature and lack of analysis of fracture location.

It may be concluded from these studies that arch height plays a role in stress fractures of the tibia, femur, and metatarsals, but the mechanisms are clearly different. Moreover, manipulation of stress fracture incidence by using energy absorbing orthotics might change the anatomic distribution of the stress fractures without causing an overall decrease. In theory, therefore, the arch height of each subject should be considered, together with the risk for each type of fracture, and the importance attributable to each entity (femoral stress fractures are obviously a greater health and training predicament than metatarsal ones).

CUSTOM-MADE ORTHOTICS

An obvious question is whether training in custom-made shoe orthotics can affect stress fracture incidence. There are two relatively common methods of producing custom-made orthotics, and each method characteristically uses its own type of materials. In the following discussion they will be referred to as "soft" orthotics and "semi-rigid" orthotics.

"Soft" or "accommodative" orthotics are usually made from Plastazote® (Zotefoams, Inc., 319 Airport Road, Hackettstown, NJ, 07840). This is a thermoplastic polyethylene foam, which utilizes pure nitrogen as a blowing agent to produce a uniform closed cell structure, and according to the volume of bubbles, different grades of hardness are created. The types of material are usually related to by their specific gravity. The foot is held by the orthotist with the subject in a sitting position. Foot prints are made into Biofoam®, a compliant synthetic material that deforms when pressure is applied to it, and then "remembers" the shape of the foot sole. The orthotist might hold the subtalar joint in "neutral position", but this is not always performed — not all personnel making orthotics are qualified. Pressure is applied by the orthotist from above the knee, thus giving a partial weight-bearing effect. Plaster of Paris is poured into the imprints, which, on setting, creates a positive model of the sole. Layers of Plastazote are applied over the sole model. They accept the form of the sole when heated, and by doing so provide a well fitted orthotic that equalizes the pressure under various areas of the foot. This type of orthotic extends the whole length of the foot. Because of the relative softness of the Plastazote, these orthotics are not really suitable for angular corrections. There is serious doubt whether this material is appropriate for making insoles.[11,33]

"Semi-rigid" orthotics are fabricated using more standardized techniques, but here also, methods vary. The basic concept of these orthotics was presented by Root et al.,[34,35] and relates to modifying the foot biomechanics so that the subtalar joint will be in the so-called neutral position. With the patient supine and the foot supported from the upper hind leg, the subtalar joint is manipulated into neutral position, determined by the relationship of the talus to the navicular. Plaster of Paris is applied to the foot, while the foot is kept in neutral subtalar position, and the plaster is allowed to set, creating a slipper cast. Markings are made on the midline of the soleus-gastrocnemius complex and midline of the posterior aspect of the calcaneus. This line is also carried on to the slipper cast, and the angle between the leg and hind-foot is noted, with neutral subtalar joint. These measurements are helpful in positioning the orthotic with relation to the horizontal. From this point, development relies on two main methods: manual and computer assisted. Manually, once the slipper cast has set completely, a model of the foot is created by pouring plaster of Paris into the slipper cast and letting it set. Firm material is set over the model, and using the measurements described above, the model and orthotic unit are balanced so that the subtalar joint will be in neutral position when weight bearing. The computer assisted method scans the slipper cast, and, using various measurements, creates a semi-rigid orthotic using CAD-CAM milling techniques. Thickness of the orthotic is determined by the subject's weight. The main functional part of these orthotics relates to the hind-foot, and the rigid part of the orthotic therefore usually only goes as far as the middle of the metatarsals. This orthotic may be covered with a full length piece of leather or similar material. In the future, optical scanning of the foot may replace casting as a means of making a negative of the foot.

In a prospective study of the effect of custom-made orthotics on stress fracture incidence among elite Israeli infantry recruits, Finestone et al. randomly dispensed three types of orthotics to a group of 404 recruits. Semi-rigid orthotics, manufactured using CAD-CAM milling techniques[36,37] (ProLab Orthotics, San Francisco, CA) were issued to 132 recruits. The orthotic was ¾ length polypropelene module, without a top covering. Soft custom-made orthotics were issued to 128 recruits. The orthotics were molded from three layers of Pelite® of different densities (upper layer: 80, middle layer: 60, lower layer: 80). The control group consisted of two subgroups: 126 recruits were issued sham orthotics (without supportive or shock absorbing qualities), and 18 recruits with no insoles. The recruits were followed carefully during 14 weeks of basic training. There was a significant reduction in stress fractures of the long bones in both groups of recruits using custom-made orthotics compared to the sham orthotic group ($P < 0.02$). When the custom-made orthotics were not grouped, the group with the "soft" orthotics demonstrated the most significant reduction in stress fracture incidence (Figure 4). Soft orthotics were clearly better tolerated than the semi-rigid, as demonstrated by the recruits evaluation and the dropout rate (Figure 5). There was similarity between the patterns of stress fracture incidence and comfort (discomfort), possibly indicating some effect of discomfort on stress fracture incidence. Direct conclusions are difficult to draw, as comfort data included recruits who dropped from the study. This was relevant for general appraisal of the orthotics but irrelevant to the effect of the orthotics on recruits who used them throughout the 14 week period (Figure 6). It can therefore be stated that in this study, discomfort was not an independent contributor to the risk for stress fracture. Even so, the comfort variable cannot be dismissed, and recently it has gained increasing attention.[38]

The main findings of the study were that training with soft and semi-rigid biomechanical custom-made orthotics was associated with fewer stress fractures. This reduction in stress fracture incidence was greater with the "soft" orthotics. There are several problems encountered when interpreting the results. Most important is the fact that even though the results are significant, no mechanism for the effect was identified. It is also not clear whether the orthotics affected the whole population

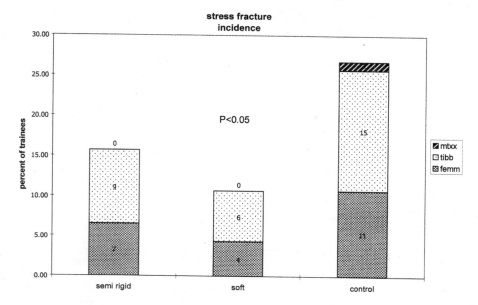

Figure 4 Stress fracture incidence by type of orthotic.[37] Number of recruits is marked in each box. Overall significance: P < 0.05. When custom made orthotics are grouped together, P < 0.02. mtxx = metatarsal stress fractures; tibb = tibia; femm = femoral

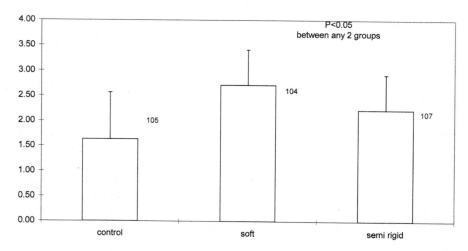

Figure 5 Comfort scores for orthotics, corrected data, dropouts given zero score.[37] Number of recruits is marked by each box. P < 0.05 for every set of paired groups.

or just a subgroup. It might be claimed that walking with orthotics which correct the position of the subtalar joint to neutral makes for better walking biomechanics. This might be so, but the "soft" orthotics were less accurately positioned with respect to

comfort scores

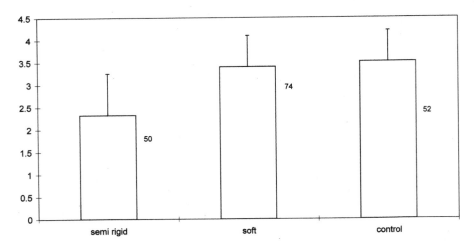

Figure 6 Comfort scores for orthotics, raw data, not including dropouts.[37] Number of recruits is marked by each box. Semi-rigid orthotics were significantly less comfortable than both other groups (P < 0.05).

neutral subtalar position, and because they were soft, their ability to hold the foot in neutral position was limited. The semi-rigid orthotics used in the study were relatively uncomfortable. This was partially due to the fact that the orthotics were only three-quarters the length of the foot, extending from the heel to toe end, just before the toes, and weren't covered with a soft material. Had they been fabricated with top covers, compliance would certainly have improved, and also perhaps their effect on stress fractures. Semi-rigid orthotics are dispensed according to the biomechanical theory that the subtalar joint should be in neutral position, and the orthotics are fabricated to correct deviations from neutral, but there is no conclusive proof of this.

There has also been some controversy recently regarding the angle of correction.[39] Pierrynowski et al.,[40] following Scott et al.[41] claimed that the subtalar neutral position is irrelevant, and suggested that a more appropriate measurement would be the "resting standing foot position" (defined as the position of a subject who is standing comfortably with feet apart, knees extended, and the heel and second toe aligned with the plane of progression). This difference in measuring subtalar joint position and motion has been clearly described,[42] with neutral measured by aligning the talus and navicular, giving about 3° varus (inversion) of the heel to the tibia in normal subjects. The difference between the two approaches might only be several unmeasurable degrees, but this demonstrates lack of precision in the field. The failure to find a significant effect on biomechanical parameters such as maximal pronation also causes some doubt regarding the effect of orthotics. Brown et al. measured pronation and calcaneal inversion in subjects with forefoot varus deformity. Biomechanical custom made orthotics, arch supports, and no orthotics were compared, and failed to control pronation.[43]

Further research into the mechanism of the effect of biomechanical orthotics is necessary. This could indicate which population subgroups might benefit from biomechanical orthotics, which would benefit from standard orthotics (possibly one of several standard orthotics with different arch supports), and which would need no orthotics. In this manner, better cost effective predictions could be made.

SUMMARY

Better shock absorbency of shoes is likely to reduce incidence of metatarsal stress fracture, but even though orthotics may be helpful, modification of the soles would probably be the better approach. Use of standard orthotics (not custom made) might play a role in modifying stress fracture morbidity, possibly by dispensing different types of orthotics to different subjects, but this requires knowledge of the arch height, so it might not be practical. Moreover, the effect is relatively complicated, and more research would need to be invested before any recommendations could be made.

Making custom orthotics for patient comfort is more an art than a science. This makes comparative studies difficult to perform, and comparing studies performed in a variety of settings by different teams, each using its own methods must be done with great care. Taking this into account, though, the present body of information justifies prophylactic custom-made orthotic issue. More research into the mechanism of the effect is necessary for better and more standardized production, and for defining sub-population effects.

REFERENCES

1. Wosk, J. and Voloshin, A., Wave attenuation in skeletons of young healthy persons, *J. Biomech.,* 14, 261, 1981.
2. Voloshin, A., Wosk, J., and Brull, M., Force wave transmission through the human locomotor system, *J. Biomech. Eng.,* 103, 49, 1981.
3. Voloshin, A. and Wosk, J., Influence of artificial shock absorbers on human gait, *Clin. Orthop.,* 160, 52, 1981.
4. Wosk, I., Folman, Y., and Liberty, S., Effect of artificial shock absorbers on heel-strike transients, *Harefuah,* 108, 128, 1985.
5. Gardner, L.I., Dziados, J.E., Jones, B.H., Brundage, J.F., Harris, J.M., Sullivan, R., and Gill, P., Prevention of lower extremity stress fractures: a controlled trial of a shock absorbent insole, *Am. J. Public Health,* 78, 1563, 1988.
6. Cinats, J., Reid, D.C., and Haddow, J.B., A biomechanical evaluation of sorbothane, *Clin. Orthop.,* 222, 281, 1987.
7. Schwellnus, M.P., Jordaan, G., and Noakes, T.D., Prevention of common overuse injuries by the use of shock absorbing insoles. A prospective study, *Am. J. Sports Med.,* 18, 636, 1990.
8. Sherman, R.A., Karstetter, K.W., May, H., and Woerman, A.L., Prevention of lower limb pain in soldiers using shock-absorbing orthotics, *J. Am. Podiatr. Med. Assoc.,* 86, 117, 1996.

9. Cook, S.D., Kester, M.A., and Brunet M.E., Shock absorption characteristics of running shoes, *Am. J. Sports Med.*, 13, 248, 1985.

10. Cook, S.D., Kester, M.A., Brunet, M.E. and Haddad R.J. Biomechanics of running shoe performance, *Clin. Sports Med.*, 4, 619, 1985.

11. Pratt, D.J., Long term comparison of some shock attenuating insoles, *Prosthet. Orthot. Int.* 14, 59, 1990.

12. Finestone, A.S., The effect of improved shoe shock attenuation on the incidence of stress fractures in infantry recruits in the I.D.F., MD thesis, Hebrew University, Jerusalem, 1990.

13. Milgrom, C., Finestone, A., Shlamkovitch, N., Wosk, J., Laor, A., Voloshin, A., and Eldad, A., Prevention of overuse injuries of the foot by improved shoe shock attenuation. A randomized prospective study, *Clin. Orthop.*, 281, 189, 1992.

14. Giladi, M., Milgrom, C., Simkin, A., Stein, M., Kashtan, H., Margulies, J., Rand, N., Chisin, R., Steinberg, R., Aharonson, Z., Kedem, R., and Frankel, V.H., Tibial bone width: a risk factor for stress fractures. Stress fractures and tibial bone width, *J. Bone Jt. Surg.*, 69B, 326, 1987.

15. Milgrom, C., Giladi, M., Simkin, A., Rand, N., Kedem, R., Kashtan, H., Stein, M., and Gomori, M., The area of inertia of the tibia: a risk factor for stress fractures, *J. Biomechan.*, 22, 1243, 1989.

16. Milgrom, C., Giladi, M., Simkin, A., Rand, N., Kedem, R., Kashtan, H., and Stein, M., An analysis of the biomechanical mechanism of tibial stress fractures among Israeli infantry recruits. A prospective study, *Clin. Orthop.*, 231, 216, 1988.

17. Finestone, A., Shlamkovitch, N., Eldad, A., Wosk, J., Laor, A., Danon, Y.L., and Milgrom, C., Risk factors for stress fractures among Israeli infantry recruits, *Mil. Med.*, 156, 528, 1991.

18. Finestone, A., Shlamkovitch, N., Eldad, A., Karp, A., and Milgrom, C., A prospective study of the effect of the appropriateness of foot-shoe fit and training shoe type on the incidence of overuse injuries among military recruits, *Mil. Med.*, 157, 489, 1992.

19. Bensel, C.K., The effects of tropical and leather combat boots on lower extremity disorders among US Marine Corps recruits, U.S. Army Natick R&D Command, TR 76-49-CEMEL, 1976.

20. Bensel, C.K. and Kish, R.N., Lower extremity disorders among men and women in army basic training and effects of two types of boots, U.S. Army Natick R&D Laboratories, NATICK/TR-83/026, 1983.

21. Milgrom, C., Burr, D., Fyhrie, D., Hoshaw, S., Finestone, A., Nyska, M., Davidson, R., Mendelson, S., Giladi, M., Liebergall, M., Lehnert, B., Voloshin, A., and Simkin, A., A comparison of the effect of shoes on human tibial axial strains recorded during dynamic loading, *Foot Ankle,* 19, 85, 1998.

22. Milgrom, C., Simkin, A., Eldad, A., Nyska, M., and Finestone, A., Using bone's adaptation ability to lower the incidence of stress fractures, *Am. J. Sports Med.*, accepted, 1999.

23. Jones, B.H., Harris, J.McA., Vinh, T.N., and Rubin, C., Exercise induced stress fractures and stress reactions of bone: epidemiology, etiology and classification, in *Exercise and Sport Sciences Reviews,* Padolf, K.B., Ed., Williams & Williams, Baltimore, Vol. 11, 1989, 379.

24. Meyerding, H.W. and Pollock, G.A., March fracture, *Surg. Gynec. Obstet.*, 67, 234, 1938.

25. Montgomery, L.C., Nelson, F.R.T., Norton, J.P., and Deuster, P.A., Orthopedic history and examination in the etiology of overuse injuries, *Med. Sci. Sports Exerc.*, 21, 237, 1989.

26. Viitasalo, J.T. and Kvist, M., Some biomechanical aspects of the foot and ankle in athletes with and without shin splints, *Am. J. Sports Med.*, 11, 125, 1983.

27. Giladi, M., Milgrom, C., Simkin, A., Stein, M., Kashtan, H., Margulies, J., Chisin, R., Steinberg, R., and Aharonson, Z., The low arch. A protective factor against stress fractures, *Orthop. Rev.*, 14, 81, 1985.

28. Simkin, A., Leichter, I., Giladi, M., Stein, M., and Milgrom, C., Combined effect of foot arch and an orthotic device on stress fractures, *Foot Ankle,* 10, 25, 1989.

29. Clark K.C., *Positioning in Radiography,* 9th ed., Year Book Medical Publishers, Chicago, 1973, 87.

30. Milgrom, C., Giladi, M., Kashtan, H., Simkin, A., Chisin, R., Margulies, J., Steinberg, R., Aharonson, Z., and Stein, M., A prospective study of the effect of a shock-absorbing orthotic device on the incidence of stress fractures in military recruits, *Foot Ankle,* 6, 101, 1985.

31. Simkin, A. and Leichter, I., Role of the calcaneal inclination in the energy storage capacity of the human foot, *Med. Biol. Eng. Comput.*, 28, 149, 1990.

32. Brosh, T. and Arkan, M., Towards early detection of the tendency to stress fractures, *Clin. Biomech.*, 9, 111, 1994.

33. Pratt, D.J., Medium term comparison of shock attenuating insoles using a spectral analysis technique, *J. Biomed. Eng.*, 10, 426, 1988.

34. Root, M.L., Orien, W.P., Weed, J.H., and Hughes, R.J., *Biomechanical Examination of the Foot,* Vol. I, Clinical Biomechanics, Los Angeles, 1971.

35. Root, M.L., Orien, W.P., and Weed, J.N., Normal motion of the foot and leg in gait, in *Normal and Abnormal Function of the Foot: Clinical Biomechanics,* Vol. II, Clinical Biomechanics, Los Angeles, 1977.

36. Finestone, A., Giladi, M., Elad, H., Salmon, A., Mendelson, S., Eldad, A., and Milgrom, C., Prevention of stress fractures using custom biomechanical shoe orthoses, *Clin. Orthop.,* 360, 182, 1999.

37. Finestone, A.S., Poliack, G., Salmon, A., Elad, H., Mandel, D., and Milgrom C., The effect of custom made orthotics on stress fractures and overuse injuries in infantry recruits, *IDF Report Shloshet Regalim*, October, 1996.

38. Nigg, B.M., Nurse, M.A., and Stefanyshyn, D.J., Shoe inserts and orthotics for sports and physical activities, *Med. Sci. Sports Exerc.*, 31S, 421, 1999.

39. Sobel, E. and Levitz, S.J., Reappraisal of the negative impression cast and the subtalar joint neutral position, *J. Am. Pod. Med. Ass.*, 87, 32, 1997.

40. Pierrynowski, M.R. and Smith, S.B., Rear foot inversion/eversion during gait relative to the subtalar joint neutral position, *Foot Ankle*, 17, 406, 1996.

41. Scott, S.H. and Winter, D.A., Talocrural and talocalcaneal joint kinematics and kinetics during the stance phase of walking, *J. Biomech.*, 24, 743, 1991.

42. Milgrom, C., Giladi, M., Simkin, A., Stein, M., Kashtan, H., Margulies, J., Steinberg, R., and Aharonson, Z., The normal range of subtalar inversion and eversion in young males as measured by three different techniques, *Foot Ankle*, 6, 143, 1985.

43. Brown, G.P., Donatelli, R., Catlin, P.A., and Wooden, M.J., The effect of two type of foot orthoses on rearfoot mechanics, *J. Orthop. Sports Phys. Ther.*, 21, 258, 1995.

CHAPTER 16

Exercise Programs That Prevent or Delay the Onset of Stress Fracture

Charles Milgrom and Richard Shaffer

CONTENTS

Introduction 247
Prior Training Activities Associated with Stress Fracture Risk 248
Bone Strengthening Exercises in the Israeli Infantry Recruit Model 248
Measurement of In Vivo Tibial Strains During Exercises 250
Bone Strengthening in the American Military 253
Home Exercises That Can Strengthen Bone and Thereby Limit Stress
    Fractures 255
Conclusion 255
References 256

INTRODUCTION

In ideal medicine, prevention is the ultimate goal for disease control. According to this ideal, effective treatment is only necessary for individuals who fall through the prevention safety net. Strategies for stress fracture prevention include strengthening bone appropriately before training, altering training to change bone's exposure to cyclic loading, and identification of risk factors for stress fracture.[1] The focus of this chapter is on the first two strategies. Most of the related data come from studies of military recruits rather than athletes. The recruit model has the advantage of uniform training, central control, and predictable high stress fracture incidences.

PRIOR TRAINING ACTIVITIES ASSOCIATED
WITH STRESS FRACTURE RISK

Can stress fractures be prevented by programs of early bone strengthening exercises? Gilbert and Johnson first alluded to this possibility in their recollections of 12 years experience in the American military.[2] They noted that recruits who led sedentary existences prior to basic training were at a high risk for developing stress fractures; those who participated in varsity sports were protected. Leabhart,[3] and Provost and Morris[4] made similar observations from retrospective studies. Greaney et al.,[5] found in a review of bone scans that marine recruits who participated in long distance running before military induction had fewer scintigraphic foci indicating stress fracture than did non runners. They, however, did not identify other types of physical exercise that protected against stress fracture.

To test the hypothesis that bone strengthening exercises can prevent stress fracture, Mustajoki et al.[6] undertook a controlled prospective study of the effect of pre-training physical fitness and sport activities on the incidence of stress fracture in a group of Finnish military recruits. Their results were disappointing in that they found no correlation between previous physical activity and stress fracture risk in their military study population; this included long distance running.

A similar prospective study was performed on a population of elite Israeli infantry recruits during 14 weeks of basic training.[7] Prior to beginning training, each recruit was questioned about his participation in sports activities. This participation was evaluated according to parameters of duration of participation, number of training sessions per week, duration of each training session, distance of training, and level of competition. The aerobic fitness of recruits was assessed by calculating VO_2 max. Like the Mustajoki study, no correlation was found between the recruits' prior participation in sports or their aerobic fitness and the incidence of stress fractures in basic training.

These studies of Swissa et al.[7] and Mustajoki et al.[6] seem to contradict what one would expect according to the so-called law formulated by Wolff in 1892: "Every change in the form or function of bone or of their function alone is followed by certain definite changes in their internal architecture, and equally definite alteration in their external conformation, in accordance with mathematical laws." Milgrom et al. observed in a subsequent study that while the incidence of stress fracture is high during Israeli infantry basic training, it is much lower in subsequent training courses in spite of higher physical demands on the same recruits.[8] This supports the concept of bone as a material which adapts to its strain environment, strengthening itself when strains and strain rates are high if given adequate time.

BONE STRENGTHENING EXERCISES IN THE ISRAELI
INFANTRY RECRUIT MODEL

The Israeli Army Medical Corps has one of the largest and most complete stress fracture data banks in the world. This includes data from a series of prospective

Table 1   Incidence of Stress Fracture Among Recruits Who Played Ball Sports 2 Years Before Induction Versus Those Who Didn't (1988 Infantry Induction Group)

| | Stress Fracture | Number of Army Recruits | | | Significance of Difference in Incidence |
		No Ball Sports Played	Ball Sports Played	Total	
All	Present	76	17	93	p = 0.001
		28.90%	13.18%	23.72%	
	Absent	187	112	299	
		71.10%	86.82%	76.27%	
Tibial	Present	61	6	67	p = 0.001
		23.19%	4.65%	17.09%	
	Absent	202	123	325	
		76.81%	95.35%	82.9%	
Femoral	Present	28	10	38	p = 0.363
		10.65%	7.75%	9.69%	
	Absent	235	119	354	
		89.35%	92.25%	90.3%	

stress fracture and overuse injury epidemiology, and from intervention studies done over the past 15 years. Most of these studies were done on the same military base using a standard experimental protocol with only minor variations. Because of this, the Israeli infantry recruit is an ideal model for the study of stress fracture. In the first epidemiological study in 1983, no correlation was found between pre-training sport activity and stress fractures.[1] The frequency of stress fractures was almost identical (31%) among those who participated and those who did not participate in sport activities prior to basic training. When results were analyzed for specific sport activities and stress fracture incidence, no correlation was found.

In a subsequent 1988 prospective study,[9] the first evidence that pre-training sports activities could lower the incidence of stress fractures in infantry recruits was found (Table 1). Recruits who played ball sports at least three times a week for more than two years prior to basic training were found to sustain a 13% incidence of stress fractures in basic training versus 28% among recruits who did not play ball sports (p = 0.001). Why the discrepancy between the findings of this and the previous study? The answer given was the increased popularity in Israel of basketball over soccer. By 1998 basketball replaced soccer as the number one ball sport among recruits.

In a subsequent 1990 Israeli study, this significant association was noted again (Table 2). Recruits who played ball sports sustained a 17% incidence of stress fractures in basic training compared to 27% among those who did not play ball sports (p = 0.046). Again, participation in other types of sports including long distance running was not found to lower the risk for stress fracture. By 1995 the full effect of the Michael Jordan phenomenon could be seen. In a 1995 study, 90% of recruits who played ball sports played basketball as their first sport. The incidence of stress fractures among those who played ball sports was 3.6% and among those who did not play ball sports was 18.8% (p = 0.005). There was also a statistically significant relationship when stress fractures were categorized anatomically to tibia and femur.

Table 2   Incidence of Stress Fracture Among Recruits Who Played Ball Sports 2 Years Before Induction Versus Those Who Didn't (1990 Infantry Induction Group)

| | Stress Fracture | Number of Army Recruits | | | Significance of Difference in Incidence |
		No Ball Sports Played	Ball Sports Played	Total	
All	Present	82	15	97	p = 0.046
		26.97%	16.67%	24.62%	
	Absent	222	75	297	
		73.03%	83.33%	75.38%	
Tibial	Present	63	11	74	p = 0.07
		20.72%	12.22%	18.78%	
	Absent	241	79	320	
		79.28%	87.78%	81.22%	
Femoral	Present	21	1	22	p = 0.035
		6.91%	1.11%	5.58%	
	Absent	283	89	272	
		93.09%	98.89%	94.42%	

Table 3   Incidence of Stress Fractures Among Recruits Who Played Ball Sports 2 Years Before Induction Versus Those Who Didn't (1995 Infantry Induction Group)

| | Stress Fracture | Number of Army Recruits | | | Significance of Difference in Incidence |
		No Ball Sports Played	Ball Sports Played	Total	
All	Present	52	2	54	p = 0.005
		18.77%	3.64%	16.26%	
	Absent	225	53	278	
		81.23%	96.36%	83.73%	
Tibial	Present	41	2	43	p = 0.024
		14.80%	3.64%	12.95%	
	Absent	236	53	289	
		85.20%	96.36%	87.04%	
Femoral	Present	28	0	28	p = 0.014
		10.11%	0%	8.43%	
	Absent	249	55	304	
		89.89%	100%	91.56%	

MEASUREMENT OF *IN VIVO* TIBIAL STRAINS DURING EXERCISES

To understand why playing basketball decreases stress fracture risk and running does not, it is important to consider the *in vivo* strain and strain rates that occur during basketball and compare them to walking and running. Lanyon et al., in their pioneering work, measured *in vivo* strains on the anteromedial tibial midshaft of a 35 year-old male during treadmill walking.[10] Their work demonstrated that the development of strain in bone during gait consists of a series of discrete events in which bone is deformed from a particular direction, released, then loaded from

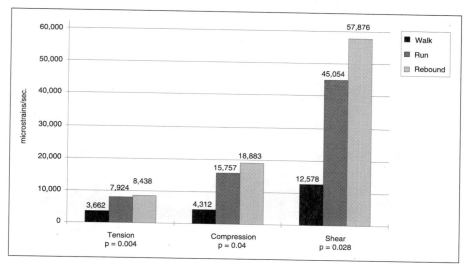

Figure 1 Comparison of *in vivo* maximal tibial strain rates during different activities.

another direction. This suggests that during gait there is an alteration in muscle force and direction of pull that quickly varies the strain on a given site. Because of the technological restraints of that time, Lanyon et al.[10] could not perform mobile strain recordings during vigorous exercises. Subsequently, Burr et al.,[11] using a portable recording system, measured *in vivo* tibial strains in a 49 year-old during vigorous physical activity that mimicked military training. They found the highest tibial strain and strain rates occurred during sprinting on a level surface and during zigzag running uphill and downhill. The strain levels during these activities were two to three times higher than strains recorded during walking. Strain rates during basketball were not measured in the Burr et al.[11] study.

Milgrom et al., using percutaneous strain gaged staples mounted in a rosette pattern, measured principal compression and tension strains and shear strains as well as strain rates in three subjects during walking, running, and playing basketball.[9] The principal compression strain was 48% higher, the principal tension strain 15% higher, and the shear strain 64% higher during basketball rebounding than during running. The compressive strain rate was 20% higher, the tension strain rate 6% higher, and the shear strain rate 28% higher during basketball rebounding than during running (Figure 1).

On the basis of the strain measurements in the Milgrom et al.[9] experiment, basketball would seem to have the highest potential to influence adaptive remodeling and strengthen lower extremity long bones. Another reason may be because it is an exercise which is multidirectional, with multiple shifts of vectors. Running generally involves monotonous repetition of the same pattern of activity. Exercises that change the strain distribution are likely to be potent osteogenic stimuli. Lanyon proposed the strain error distribution hypothesis.[12] According to this hypothesis, the more unusual the strain distribution, the more potent is its osteogenic potential.

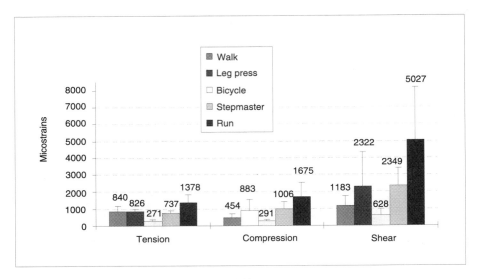

Figure 2 Principal strains during exercise activities.

Animal experiments suggest that the amount of strain and strain rate change are major determinants of the adaptive response of growing bone to dynamic loading.[13,14] It is probable that the high strains and strain rates that occur during basketball can elicit maximal bone adaptation. For the adapted stiffer bone of recruits who played basketball at least two years prior to basic training the high bone stresses of Israeli basic training, most likely resulted in lower bone strains for a given activity than for recruits who did not play basketball. As a result, the basketball players had less bone damage and a lower incidence of stress fractures during basic training.

Milgrom et al., in another work, compared the *in vivo* tibial strains in six subjects during exercises commonly performed in health clubs.[15] The measurements were made during treadmill walking, during exercise bicycling, while performing leg presses, using a stepmaster, and during running. Running was found to have the highest strain and strain rates (Figures 2 and 3), indicating that it has the highest potential of the exercises tested to initiate bone's remodeling response and strengthen the tibia. It should be remembered that while these *in vivo* strain measurements are important, their validity is limited to the specific site of strain measurement on the tibia. The results may not necessarily be valid for the femur, or even for other anatomical portions of the tibia.

On the basis of the epidemiologic study of Milgrom et al.[9] as well as their measurements of *in vivo* tibial strains, a logical strategy for lowering the incidence of stress fractures in military recruits and athletes would be to adapt their bones before they begin their formal training by a pre-training program, with at least two years of properly applied high strain and strain rate-generating exercises that mimic those that occur during basketball. Such a program would ideally stiffen the bone and not lead to stress fractures during this adaptation period.

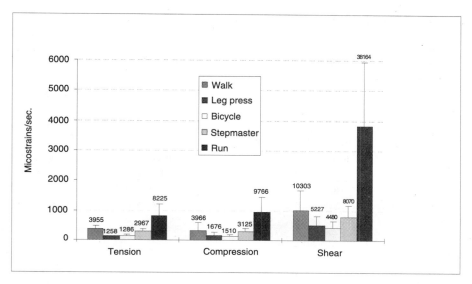

Figure 3 Principal strain rates during exercise activities.

BONE STRENGTHENING IN THE AMERICAN MILITARY

Another well characterized stress fracture model is the U.S. Marine recruit.[16] This model is different from the Israeli infantry model in the duration, intensity, and plan of training as well as the climate, terrain, shoe gear, and the characteristics of the recruit population.[17] The basis of diagnosis of stress fracture is also different between the two models. In the Israeli model, the primary diagnostic tool is bone scan, while bone scan is used less frequently in the U.S. Marine model.

A tactic used in U.S. Marine training to minimize stress fracture risk has been to reduce "training errors" when designing the basic training regimen.[18] Training error is defined as an exercise program which prescribes inappropriate frequency, intensity, time, or type (FITT) of exercise for the physical condition of the individuals. Training error can also occur when abrupt changes are made to an exercise regimen. Consequently, the prevention of training error requires knowledge of the physical condition of the individual trainee or population. The overall goal is to reach the desired fitness and training levels at the end of the training while minimizing risk for stress fracture.

In an epidemiologic study among U.S. Marine recruits, it was found that stress fracture risk during marine training is increased by poor physical fitness and low levels of physical activity prior to basic training.[18] The basis for assigning recruits to high or low risk groups for stress fracture was a short five question questionnaire, which is a self-assessment of physical fitness. Recruits in the high risk group were 2.45 times (CI 1.36 to 4.42) more likely to suffer from a stress fracture during basic training than individuals in the low risk category. In a further refinement, recruit baseline physical fitness scores on an initial strength test which includes a 2.4 km maximal effort run were added to the physical fitness self–assessment scores to categorize recruits into high and low stress fracture risk groups. Using these combined parameters, it was found that risk for stress fracture was 3.26 times greater for the high risk group.

On the basis of these data, the U.S. Marines decided to alter the basic training regime. They had the benefit of previous American military experiences. Scully and Besterman reported in 1982 that "cyclic training" lowered the incidence of stress fractures in U.S. Army recruits.[19] The concept of cyclic training is that instead of linearly increasing training increments each week, the increase is by progressive cycles. In each cycle the training level first increases, then decreases, then increases again. This concept was later discredited and is not used currently in the U.S. Army.

The revised U.S. Marine training that was developed is based on the following principles:

1. Balanced total body work-out
2. Gradual overload and progression
3. Emphasis on aerobic activity early in training and slowly incorporating strength training
4. Warm-up and cool-down
5. Specificity of exercise
6. Training of trainers in proper exercise technique.

This revised exercise program was evaluated for reduction of stress fracture incidence in three groups of marine recruits that were followed for twelve weeks of basic training. All three groups were homogeneous for incoming physical activity and fitness status. The first group used the traditional training program. The second and third groups used the revised training program. However, the third group performed fewer running miles (33 versus 41 miles in 12 weeks). At the end of the training program, there were significantly fewer stress fractures in the third group (Table 4). Importantly, the effect of the revised training program was greatest in the high risk recruits, with reduction from 10% in the traditional training regimen to 3% in the revised training program with the fewest running miles. The onset of the first stress fractures was also delayed until more than halfway through the training. Just as important is that at the end of the training programs all three groups had reached equal physical fitness levels.

Table 4   Evaluation of Running Mileage, Stress Fracture Incidence, and Final Fitness among Male Recruits

	Mileage*	% Stress fracture	Final 3-mile Time (mean)
Group 1 (n = 1136)	55	3.7	20:20
Group 2 (n = 1050)	41	2.7	20:44
Group 3 (n = 1036)	33	1.7	20:53

* Total organized running during basic training.

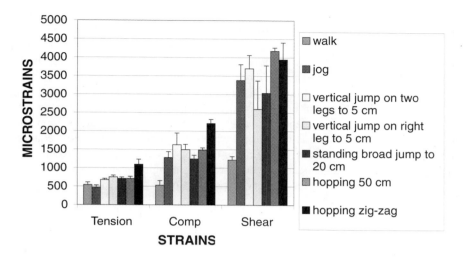

Figure 4 Principal strains versus activity for female subject.

HOME EXERCISES THAT CAN STRENGTHEN BONE
AND THEREBY LIMIT STRESS FRACTURES

The finding of Milgrom et al.[9] that playing basketball regularly prior to basic training protected infantry recruits for stress fractures is an important key to developing stress fracture prevention exercises. However, sending everyone to play basketball is not a realistic program. Milgrom et al. sought to develop a program of exercises to strengthen bone and prevent stress fractures that can be done at home without special equipment. Their strategy was to identify exercises that generated strain and strain rates of the magnitude of basketball. Figure 4 shows the *in vivo* tibial strains for a female subject during various hopping and jumping exercise activities compared with walking and jogging. Zigzag hopping had statistically significantly higher tension and compression strains than the other exercises, and along with 50 cm hopping, the highest shear strains. These preliminary data suggest that a home program of hopping and zigzag hopping can strengthen bone and thereby prevent stress fracture in subsequent training.

CONCLUSION

The sports literature lacks studies specifically related to the issue of bone strengthening stress fracture prevention exercises. Therefore, our knowledge of this topic is limited to military studies and *in vivo* bone strain gage experiments. From the Israeli infantry and U.S. Marine stress fracture models, we can see that proper exercise programs can prevent or delay the onset of stress fracture. The goal of these programs is stress fracture prevention without compromising the end training goals of achieving a fit combat soldier or competitive athlete. Strengthening of bone before the formal training program evidently takes considerable time and therefore requires prior knowledge of who the trainees will be. The Israeli data suggest that a time interval of two years is necessary for bone strengthening to occur. During this period there must be gradual exposure of bone to both high strain and strain rates, and varied strain distributions. Playing basketball or following a program of hopping, zigzag hopping, and vertical jumps would seem ideal activities. The other tactic for reducing stress fracture incidence is to alter the training program to fit the population of trainees. By reducing training errors, which prescribe inappropriate frequency, intensity, time, or type of exercises for the training population, stress fracture incidence can be lowered. This can be done without compromising the end physical fitness goals, and there is "less pain with equal gain".

REFERENCES

1. Giladi, M., Milgrom, C., Simkin, A., and Danon, Y.L., Stress fractures. Identifiable risk factors, *Am. J. Sports Med.*, 19, 647, 1991.
2. Gilbert, R.S. and Johnson, H.A., Stress fractures in military recruits — a review of twelve years' experience, *Mil. Med.*, 131, 716, 1966.
3. Leabhart, J.W., Stress fractures, *Med. Newsl.*, 32, 3, 1958.
4. Provost R.A. and Morris, J.M., Fatigue fracture of the femoral shaft. *J. Bone Jt. Surg.*, 51A, 487, 1969.
5. Greaney, R.B., Gerber, F.H., Laughlin, R.L., Kmet, J.P., Metz, C.D., Kilcheski, T.S., Rao, B.R., and Silverman, E.D., Distribution and natural history of stress fractures in U.S. Marine recruits. *Radiology*, 146, 339, 1983.
6. Mustajoki, P., Laapio, H., and Meurman, K., Calcium metabolism, physical activity and stress fracture (Let), *Lancet*, 2, 797, 1983.
7. Swissa, A., Milgrom, C., Giladi, M., Kashtan, H., Stein, M., Margulies, J., Chisin, R., and Aharonson, Z., The effect of pre-training sport activity on the incidence of stress fracture among military recruits. A prospective study. *Clin. Orthop.*, 245, 256, 1989.
8. Giladi, M., Milgrom, C., Kashtan, H., Stein, M., Chisin, R., and Dizian, R., Recurrent stress fractures in military recruits. A long term follow-up of sixty-six recruits with stress fractures, *J. Bone Jt. Surg.*, 68B, 439, 1986.
9. Milgrom, C., Simkin, A., Eldad, A., Benjuya, N., Edenman, I., Nyska, M., and Finestone, A., Using bone's adaptation ability to lower the incidence of stress fractures. *Am. J. Sports Med.*, 28, 245, 2000.
10. Lanyon L.E., Hampson G.J., Goodship A.E., and Shah J.S., Bone deformation recorded in vivo from strain gages attached to the human tibial shaft, *Acta Orthop. Scand.*, 46, 256, 1975.
11. Burr, D. B., Milgrom, C., Fyhrie, D., Forwood, M., Nyska, M., Finestone, A., Hoshaw, S., Saiag, E., and Simkin, A., *In vivo* measurement of human tibial strains during vigorous activity, *Bone,* 18, 405, 1996.
12. Lanyon, L.E., Using functional loading to influence bone mass and architecture: objectives, mechanisms, and relationship with estrogen of the mechanically adaptive process in bone, *Bone*, 18, 37s, 1996.

13. Mosley, J.R. and Lanyon, L.E., Strain rate as a controlling influence on adaptive modeling in response to dynamic loading of the ulna in growing male rats, *Bone,* 23, 313, 1998.
14. Turner, C.H, Owan, I., and Takano, Y., Mechanotransduction in bone: role of strain rate, *Am. J. Physiol.,* 269, E438, 1995.
15. Milgrom, C., Finestone, A., Simkin, A., Ekenman, I., Mendelson, S., Millgram, M., Nyska, M., Larsson, E., and Burr, D., *In vivo* strain measurements to evaluate the tibial bone strengthening potential of exercises, *J. Bone Jt. Surg.,* 82B, 591, 2000.
16. Beck, T.J., Ruff, C.B., and Mourtada, F.A., Dual-energy x-ray absorptiometry derived structural geometry for stress fracture prediction in male US Marine Corps recruits, *J. Bone Miner. Res.,* 11, 645, 1996.
17. Milgrom, C., Giladi, M., Stein, M., Kashtan, H., Margulies, J., Chisin, R., Steinberg, R., and Aharonson, Z., Stress fractures in military recruits. a prospective study showing an unusually high incidence, *J. Bone Jt. Surg.,* 67B, 732, 1985.
18. Shaffer, R.A., Brodine, S.K., Almeida, S.A., Williams, K.M., and Ronaghy, S., Use of simple measures of physical activity to predict stress fractures in young men undergoing a rigorous physical training program, *Am. J. Epidemiol.,* 149, 236, 1999.
19. Scully, T.J. and Besterman, G., Stress fractures — a preventable training injury, *Mil. Med.,* 147, 285,1982.

CHAPTER 17

Pharmaceutical Treatments That May Prevent or Delay the Onset of Stress Fractures

David B. Burr

CONTENTS

Introduction...259
Potential Pharmaceutical Treatments to Prevent Stress Fracture 262
    Bisphosophonates 262
    Indomethacin and NSAIDS...264
Potential Pharmaceutical Therapies to Enhance the Healing of Stress
    Fractures..265
Conclusion 266
References...267

INTRODUCTION

Attempts to prevent stress fractures have focused on improvements in the design of training equipment (see Chapter 15), the development of training regimes that gradually increase workloads without overloading the skeleton,[1-5] and only to a small extent on nutrition and diet.[1] However, these approaches are often ineffective.[6] Pharmaceutical therapies have not been devised, although there are several that have the potential to either prevent stress fractures or accelerate the recovery from a stress fracture. Currently, pharmaceutical agents are prescribed only for the treatment of inflammation and pain rather than to promote more rapid healing of the fracture.[4]

The slow progress in the development of useful pharmaceutical treatments may stem from many causes, including reluctance to use drug therapies for a condition that will heal on its own with a few weeks of rest. However, it is also true that the usefulness of a pharmaceutical treatment for stress fracture depends on the etiology of the fracture, which is controversial.

One hypothesis about the pathogenesis of stress fractures is that they are solely a mechanical result of repeated large-magnitude loads on the bone, i.e., many loading cycles will lead to fatigue failure of the structure. This seems unlikely in view of the recent *in vivo* human strain data which show that strains at a stress fracture site rarely or never exceed 2000 με,[7-11] a magnitude that is too low to cause fractures within a physiologically reasonable period of time.[9,12]

A second scenario for the pathogenesis of stress fractures is that the "adaptive" response to overloading — bone remodeling — transiently reduces bone mass. Each time a new remodeling unit is started, it temporarily creates a new resorption space, increasing porosity and reducing bone mass.[13] The transient reduction in bone mass caused by the acceleration of remodeling decreases bone strength exponentially.[14-16] Because there is less bone to sustain loading, strains on the remaining bone increase; a new remodeling cycle can begin and more bone is lost. Over time, this leads to a gradual loss of bone and eventually to increased fragility and fracture.

Martin[17] simulated the effects of positive feedback between (a) increased porosity associated with increased activation frequency for remodeling as the bone attempts to adapt to the overload; (b) the increased strain that occurs because of increased porosity/reduced bone mass; and (c) increased microdamage accumulation that follows an increased number of cycles of repetitive loading. The computational model shows that as strain magnitude or the number of load cycles per day increases, a critical threshold is reached at which porosity, damage, and strain begin to increase at a rapidly accelerating and uncontrollable rate. This results in an unstable situation in which a fracture can occur. Although periosteal woven bone, in some instances the only radiographic evidence that a stress fracture has occurred, can strengthen the bone, this new bone does not remove the instability. The model shows that porosity introduced by remodeling can contribute via a positive feedback mechanism to an unstable situation in which a stress fracture will occur. The model also predicts that suppression of bone remodeling, which prevents the increased porosity associated with remodeling and maintains lower strains on the bone, can prevent the stress fracture.

Experimental studies with the rabbit impulsive loading model (see Chapters 11 and 14) also suggest that positive feedback between loading and remodeling may be a feature of the pathogenesis of stress fractures in this model. Rabbits loaded for 32,400 cycles over the course of one day showed no biological evidence of skeletal damage.[18] Rabbits loaded for 37,500 cycles over three weeks also did not have a significant accumulation of bone microdamage, but did have a significantly increased activation of new bone remodeling and increased porosity. Uptake of [99m]technetium was increased in 80% of these rabbits, while 48% showed evidence of overt stress fracture by three weeks.[19] By 6 weeks of loading, activation of new bone remodeling had increased further still, and bone microdamage (measured as crack density) was increased by more than 10 times. The incidence of overt stress fractures in these animals had increased to 68%, while fewer than 10% of the rabbits showed no evidence of change after 6 weeks. These data suggest that overloading first creates a biological remodeling response, that this remodeling response can be associated with early signs of a stress fracture, and that continued loading will cause acceleration of bone microdamage accumulation that will further increase the incidence of stress fracture, perhaps through a positive feedback mechanism between bone remodeling and damage accumulation. This pathogenesis suggests that the incidence of stress fractures could be significantly reduced by agents that suppress the bone remodeling response to high acute levels of activity.

The view that stress fractures are the result of positive feedback mechanisms between the mechanical environment and the biological response to it is consistent with the epidemiologic data that exist. Where it is possible to tell, most stress fractures begin within three to seven weeks after the initiation of vigorous training.[20-22] This is coincident with the period when the first phase of bone remodeling (resorption) occurs following the introduction of a higher than usual strain stimulus, but before new bone formation is well established. Generally, after a change in a training regimen, the activation of new remodeling requiring the proliferation and recruitment of new cells will take five to seven days. The resorption period follows for about three weeks, while the formation phase occurs over the following three months.[23] Thus, fractures occurring between three and seven weeks would be well into the resorption phase of bone remodeling before formation and mineralization caused by the accelerated activity is complete.

One would expect that an increase in bone turnover would be accompanied by an elevation of serum or urine biochemical markers reflective of turnover. In a 12 month prospective study of young athletes, about 20% of whom developed stress fractures, Bennell et al.[24] reported 5 to 35% increases in turnover markers without, however, demonstrating statistical significance. Bone turnover in athletes who developed stress fractures was not different from those who did not develop stress fractures at baseline, or either immediately prior or subsequent to the beginning of bone pain. One prospective study did detect a significant increase in plasma hydroxyproline during the first week of military training in a group of recruits who subsequently presented with a stress fracture, compared to those who did not.[25] In this study of 104 males in training to be Navy Seals, mean basal hydroxyproline values were 40% higher in those who subsequently presented with stress fractures compared to the total population of trainees (Figure 1). This suggests that an initially higher bone turnover rate is a risk factor for subsequent fracture. Others also report increased collagen turnover in exercising mice[26] and in ultramarathon runners.[27] Failure to detect increased bone turnover either prior to or following the onsent of stress fractures in athletes[24] may stem from the measurement of serum and biochemical markers of bone remodeling that reflect overall total body bone remodeling and are not sufficiently sensitive to detect locally accelerated bone turnover.

Therefore, one approach to preventing stress fractures may be to suppress the initial biological reaction (i.e., bone remodeling) to overloading of the bone.

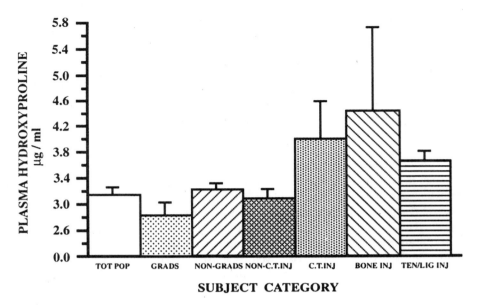

Figure 1   Basal hydroxyproline levels in Navy recruits who subsequently presented with bone or connective tissue injuries. Basal hydroxyproline levels were significantly higher in those who presented with significant connective tissue injuries (C.T. INJ) and subjects who fractured (BONE INJ). Levels were also slightly raised, though not significantly, in those who presented with tendon or ligament injuries (TEN/LIG INJ) compared to those who were not injured (NON–C.T. INJ) or the total population (TOT POP). GRADS and NON-GRADS refer to those subjects who completed or didn't complete the training program. (From Murguia, M.J. et al., *Am. J. Sports Med.,* 16, 660, 1988. With permission).

POTENTIAL PHARMACEUTICAL TREATMENTS
TO PREVENT STRESS FRACTURE

Several pharmaceutical agents offer the potential to prevent or delay the onset of stress fractures. These compounds suppress bone turnover, preventing the initial loss of bone that may contribute to the onset of the fracture.

Bisphosophonates

Bisphosphonates (BP) are compounds that significantly reduce the activation frequency for bone remodeling. Histologically, bisphosphonates reduce resorption depth[28,29] and reduce activation frequency.[30] Depending on dosage, activation frequency with the newer generation bisphosphonates can be reduced as much as 80 to 90%.[31] Alendronate at 10 mg/day has been shown to reduce bone resorption by about 50% between one and three months,[32] but does not cause further decreases in biochemical markers over the subsequent six months of treatment. This suggests that alendronate does not have a cumulative effect on bone remodeling suppression even with long-term administration.[33] Although earlier bisphosphonates such as etidronate inhibited mineralization of new bone,[34-36] the newer, more potent BPs have an anti-resorptive effect at lower doses without preventing normal mineralization.

In humans, absorption of an oral dose of alendronate is ~1%, and occurs mainly in the upper gastrointestinal tract. Absorption is linear within the dosing range of 5 to 80 mg.[37]

One concern with BPs is that they are retained in bone and might have long-term effects. For example, Kasting and Francis[38] projected that an intermittent cyclic treatment of etidronate (14 days of 400 mg/day orally followed by 76 days without drug) would result in retained mass of 300 to 600 mg for a daily absorbed dose of 12 mg. This would be distributed over the bone surface so that it would affect only a few percent of the potentially active surface. The more recent generations of bisphosphonates, because they are more potent, would affect even less of the bone surface. Chennekatu et al.[39] showed that the total skeletal alendronate content of bone in an average dog following three years of treatment at five times the clinical dose for osteoporosis was only 0.001% of the total bone mass. The effects of bisphosphonates are likely transient, and may disappear once the drug is withdrawn.[40] Therefore, short term exposure to bisphosphonates over the course of a 14 week basic training period would not be expected to cause long-term deleterious effects on the skeleton.

The pharmacologic activity of BPs are retained for a period of time after cessation of treatment. Decreased bone turnover (evaluated by serum and urinary biomarkers) was observed for one year after discontinuation of a two year program of either 5 or 10 mg/day treatment with alendronate. Although the terminal half-life of bisphosphonate activity in humans is approximately 10 years, the pharmacalogic half-life of bisphosphonate activity is much shorter.[37] The pharmacologic activity of BPs in bone is retained only until new bone has been laid down over the exposed surface.[41,42]

Studies showing the effects of bisphosphonates on bone biomechanics generally indicate that the nature of the effects are dose- and species-dependent.[43] For example, doses of pamidronate up to 1.0 mg/kg/day sc given to immature mice improved the ultimate strength of the femoral diaphysis in bending,[44] but higher doses (>4.5 mg/kg/day) given to growing rats depressed diaphyseal strength and stiffness.[45] Similar results have been reported for alendronate.[46]

Bisphosphonates have a greater effect on mechanical strength of trabecular bone than cortical bone, as might be expected from the higher turnover rate in trabecular bone. Oral doses of alendronate (2 to 8 mg/kg/day) given to adult beagles for six months had no effect on torsional stiffness, strength, or energy absorption in the femur.[46] Lower doses of alendronate given IV (0.05 to 0.25 mg/kg every two weeks) also had no effect on cortical bone from the femur, but the strength of trabecular cylinders taken from L_4 of the high-dose animals was twice as great as that from vehicle-treated animals.[30] Trabecular bone from the femur showed no change in strength in that study.

There are several potential advantages of bisphosphonates for prevention of stress fractures. They appear to have few side effects, and no associated mortality. Because they have been widely tested and have been used for treatment of osteoporosis, the relationship between oral dosage and the amount of remodeling suppression is relatively well known.[47] Therefore, dosage could be modulated depending on the amount of remodeling suppression one would like to achieve.

On the other hand, bisphosphonates are known to cause gastrointestinal disturbances in some people, leading in some cases to esophageal or gastric ulceration.[37,48,49] Also, it is possible that there may be some retention of the bisphosphonates in the bone for a period of time after withdrawal, and that they could continue to suppress remodeling slightly in the post-training period. However, with the more potent bisphosphonates, the risk for this is reduced and is not considered a signficant drawback to their use.

Indomethacin and NSAIDS

Prostaglandin synthesis is associated with enhanced bone formation and accelerated bone turnover, both following fracture[50,51] and when administered exogenously on an intermittent basis.[52,53] Prostaglandins may also be produced in response to mechanical strain without the presence of a fracture.[54,55] Prostaglandins are associated with increased intracortical bone turnover, which results in greater cortical porosity.[53] Indomethacin and other nonsteroidal anti- inflammatory drugs (NSAIDS) inhibit cyclooxygenase synthesis, which is necessary to produce prostaglandins, and have been shown to suppress cortical bone remodeling[56-58] without destroying the coupling between bone resorption and bone formation.[59] This suggests that indomethacin acts as an inhibitor of remodeling activation,[60] similar to the bisphosphonates, and may accomplish this by disrupting osteoclast recruitment and/or activity.[61]

Regardless of the cause, the etiology for stress fractures involves localized increased intracortical bone turnover. This phenomenon was termed the regional acceleratory phenomenon (RAP) by Frost.[62] Following osteotomy[59] or cortical drilling,[60] indomethacin inhibits the RAP, reduces the number of resorption and formation sites, and prevents the increased porosity that would normally accompany the RAP. This suggests that indomethacin may have potential utility for the prevention of stress fractures by suppressing the biological response to damage. However, there is evidence that prostaglandins may actually enhance the RAP in experimentally produced overt fractures by increasing both resorption and formation, but may delay healing by suppressing full mineralization of the new bone.[50,51] Although some have suggested that the suppressive effects of indomethacin may depend on the extent of trauma[57] without affecting normal turnover processes in nonfractured bone,[57,59] it is likely that its effect is dose dependent.[63]

NSAIDS prevent bone loss that occurs following decreased mechanical usage,[58,64,65] suggesting that they may also be able to prevent the loss that accompanies mechanical overuse.[63] However, another effect of mechanical usage is to stimulate apposition of new bone to the periosteal surface. This new bone is mechanically advantageous, as it has a greater effect on the structural rigidity of a long bone than does addition of bone to the endocortical surface. Periosteal apposition is prostaglandin mediated[52] and the administration of indomethacin will suppress some of the new bone formation that mechanical loading would otherwise produce.[66]

One advantage of indomethacin, or any NSAID, for treating overuse injuries is that because they inhibit cyclooxygenases, they will also control inflammatory processes that may accompany injury or overload. Therefore, they may not only prevent or delay the development of a fracture, but also may reduce the pain associated with the injury, or with other traumatic events related to the overloading (e.g., periosteal inflammation without stress fracture).

However, there may also be several disadvantages. Indomethacin reduces the amount of periosteal apposition, and therefore could prevent the normal adaptation of bone to greater loads and higher levels of activity. Although indomethacin benefits the bone by preventing loss, it also may prevent some of the bone gain, particularly in regions where it is mechanically most advantageous. However, not all NSAIDS have this effect. Flurbiprofen, for example, reduces bone turnover rate but can simultaneously enhance direct apposition of lamellar bone to the periosteal surface of cortical bone,[67-69] although it does not intensify bone formation on trabecular surfaces. Nevertheless, it would allow and in fact promote the reinforcement of bone strength that mechanically-stimulated periosteal apposition produces. As with the bisphosphonates, some NSAIDS are also known to promote gastric ulceration and must be taken with meals. Because of these disadvantages, the potential use of NSAIDs to prevent stress fractures requires additional testing and evaluation.

The use of selective cyclooxygenase-2 (COX-2) inhibitors has overcome the problem of gastric ulceration. COX-2 inhibitors do not have to be taken after meals. The effect of this new class of compound also requires additional study.

POTENTIAL PHARMACEUTICAL THERAPIES TO ENHANCE THE HEALING OF STRESS FRACTURES

Potential therapies to delay the occurrence of stress fractures rely on disruption of the positive feedback between bone remodeling and mechanical overload through suppression of new remodeling events. Stress fractures that have already occurred are more likely to benefit from treatment with agents that accelerate repair and remodeling.

Intermittently administered parathyroid hormone (PTH) is one agent known to accelerate intracortical bone turnover without having a long term negative effect on bone mass or short or long term negative effects on bone strength. Studies in rabbits[70,71] and monkeys[72] show that PTH increased intracortical bone turnover even at doses as low as 1 to 10 ug/kg/day. Although the increased turnover might be expected initially to reduce the overall strength and stiffness of the bone, increased apposition of bone to both periosteal and endocortical surfaces more than compensates for the transient loss of bone intracortically, resulting in significant improvement in the structural strength, stiffness, and work to failure of the bone. Because of the increased bone turnover and larger cortical porosity, the stiffness of the whole bone is reduced but the tissue elastic modulus is not changed, so the new bone is just as capable of weight bearing as the bone it replaces. This has been confirmed by scanning acoustic microscopic studies of bone matrix following treatment with PTH.[70]

Mechanical compensations for the transient intracortical loss occur early, within the first month of treatment.[71] In a study of the short term effects of PTH on cortical bone turnover in rabbits, PTH increased the activation frequency for new remodeling in the tibia by two to three times without increasing intracortical porosity or compromising mechanical strength.[71] The mild increase in bone turnover would be sufficient to accelerate healing, but is not elevated so much that it would increase cortical porosity. This suggests that PTH could be used to accelerate the repair of damage related to a stress fracture without further compromising the strength of the bone. Given at higher doses, PTH increases cortical porosity in a dose-dependent manner,[72,73] so it is important to titrate the dose to maximize healing and minimize further loss of bone through elevated remodeling.

Following withdrawal of PTH treatment at low doses (e.g., 1 µg/kg/day), porosity will return to normal as the remodeling space is refilled.[72] For short term treatments (one to two months), the remodeling space should be refilled within one formation period (~90 days in adult humans). Prolonged treatment might require two to three remodeling periods to normalize,[72] but longer treatment periods should not be necessary to treat a stress fracture. At low doses, the effect on intracortical porosity is transient and can be reversed with a short duration of withdrawal.

Because intermittently administered PTH stimulates the apposition of bone periosteally, there may be long term beneficial effects on bone strength even after withdrawal of treatment. Periosteal bone does not appear to be removed even when PTH treatment is discontinued,[72] so the increased bending rigidity caused by the larger bone cross-sectional moment of inertia will result in lasting improvement of the mechanical properties of bone when the subject returns to strenuous activity. Refilling of the remodeling space over the one to two remodeling periods following withdrawal of PTH therapy, in combination with the new bone periosteally, should result in continuously increasing bone strength over the three to six months following treatment. This could have additional benefits to the active athlete or training soldier. Whereas the prescription for rest following the onset of a stress fracture will result in continued bone loss, and subsequent activity following convalescence can only be expected to achieve pre-fracture bone strength values, treatment with intermittently administered PTH would be expected to result in a stronger bone and a reduced risk for future fracture.

CONCLUSION

The potential for pharmaceutical treatments that can delay or prevent the onset of stress facture, or that can accelerate healing of stress fracture once it has occurred, has been understudied. However, there are several drug treatments that may have the capacity to reduce the risk for fracture or improve the potential for early return to activity. These drugs are approved for treatment of other conditions in humans, and their adverse effects are well known and not serious. Use of these drugs for short periods of time, either during a transient but sudden increase in activity like that found among military trainees, or for short-term treatment following the presentation of a stress fracture, are likely to have beneficial effects without adverse side effects.

REFERENCES

1. Grimston, S.K. and Zernicke, R.F., Exercise-related stress responses in bone, *J. Appl. Biomech.*, 9, 2, 1993.
2. Clement, D.B., Tibial stress syndrome in athletes, *J. Sports Med.*, 2, 81, 1974.
3. Matheson, G.O., Clement, D.B., McKenzie, D.C., Taunton, J.E., Lloyd-Smith, D.R., and Macintyre, J.G., Stress fractures in athletes: a study of 320 cases, *Am. J. Sports Med.*, 15, 46, 1987.
4. Knapp, T.P. and Garrett, W.E., Jr., Stress fractures: general concepts, *Clin. Sports Med.*, 16, 339, 1997.
5. Pope, R.P., Prevention of pelvic stress fractures in female army recruits, *Mil. Med.*, 164, 370, 1999.
6. Andrish, J.T., Bergfeld, J.A., and Walheim, J., A prospective study on the management of shin splints, *J. Bone Jt. Surg.*, 56A, 1697, 1974.
7. Burr, D.B., Milgrom, C., Fyhrie, D., Forwood, M., Nyska, M., Finestone, A., Hoshaw S., Saiag, E., and Simkin A., *In vivo* measurement of human tibial strains during vigorous activity, *Bone*, 18, 405, 1996.
8. Milgrom, C., Burr, D., Fyhrie, D., Forwood, M., Finestone, A., Nyska, M., Giladi, M., Liebergall, M., and Simkin, A., The effect of shoe gear on human tibial strains recorded during dynamic loading: a pilot study, *Foot Ankle Int.*, 17, 667, 1996.
9. Burr, D.B., Bone, exercise, and stress fractures, *Exerc. Sport Sci. Rev.*, 25, 171, 1997.
10. Fyhrie, D.P., Milgrom, C., Hoshaw, S.J., Simkin A., Car, S., Drumb, D., and Burr, D.B., Effect of fatiguing exercise on longitudinal bone strain as related to stress fracture in humans, *Ann. Biomed. Eng.*, 26, 660, 1998.
11. Milgrom, C., Finestone, A., Levi, Y., Simkin, A., Ekenman, I., Mendelson, S., Millgram, M., Nysak, M., Benjuya, N., And Burr. D.B., Do high impact exercises produce higher tibial strains than running?, *Br. J. Sports Med.*, 34, 195, 2000.
12. Schaffler, M.B., Radin, E.L., and Burr, D.B., Long-term fatigue behavior of compact bone at low strain magnitude and rate, *Bone*, 11, 321, 1990.
13. Parfitt, A.M., The morphologic basis of bone mineral measurements. Transient and steady state effects of treatment in osteoporosis, *Miner. Electr. Metab.*, 4, 273, 1980.
14. Carter, D.R. and Hayes, W.C., The compressive behavior of bone as a two phase porous structure, *J. Bone Jt. Surg.*, 59A, 954, 1977.
15. Rice, J.C., Cowin, S.C., and Bowman J.A., On the dependence of the elasticity and strength of cancellous bone on apparent density, *J. Biomech.*, 21, 155, 1988.
16. Schaffler, M.B. and Burr, D.B., Stiffness of compact bone: effects of porosity and density, *J. Biomech.*, 21, 13, 1988.
17. Martin, R.B., Mathematical model for repair of fatigue damage and stress fracture in osteonal bone, *J. Orthop. Res.*, 13, 309, 1995.
18. Schaffler, M.B. and Boyd, R.D., Bone remodeling and microdamage accumulation in experimental stress fracture, *Trans. Orthop. Res. Soc.*, 22, 113, 1997.
19. Burr, D.B., Milgrom, C., Boyd, R.D., Higgins, W.L., Robin, G., and Radin, E.L., Experimental stress fractures of the tibia. Biological and mechanical aetiology in rabbits, *J. Bone Jt. Surg.*, 72B, 370, 1990.
20. Garcia, J.E., Grabhorn, L.L., and Franklin, K.J., Factors associated with stress fractures in military recruits, *Mil. Med.*, 152, 45, 1987.
21. Kowal, D.M., Nature and causes of injuries in women resulting from an endurance training program, *Am. J. Sports Med.*, 8, 265, 1980.
22. Sullivan, D., Warren, R.F., Pavlov, H., and Kelman, G., Stress fractures in 51 runners, *Clin. Orthop. Rel. Res.*, 187, 188, 1984.

23. Parfitt, A.M., The cellular basis of bone remodeling: the quantum concept reexamined in light of recent advances in the cell biology of bone, *Calcif. Tissue Int.*, 36 (Suppl. 1), S37, 1984.

24. Bennell, K.L., Malcolm, S.A., Brukner, P.D., Green, R.M., Hopper, J.L., Wark, J.D., and Ebeling, P.R., A 12-month prospective study of the relationship between stress fractures and bone turnover in athletes, *Calcif. Tissue Int.*, 63, 80, 1998.

25. Murguia, M.J., Vailas, A., Mandelbaum, B., Norton, J., Hodgdon, J., Goforth, H., and Riedy, M., Elevated plasma hydroxyproline. A possible risk factor associated with connective tissue injuries during overuse, *Am. J. Sport Med.*, 16, 660, 1988.

26. Heikkinen, E. and Vuori, I., Effect of physical activity on the metabolism of collagen in aged mice, *Acta Physiol. Scand.*, 84, 543, 1972.

27. Takala, T.E.S., Vuori, J., Anttinen, H., Väänänen, K., and Myllylä, R., Prolonged exercise causes an increase in the activity of galactosylhydroxylsyl glucoyltransferase and in the concentration of type III procollagen aminopropeptide in human serum, *Pfluegers Arch.*, 407, 500, 1986.

28. Steiniche, T., Hasling, C., Charles, P., Eriksen, E.F., Melsen, F., and Mosekilde, L., The effects of etidronate on trabecular bone remodeling in postmenopausal spinal osteoporosis: a randomized study comparing intermittent treatment and an ADFR regime, *Bone,* 12, 155, 1991.

29. Boyce, R.W., Paddock, C.L., Gleason, J.R., Sletsema, W.K., [sic] and Eriksen, E.F., The effects of risedronate on canine cancellous bone remodeling: three-dimensional kinetic reconstruction of the remodeling site, *J. Bone Miner. Res.*, 10, 211, 1995.

30. Balena, R., Toolan, B.C., Shea, M., Markatos, A., Myers, E.R., Lee, S.C., Opas, E.E., Seedor, J.G., Klein, H., Frankenfield, D., Quartuccio, H., Fioravanti, C., Clair, J., Brown, E., Hayes, W.C., and Rodan, G.A., The effects of a 2-year treatment with the aminobisphosphonate alendronate on bone metabolism, bone histomorphometry, and bone strength in ovariectomised nonhuman primates, *J. Clin. Invest.*, 92, 2577, 1993.

31. Forwood, M.R., Burr, D.B., Takano, Y., Eastman, D.F., Smith, P.N., and Schwardt, J.D., Risedronate treatment does not increase microdamage in the canine femoral neck, *Bone*, 16, 643, 1995.

32. Garnero, P., Shih, W.J., Gineyts, E., Karpf, D.B., and Delmas, P.D., Comparison of new biochemical markers of bone turnover in late postmenopausal osteoporotic women in response to alendronate treatment, *J. Clin. Endocrinol. Metab.*, 79, 1693, 1994.

33. Chesnut, C.H., McClung, M.R., Ensrud, K.E., Bell, N.H., Genant, H.K., Harris, S.T., Singer, F.R., Stock, J.L., Yood, R.A., Delmas, P.D., Kher, U., Pryor-Tillotson, S., and Santora, A.C., Alendronate treatment of the postmenopausal osteoporotic woman: effect of multiple dosages on bone mass and bone remodeling, *Am. J. Med.*, 99, 144, 1995.

34. Flora, L., Hassing, G.S., Parfitt, A.M., and Villanueva, A.R., Comparative skeletal effects of two diphosphonates in dogs, *Metab. Bone Dis. Relat. Res.*, 2 (Suppl.), 389, 1980.

35. Gibbs, C.J., Aaron, J.E., and Peacock, M., Osteomalacia in Paget's disease treated with short term, high dose sodium etidronate, *Br. Med. J.*, 292, 1127, 1986.

36. Geddes, A.D., D'Souza, S.M., Ebetino, F.H., and Ibbotson, K.J., Bisphosphonates: structure-activity relationships and therapeutic implications, *Bone Miner. Res.*, 8, 265, 1994.

37. Yates, A.J. and Rodan, G.A., Alendronate and osteoporosis, *DDT*, 3, 69, 1998.

38. Kasting, G.B. and Francis, M.D., Retention of etidronate in human, dog, and rat, *J. Bone Miner. Res.*, 7, 513, 1992.

39. Chennekatu, P.P., Guy, J., Shea, M., Bagdon, W., Kline, W.F., and Hayes, W.C., Long-term safety of the aminobisphosphonate alendronate in adult dogs. I. General safety and biomechanical properties of bone, *J. Pharmacol. Exper. Ther.,* 276, 271, 1996.

40. Geusens, P., Nijs, J., van der Perre, G., van Audekercke, R., Lowet, G., Goovaerts, S., Barbier, A., Lacheretz, F., Remandet, B., Jiang, Y., and Dequeker, J., Longitudinal effect of tiludronate on bone mineral density, resonant frequency, and strength in monkeys, *J. Bone Miner. Res.,* 7, 599, 1992.

41. Sato, M., Grasser, W., Endo, N., Akins, R., Simmons, H., Thompson, D.D., Golub, E., and Rodan, G.A., Bisphosphonate action. Alendronate localization in rat bone and effects on osteoclast ultrastructure, *J. Clin. Invest.,* 88, 2095, 1991.

42. Rodan, G.A. and Balena R., Bisphosphonates in the treatment of metabolic bone diseases, *Ann. Med.,* 25, 373, 1993.

43. Ferretti, J.L., Effects of bisphosphonates on bone biomechanics, in *Bisphosphonate Therapy in Acute and Chronic Bone Loss,* Bijvoet, A.M., Caufield, R., Fleisch, H., and Russell, R.G.G., Eds., Elsevier, Amsterdam, 1993.

44. Glatt, M., Pataki, A., Blättler, A., and Reife, R., APD long-term treatment increases bone mass and mechanical strength of femora of adult mice, *Calcif. Tiss. Int.,* 39, A72, 1986.

45. Ferretti, J.L., Cointry, G., Capozza, R., Montuori, E., Roldán, E. and Pérez, L.A., Biomechanical effects of the full range of useful doses of (3-amino-1-hydroxypropy-lidene)-1,1-bisphosphonate (APD) on femur diaphyses and cortical bone tissue in rats, *Bone Miner.,* 11, 101, 1990.

46. Einhorn, T., Peter, C.P., Clair, J., Rodan, G.A., and Thompson, D.D., Effect of alendronate on mechanical properties of bone in rats and dogs, *J. Bone Miner. Res.,* 5 (Suppl. 1), S97, 1990.

47. Mashiba, T., Turner, C.H., Hirano, T., Forwood, M.R., Johnston, C.C., and Burr, D.B., The effects of suppressed bone turnover by bisphosphonates on microdamage accumulation and biomechanical properties in clinically relevant sites in beagles, *Bone,* (submitted).

48. Black, D.M., Cummings, S.R., Karpf, D.B., Cauley, J.A., Thompson, D.E., Nevitt, M.C., Bauer, D.C., Genant, H.K., Haskell, W.L., Marcus, R., Ott, S.M., Torner, J.C., Quandt, S.A., Reiss, T.F., and Ensrud, K.E., Randomised trial of effect of alendronate on risk of fracture in women with existing vertebral fractures, *Lancet,* 348, 1535, 1996.

49. Cummings, S.R., Black, D.M., Thompson, D.E., Applegate, W.B., Barrett-Connor, E., Musliner, T.A., Palermo, L., Prineas, R., Rubin, S.M., Scott, J.C., Vogt, T., Wallace, R., Yates, A.J., and LaCroix, A.Z., Effect of alendronate on risk of fracture in women with low bone density but without vertebral fractures, *JAMA,* 280, 2077, 1998.

50. Shih, M-S. and Norrdin, R.W., Effects of prostaglandins on regional remodeling changes during tibial healing in beagles. A histomorphometric study, *Calcif. Tiss. Int.,* 39, 191, 1986.

51. Shih, M-S. and Norrdin, R.W., Effects of prostaglandin E_1 on regional haversian remodeling in beagles with fractured ribs: a histomorphometric study, *Bone,* 8, 87, 1987.

52. Li, X.J., Jee, W.S.S., Li, Y.L., and Patterson-Buckendahl, P., Transient effects of subcutaneously administered prostaglandin E_2 on cancellous and cortical bone in young adult dogs, *Bone,* 11, 353, 1990.

53. Jee, W.S.S., Mori, S., Li, X.J., and Chan, S., Prostaglandin E_2 enhances cortical bone mass and activates intracortical bone remodeling in intact and ovariectomized female rats, *Bone,* 11, 253, 1990.

54. Yeh, C.-K. and Rodan, G.A., Tensile forces enhance prostaglandin E synthesis in osteoblastic cells grown on collagen ribbons, *Calcif. Tissue Int.,* 36, S67, 1984.

55. Binderman, I., Shimshini, Z., and Somjen, D., Biochemical pathway involved in the translation of physical stimulus into biological message, *Calcif. Tissue Int.,* 36, S82, 1984.

56. Sudmann, E. and Bang, G., Indomethacin induced inhibition of haversian remodelling in rabbits, *Acta Orthop. Scand.,* 50, 621, 1979.

57. Keller, J., Kjærsgaard-Andersen, P., Bayer-Kristensen, I., and Melsen, F., Indomethacin and bone trauma. Effects on remodeling of rabbit bone, *Acta Orthop. Scand.,* 61, 66, 1990.

58. Norrdin, R.W., Jee, W.S.S., and High, W.B., The role of prostaglandins in bone *in vivo, Prostaglandins, Leukotrienes Essential Fatty Acids,* 41, 139, 1990.

59. Keller, J., Bayer-Kristensen, I., Bak, B., Bünger, C., Kjærsgaard-Andersen, P., Lucht, U., and Melsen, F., Indomethacin and bone remodeling. Effect on cortical bone after osteotomy in rabbits, *Acta Orthop. Scand.,* 60, 119, 1989.

60. Saffar, J.L. and Leroux, P., Role of prostaglandins in bone resorption in a synchronized remodeling sequence in the rat, *Bone,* 9, 141, 1988.

61. Van Tran, P., Vignery, A., and Baron, R., Cellular kinetics of the bone remodeling sequence in the rat, *Anat. Rec.,* 202, 445, 1982.

62. Frost, H.M., The regional acceleratory phenomenon: a review, *Henry Ford Hosp. Med. J.,* 31, 3, 1983.

63. Leroux, P. and Saffar, J.L., Dose-effect and evidence of escape of inhibition after indomethacin treatment in a synchronized model of bone resorption, *Agents Actions,* 38, 290, 1993.

64. Thompson, D.D. and Rodan, G.A., Indomethacin inhibition of tenotomy-induced bone resorption in rats, *J. Bone Miner. Res.,* 3, 409, 1988.

65. Schoutens, A., Verhas, M., Dourov, N., Bergmann, P., Caulin, F., Verschaeren, A., Mone, M., and Heilporn, A., Bone loss and bone blood flow in paraplegic rats treated with calcitonin, diphosphonate, and indomethacin, *Calcif. Tiss. Int.,* 42, 136, 1988.

66. Pead, M.J. and Lanyon, L.E., Indomethacin modulation of load-related stimulation of new bone formation *in vivo, Calcif. Tiss. Int.,* 45, 34, 1989.

67. Aufdemorte, T.B., Fox, C., McGuff, H.S., and Holt, G.R., Flurbiprofen enhances lamellar bone formation and decreases resorption in the baboon endosseous bone wound healing model, *J. Bone Miner. Res.,* 6 (Suppl. 1), S126, 1991.

68. Jee, W.S.S., Li, X.J., and Li, Y.L., Flurbiprofen-induced stimulation of periosteal bone formation and inhibition of bone resorption in older rats, *Bone,* 9, 381, 1988.

69. Li, X.J., Jee, W.S.S., and Li, Y.L., Flurbiprofen enhances growth and cancellous and cortical bone accumulation in rapidly growing long bones, *Bone,* 10, 35, 1989.

70. Hirano, T., Burr, D.B., Turner, C.H., Sato, M., Cain, R.L., and Hock, J.M., Anabolic effects of human biosynthetic parathyroid hormone fragment (1-34), LY333334, on remodeling and mechanical properties of cortical bone in rabbits, *J. Bone Miner. Res.,* 14, 536, 1999.

71. Mashiba, T., Burr, D.B., Turner, C.H., Sato, M., Cain, R.L., and Hock, J.M., Effects of human PTH (1-34), LY333334, on bone mass, remodeling and mechanical properties of cortical bone during the first remodeling cycle in rabbits, *Bone* (submitted).

72. Burr, D.B., Hirano, T., Turner, C.H., Hotchkiss, C., Brommage, R., and Hock, J.M., Intermittently administered hPTH (1-34) treatment increases intracortical bone turnover and porosity without reducing bone strength in the humerus of ovariectomized cynomolgus monkeys, *J. Bone Miner. Res.,* (in press).

73. Hirano, T., Burr, D.B., Cain, R.L., and Hock, J.M., Changes in geometry and cortical porosity in adult, ovary-intact rabbits after 5 months treatment with LY333334 (hPTH 1-34), *Calcif. Tiss. Int.,* 66, 456, 2000.

CHAPTER 18

Physical Diagnosis of Stress Fractures

Ingrid Ekenman

CONTENTS

Introduction..271
The Stress Fracture History..272
Tibial Stress Fractures 273
Femoral Stress Fractures 273
Metatarsal Stress Fractures..275
Navicular Stress Fractures...276
Calcaneal Stress Fractures...276
Pelvic Stress Fractures...276
Be Aware..277
Summary...277
References...277

INTRODUCTION

Stress fractures are considered to be caused by cyclical overloading of bone. The amount of cyclical overloading necessary to cause a stress fracture at any specific anatomical site varies according to the individual. One extreme is the marathon trainee who develops a metatarsal stress fracture secondary to long and arduous training, and the other, the middle aged tourist who develops the same type of stress fracture while sightseeing in Paris. The usual clinical presentation of stress fracture is exertionally related bone pain. However, the type and severity of symptoms are related to the specific bone, and may be especially confusing when the femur, hip, pelvis, or navicular are involved. Additionally, tolerance and interpretation of musculoskeletal pain may vary greatly between individuals. The physical diagnosis of stress fracture as well as the differential diagnosis is different for each individual bone. Therefore, each bone will be discussed individually.

THE STRESS FRACTURE HISTORY

As in other fields of medicine, stress fracture physical diagnosis begins with a didactic history. The athlete, and to a much lesser extent the military recruit, is usually able to give a comprehensive history of the problem, which in the case of stress fracture manifests itself by the appearance of pain. Devas states that in the majority of cases there is a slow progression of symptoms over several weeks, but "occasionally pain comes on so severely and quickly that an athlete can not finish his sport".[1] When asking the standard questions as to the onset, site, duration, consistency, intensity of pain, and limitations caused by the pain, the examiner should be aware that the responses he receives may sometimes be distorted for conscious or subconscious reasons. It is important to hunt for the possible etiology of the stress fracture in the history. Athletes usually have well patterned training programs. Any unusual change in training may be the cause of the stress fracture. Devas gives the example of an athlete who usually ran on a track, but owing to exceptionally heavy rainfall had to train on a hard road instead.[1] For the non athlete there often is a history of a recent holiday away from home, with extra walking.

Of course, not every case of exertionally related bone pain represents a stress fracture. Sometimes no reason will be found, and the pain is said to be a normal consequence of training. Milgrom et al., in a prospective study, found that 41% of Israeli infantry recruits suffered from medial tibial pain during 14 weeks of basic training.[2] All the cases were evaluated by bone scintigraphy. Scintigraphic abnormalities were found in 63%, stress fractures in 46%, periostitis in 2%, and an irregular area of increased scintigraphic uptake in 15%. The latter may reflect the very early stages of a stress fracture or a remodeling response. Thus, even in the uniform training environment of this military study, the clinical suspicion of a medial tibial stress fracture was only confirmed in about half of the cases.

The differential diagnosis of exertionally related bone pain includes tumor, both benign and malignant, and infection. The underlying pathology can cover the spectrum of a benign bone cyst, aneurysmal bone cyst, osteogenic sarcoma, metastatic lesion of bone, and hematological tumor. These possibilities must always be in the back of the examiner's mind. Each of these pathologies usually has distinct age and anatomical prevalences.[3] Bilateral and symmetrical exertionally related bone pain is highly unlikely to represent tumor or infection. The anatomical location of the bone pain also can be a key. Diaphyseal femoral stress fractures occur in the medial cortex. Diaphyseal tibial stress fractures occur along the posterior medial or anterior cortices. Therefore, for example, exertionally related bone pain along the lateral cortex of these bones is not consistent with stress fractures.

Exertional bone pain at multiple sites is consistent with stress fracture as well as tumor or infection. Milgrom et al. reported on an elite infantry soldier who sustained 14 stress fractures at different anatomical sites during the course of one year of arduous training.[4] When taking a history the examiner must be aware of the possibility that multiple stress fractures exist and that the most painful stress fracture site can mask less painful areas. The subject should be asked routinely if in addition to the area of the chief complaint, there are other less painful sites. The subject may also not connect the possibility that tightness or an ache in the thigh or groin muscles may represent stress fracture.[1] This often is the only sign of a femoral stress fracture.

TIBIAL STRESS FRACTURES

The tibia is the most common site for stress fractures among athletes and military trainees. Many studies report that about 50% of all stress fractures occur in the tibia, with the most frequent locations either in the distal or middle third, along the posterior medial border.[5,6,7] The anterior cortex is involved less frequently. Because there is little soft tissue protection over the anterior and medial borders of the tibia, the periosteum in these areas has a role in protective sensation. This function necessitates a high senstivity, and may be the reason why tibial stress fractures present early with pain.[8,9]

The term shin splints confuses the diagnosis of medial tibial pain. To some, shin splints describes all medial tibial pain, to some it represents a periostitis, and to others it refers to medial tibial pain of idiopathic origin.[10-14] The differential diagnosis includes stress fracture, periostitis, musculotendinous injury, and ischemia of the medial compartment. Physical examination is the key to narrowing the differential diagnosis. The examiner palpates the posterior medial border of the tibia, applying firm finger pressure. Tenderness along the entire length or along a broad band is consistent with periostitis. Point tenderness is consistent with a stress fracture. There may be multiple stress fractures in the medial tibia, and they may be of different severity. When there is question of secondary gain, the examiner should record the point of tenderness and measure its distance from a landmark such as the medial malleolus or medial tibial plateau. If the point of tenderness is not consistent on consecutive measurements, this will raise a question about the physiology of the complaint.

Physical examination of exertional anterior compartment syndrome is time consuming. Ideally, the subject should be examined first at rest, and then sent to run a distance thought to be great enough to cause symptoms on the basis of the history. After the run, the subject is immediately examined to see if there is swelling and tenderness over the compartment.

Anterior tibial stress fractures usually have a much slower onset than medial tibial stress fractures. The physical diagnosis is very simple because there are no other relevant anatomical structures over the anterior tibia. The examiner uses finger pressure to palpate the anterior tibial border. Any localized point tenderness is consistent with stress fracture.

FEMORAL STRESS FRACTURES

The periosteum of the femur is less sensitive than the periosteum of the tibia, making it difficult to delineate between muscle and bone pain in the proximal femur.

Milgrom et al. used a bone scan as the basis for diagnosis of stress fracture, and found a high incidence of asymptomatic stress fractures of the femur in Israeli military recruits.[7] They related this phenomenon to the low sensitivity of the femoral periosteum as compared with that of the tibia. The higher levels of pain associated with a tibial stress fracture could mask that of a concomitant femoral stress fracture. Devas states that "the lack of symptoms in a stress fracture of the femur can mislead. It is unusual to have a long history of severe pain."[6] According to Devas, the symptoms can consist of either a mild aching in the thigh or a complaint of muscle stiffness in the region of the hip or knee. At the Central Military Hospital in Helsinki, Visuri and Hietaniemi found three military recruits with displaced femoral stress fractures. Before displacement, they suffered from knee and distal femoral pain for two to six weeks.[15]

Milgrom et al. have described the "fist test" as an integral part of the stress fracture examination (Figure 1).[16] They recommend that for any patient with a

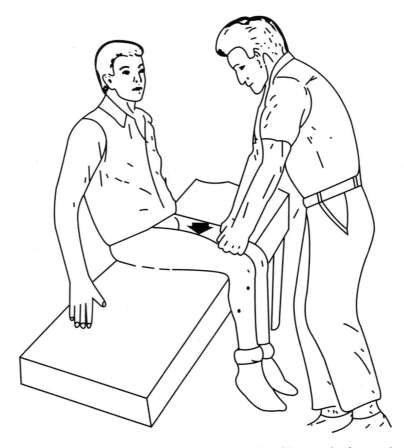

Figure 1   The "Fist Test" is performed by applying the weight of the examiner's upper torso via clenched fists over the anterior aspect of the femurs from distal to proximal. The test is positive if a difference in sensitivity or pain can be detected.

complaint consistent with stress fracture, a complete lower extremity stress fracture examination should be done automatically. For the femur, this consists of the "fist test". Because of low sensitivity of the femoral periosteum and its protection by a thick envelope of muscles, palpation by finger pressure is not sufficient. The authors recommend palpating both femurs simultaneously from proximal to distal, leaning on them with the weight of the body applied by a fist on each femur. A difference in sensitivity or pain on palpation is consistent with a femoral stress fracture.

Tenderness in the area of the hip joint and the femoral neck should alert the examiner to the possibility of a femoral neck stress fracture. Those are the most malignant of all the stress fractures. Fortunately they are not common, occurring only occasionally among athletes and military recruits. Femoral neck stress fractures also occur in the elderly in the form of insufficiency fractures. A descriptive classification based on the degree of fracture displacement was presented by Blickenstaff and Morris,[10] while Fullerton and Snowdy[17] categorized types of fracture as compression, tension, and displaced fractures. Sustaining a displaced femoral neck stress fracture is a disaster at any age, and for an elite athlete it usually means the end of the career.

Devas states that sometimes the presenting symptoms of a femoral neck stress fracture may be when the hip gives way due to a femoral neck fracture.[1] A groin ache that gradually develops and is related to the level of exertion is a more typical presentation. Sometimes the pain is so severe that activity has to be stopped. Bilateral femoral neck stress fractures have been reported and are not always of the same magnitude. A complete assessment of the hip area should be made on a stress fracture physical examination. The exam is done bilaterally, with the unaffected side used to represent the normal sensitivity of the area to exam. With the patient lying supine, the sole of his foot is hit with the clenched fist of the examiner. Any pain in the groin area secondary to this is consistent with a femoral neck stress fracture. The region of the femoral neck is then specifically palpated. Again, tenderness here is consistent with a femoral neck stress fracture. With the hip flexed to 90° the hip is passively rotated, achieving maximum internal and external rotation. Again, pain from this maneuver can represent a femoral neck stress fracture. However, it can also be secondary to a synovitis of the hip or pain from the groin muscles attached to the hip. The patient can additionally be asked to stand and alternatively perform a vertical jump on both legs, and then on the affected leg. Pain in the hip region secondary to this is consistent with a femoral neck stress fracture.

METATARSAL STRESS FRACTURES

Metatarsal stress fractures are the most well known stress fractures and are often called "march fractures", a term that refers to their first description in 1885 by Breitheupt.[18] They most often occur in the second or third metatarsal, and they usually heal without complications within three to four weeks. Their epidemiology can be quite different from that of the tibial or femoral stress fracture. Someone can be entirely asymptomatic at the beginning of an exertional activity and at the end be found to have a frank fracture of one or more of the cortices of the second or third metatarsus. On physical examination, the foot should be placed on the ground and each metatarsus palpated using finger pressure for signs of local tenderness. Pain specifically on the bone and not over the metatarsal interspace is consistent with a metatarsal stress fracture.

NAVICULAR STRESS FRACTURES

This kind of stress fracture is relatively uncommon, and symptoms often persist for an extended time before the diagnosis is made. Physical examination is again the key to diagnosis. The history is usually pain in the midfoot, which increases after exercise and at the end of the day. Often these symptoms are thought to represent ligamentous strain. The navicular should be palpated by finger pressure along its dorsal surface, its medial surface and along the inferior border of the talonavicular joint. Specific tenderness at any of these sites is consistent with stress fracture of the navicular. Routine radiographs are usually not helpful in diagnosing this fracture in the acute stages. CT is far superior to either plain radiographs or plain tomograms when diagnosing and treating these injuries. Often there is wide displacement of a complete fracture, and operation with grafting and compression screws is necessary.[19,20]

CALCANEAL STRESS FRACTURES

Most pain in the heel regions of athletes is secondary to plantar fascitis or heel spur syndrome. These conditions can be differentiated from calcaneal stress fracture by careful physical examination. Typically, in calcaneal stress fracture there is tenderness under the ball of the heel as well on each side of the body of the calcaneus at its junction with the tuberosity. This is the anatomical site of the calcaneal stress fracture. Movements of the subtalar joint are unrestricted passively and there is no tenderness on the calcaneal tuberosity. In plantar fascitis and heel spur syndrome, the pain is specifically localized to a point or region on the ball of the heel.

PELVIC STRESS FRACTURES

Pelvic stress fractures are usually confined to two types, pubic rami or sacroiliac joint. The former are more prevalent in females than males. Sacroiliac stress fractures are extremely rare, and to date have not been reported in females.[21] The physical exam of a suspected pubic stress fracture consists of direct palpation of the inferior and superior pubic rami bilaterally. A bilateral examination is essential because this area may be ordinarily sensitive, and comparison must be done with the unaffected side. The examination of a suspected sacroiliac joint stress fracture is difficult because of the anatomical depth and plane of the joint. Pain in this region may also represent back pain. Direct palpation of the joint area is attempted with finger pressure. The presence of pain on performing the Gaenslen's sign indicates that the pathology is specifically present in the sacroiliac joint.[22] This sign is performed while the patient lies supine on the examination table. The patient is instructed to draw both legs onto his chest. Then the patient is shifted to the side of the table so that the buttock of the affected side extends over the edge of the table while the other remains on it. The unsupported leg on the affected side is allowed to drop over the edge while the opposite leg remains flexed. A complaint of pain in the region of the sacroiliac joint while performing this maneuver is a positive sign.

BE AWARE

While exertionally related bone pain in the athlete or military trainee often represents a stress fracture, there is also the possibility of bone tumor. This may be benign or malignant. Bilateral and symmetrical pain virtually rules out the possibility of a bone tumor. If the pain is on the lateral cortex of the femur or the tibia, the pathology is highly unlikely to be a stress fracture. A plain x-ray centered on the clinically suspicious site is usually all that is needed to remove bone tumor from the differential diagnosis. Occasionally a bone scan will be required.

SUMMARY

The stress fracture physical examination begins with a complete history. The history not only will aid in diagnosis, but can offer hints as to errors in the specific training program. This information can be valuable for stress fracture prevention in other trainees. For anyone suspected of a stress fracture, a comprehensive stress fracture exam of the lower extremities should be done. This may unmask the unsymptomatic or barely symptomatic femoral stress fracture. Conformation of a clinical suspicion of a stress fracture is done using imaging techniques. The role of plain radiographs, bone scintigraphy, and MR in diagnosis and treatment are discussed in other chapters. One should always be aware that the primary pathology in exertionally related bone pain is not always an overuse injury. In a small number of cases it may reflect bone tumor, either benign or malignant.

REFERENCES

1. Devas, M., *Stress Fractures*, Churchill Livingston, Edinburgh, 1975.
2. Milgrom, C., Giladi, M., Stein, M., Kashtan, H., Margulies, J., Chisin, R., Steinberg, R., Swissa, A., and Aharonson, Z., Medial tibial pain, *Clin. Orthop.*, 213, 167, 1986.
3. Spjut, H.J., Dorfam, H.D., Fechner, F.E., and Ackerman, L.V., *Tumors of Bone and Cartilage*, Armed Forces Institute of Pathology, Washington, D.C., 1971.
4. Milgrom, C., Chisin, R., Giladi, M., Stein, M., Kashtan, H., Margulies, J., and Atlan, H., Multiple stress fractures — a longitudinal study of a soldier with 13 lesions, *Clin. Orthop.*, 192, 174, 1985.
5. Hulkko, A., *Stress Fractures in Athletes*, Thesis, University of Oulu, 1988.
6. Johansson, C., Ekenman, I., and Lewander, R., Stress fractures of the tibia in athletes: diagnosis and natural course, *Scand. J. Med. Sci. Sports*, 2, 87, 1992.

7. Milgrom, C., Giladi, M., Stein, M., Kashtan, H., Marguiles, J., Chisin, R., Steinberg, R., and Ahronson, Z., Stress fractures in military recruits. A prospective study showing an unusually high incidence, *J. Bone Jt. Surg.*, 67B, 732, 1985.

8. Milgrom, C., Finestone, A., Shlamkovitch, N., Giladi, M., Lev, B., Wiener, M., and Schaffler M., Stress fracture treatment, *Orthop. Int.*, 363, 1995.

9. Schaffler, M. and Boyd, R., Bone remodelling and microdamage in experimental stress fracture, 43rd Annual Meeting ORS, San Francisco, 113, 1997.

10. Blickenstaff, L.D. and Morris, J.M., Fatigue fracture of the femoral neck, *J. Bone Jt. Surg.*, 48A, 1031, 1966.

11. Clement, D.B., Taunton, J.E., Smart, G.W., and McNicol, K.L., Survey of overuse injuries, *Physician Sportsmed.*, 9, 47, 1981.

12. Friedenberg, Z.B., Fatigue fractures of the tibia, *Clin. Orthop.*, 76, 111, 1971.

13. Michael, R H. and Holder, L.E., The soleus syndrome. A cause of medial tibial stress (shin splints), *Am. J. Sports Med.*, 13, 87, 1984.

14. Styf, J., Diagnosis of exercise-induced pain in the anterior aspect of the lower leg, *Am. J. Sports Med.*, 16, 165, 1988.

15. Visuri, T. and Hietaniemi, K., Displaced stress fractures of the femoral shaft: a report of three cases, *Mil. Med.*, 157, 325, 1992.

16. Milgrom, C., Finestone, A., Shlamkovitch, N., Eldad, A., Saltzman, S., Giladi, M., Chisin, R., and Danon, Y.L., The clinical assessment of femoral stress fractures: a comparison of two methods, *Mil. Med.*, 158, 190, 1993.

17. Fullerton, L.R. and Snowdy, H.A., Femoral neck stress fractures, *Am. J. Sports Med.*, 16, 365, 1988.

18. Breitheupt, M.D., Zur pathologie des menschlichen fusses, *Med. Ztg.*, 24, 169, 1855.

19. Fitch K., Blackwell, J., and Gilmour, W., Operation for non-union of stress fracture of the tarsal navicular, *J. Bone Jt. Surg.*, 71B, 105, 1989.

20. Hulkko, A., Orava, S., Peltokallio, P., Tulikkoura, I., and Walden, M., Stress fracture of the navicular bone, *Acta Orthop. Scand.*, 56, 503, 1985.

21. Volpin, P., Milgrom, C., Goldsher, D., and Stein, H., Stress fractures of the sacrum following strenuous activity, *Clin. Orthop.*, 243, 184, 1989.

22. Hoppenfeld, H., *Physical Examination of the Spine and Extremities*, Appleton-Century–Crofts, New York, 1976.

CHAPTER **19**

The Role of Various Imaging Modalities in Diagnosing Stress Fractures

Roland Chisin

CONTENTS

Introduction 279
Plain Radiographs 280
Bone Scintigraphy 280
    Classification by Image Characteristics 283
    Soft Tissue Versus Bony Lesions 285
    Appearance of Developing and Healing Stress Fractures 286
    Diagnosis of Pelvic Stress Fractures 286
    Diagnosis of Stress Fractures of Foot and Ankle 287
    Asymptomatic Stress Fractures 289
Computed Tomography 291
Magnetic Resonance Imaging 291
Summary 291
References 292

INTRODUCTION

The first description of stress fracture was made in 1855 by Breitheupt.[1] His diagnosis was made clinically, and only subsequently confirmed radiographically. Originally, stress fractures were considered to be confined to the metatarsus in soldiers who marched. Hence, the name march fracture. Later, stress fractures were identified in athletes, and in bones of the upper as well as lower extremities. Up until the mid 1970s, plain radiographs were the only diagnostic modality available to confirm a clinical suspicion of stress fracture. The limitation of radiographs is that they can only identify a stress fracture if it has progressed to the stage of a visible macro fracture or if there is healing callus present. Since the mid 1970s, bone scintigraphy has been used for early detection of stress fracture while it still is in the microdamage stage. Recently, MRI has begun to play a role in identifying stress fractures.

The diagnosis of stress fractures is primarily clinical. The classic history of exercise-associated bone pain and typical examination findings of localized bony tenderness are consistent with a diagnosis of stress fracture. However, clinical assessment is usually not definitive. In a prospective study of stress fractures, Milgrom et al. found that in only 50% of military recruits with a clinical suspicion of tibial stress fracture, was the diagnosis confirmed by scintigraphy. [2] When the patient with a clinical suspicion of stress fracture is a competitive athlete or a soldier who wishes to continue training, early diagnosis is essential. Various imaging techniques are then available to the clinician. We shall review the application of those tools for the diagnosis of stress fractures of the lower extremities and pelvis. Detailed treatment algorithms based on imaging findings and tailored according to localization of common stress fractures of the lower extremities can be found in Chapter 20.

PLAIN RADIOGRAPHS

Plain radiographs have poor sensitivity but are highly specific for the diagnosis of stress fractures.[3] A stress fracture can be confirmed by the presence of any of the classic radiographic abnormalities: periosteal bone formation, a horizontal or oblique linear pattern of sclerosis, hazy endosteal callus formation, or a fracture line (Figures 1–3). In most patients with stress fractures, there is no obvious radiographic abnormality unless symptoms have been present for at least two or three weeks.[4] In some patients, radiographic changes never appear. For maximum resolution, the radiographs should be centered on the specific anatomical area in question. In two series of military recruits, only 18 and 20% of the scintigraphic foci representing stress fractures were positive on x-ray.[2,5] In the Zwas et al. series, the percentage of false-negative radiographs was the highest for scintigraphic Grade I lesions (96%), less for Grade II and III (79 and 24%, respectively), and non-existent for Grade IV.[5] The probability of a positive x-ray is lower for the tibia but higher for the femur or metatarsus. This is probably because tibial stress fractures present early with strong pain, and thereby prevent the trainee from continuing activity that could allow the tibial stress fracture to progress. This generally prevents medial tibial stress fractures from developing into macro stress fractures that can be seen on x-ray.

BONE SCINTIGRAPHY

Bone scintigraphy is the most sensitive indicator of bone stress, but has poor specificity. Bone scanning is almost exclusively performed using ^{99m}Tc-labeled disphosphonates. Methylene diphosphonate (MDP) is still the most widely used agent;

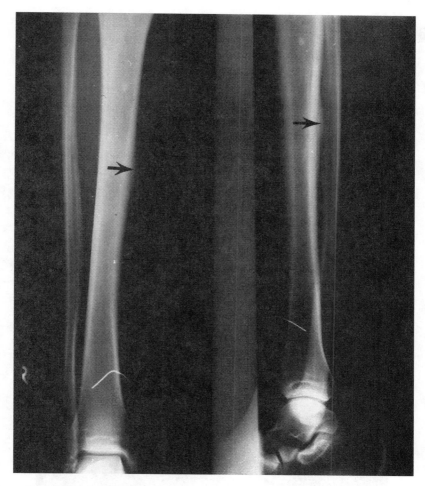

Figure 1 Radiograph of the tibia demonstrates the healing callus of a stress fracture in the medial aspect of the middle third (arrows).

hydroxyethylidene diphosphonate (HEDP) or hydroxymethylene disphosphonate (HMDP) are less frequently used. The mechanism of tracer uptake in bone is not entirely elucidated, but it is believed that disphosphonate is adsorbed on the hydroxyapatite matrix of the bone, with particular affinity for sites of new bone formation. The immature collagen also may trap ^{99m}Tc disphosphonate. Disphosphonate uptake on bone is thought to primarily reflect osteoblastic activity, but it is generally accepted that bone tracer deposition is also dependent on bone blood flow.[6] Einhorn et al. studied the localization of ^{99m}Tc-disphosphonate in bone using micro autoradiography.[7] Four rabbits underwent operation in which two 1.5 mm drill holes were created in the subtrochanteric region of their femurs, and four rabbits underwent sham operation. After seven days, the rabbits underwent bone scans. After the scans were completed, the animals were sacrificed and their femurs histologically processed

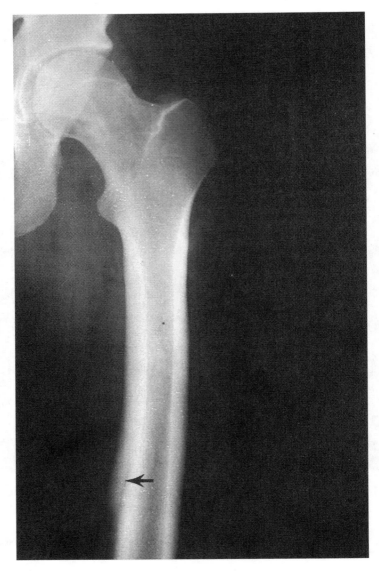

Figure 2 Radiograph of the femur shows the healing callus of a stress fracture in the medial
aspect of the mid diaphysis (arrow).

for micro autoradiography and routine histopathology. The ^{99m}Tc isotope was localized in mineralized fronts and was absent from the cytoplasm of osteoblasts and
osteoclasts. There was increased activity in the region of the drill holes.

In order to obtain a bone scan, a standard dose of 20 mCi (750 MBq) of ^{99m}Tc
MDP is used. Anterior and posterior whole body scans are performed two to
three hours after intravenous injection. Additional delayed spot views of the pelvis,

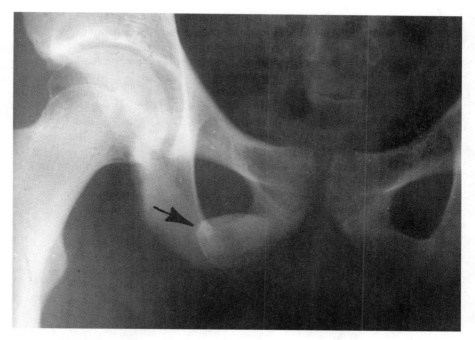

Figure 3   Radiograph of the pubis showing the healing callus of a stress fracture of the inferior pubic ramus (arrow).

femurs, knees, tibias, and feet are sometimes necessary. A comprehensive foot scintigraphic evaluation should include plantar views, which best depict the metatarsals. Single photon emission computed tomography (SPECT) imaging is most useful in a suspected pars intra-articular stress fracture, but only marginally useful in suspected long bone stress fractures.

Classification by Image Characteristics

Tibial lesions are the most common stress fractures, most frequently medial and sometimes anterior. Scintigraphic features of stress fractures relate to the focal intensity and the extent of cortical involvement. Various classifications have been proposed by Matin,[8] Zwas et al.,[5] and Milgrom et al.[9] The typical appearance of stress fracture in a long bone such as the tibia is a fusiform transverse focus that is optimally evaluated using two orthogonal views. This means that in addition to an anterior-posterior view of the relevant bone, a lateral view is required to assess the percentage of thickness involved. Matin's system ranges from stage I with involvement of up to 20% of cortical thickness through stage V (80 to 100% involvement), or a full-thickness stress fracture. Alternatively, a four-stage system may divide cortical involvement into stage I (0 to 25%) to stage IV (76 to 100%). Zwas et al. divide the range of the scintigraphic findings into four grades: ·

I. Ill-defined cortical lesion with slightly increased activity
II. Larger, well-defined elongated cortical area of moderately increased activity
III. Wide-fusiform corticomedullary area of highly increased activity
IV. Well-defined intramedullary transcortical lesion with intensely increased activity (Figures 4 and 5).[5]

Milgrom et al., in a similar way, rate the scans into Grade 1 and 2 for irregular and/or poorly defined areas of increased activity, and Grades 3 and 4 for sharply marginated — focal or fusiform — findings.[9]

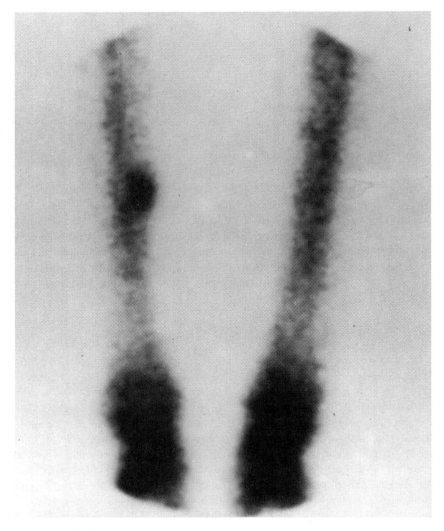

Figure 4 Anterior bone scintigraphy of the tibias with a grade III focus by the Zwas scale in the right medial tibia.[5]

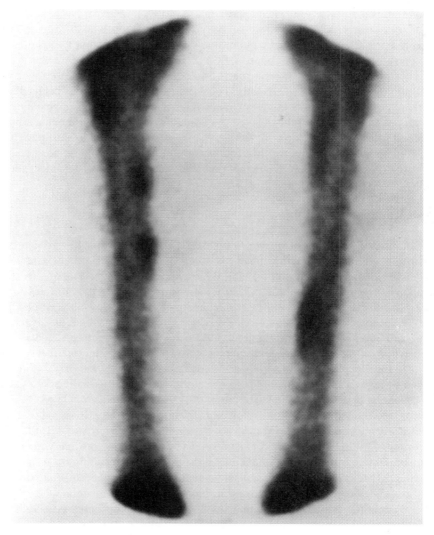

Figure 5 Anterior bone scintigraphy of tibias with multiple foci by the Zwas scale: 2 Grades II in the right tibia and a Grade IV in the left tibia.[5]

Soft Tissue Versus Bony Lesions

Using a triple-phase ^{99m}Tc MDP bone scan, one can differentiate soft tissue and bony injury.[3] In the first phase, flow images obtained immediately after the intravenous injection of the tracer show perfusion in bone and soft tissues and may demonstrate increased perfusion in acute inflammation. The second phase ("blood pool" phase), imaged one to two minutes after the injection, reflects the degree of hyperemia and capillary permeability of bone and soft tissue. It may also show increased uptake in acute inflammation. The third phase consists of delayed images taken three to four hours after injection, when approximately 50% of the tracer has concentrated in the bone matrix. All three phases can be positive in patients who have acute stress fractures. In soft tissue injuries without bony involvement, the first two phases are often positive, but the delayed phase shows no or minimal increased uptake. As the bony lesion in stress fracture heals, perfusion returns to normal, followed by blood pool normalization a few weeks later. Focal increased uptake on the delayed scan resolves last because remodeling continues after pain disappears. As healing continues, uptake intensity on the delayed scan diminishes three to six months after an uncomplicated stress fracture; sometimes the increased uptake persists longer than twelve months. Bone scans are therefore not useful in monitoring the bone healing of a stress fracture, and they should not be unduly repeated. This assessment should be based on clinical judgment.[3]

Appearance of Developing and Healing Stress Fractures

Although focal areas of increased uptake on the delayed images are generally consistent with stress fractures, the classical significance of irregular areas of increased uptake is more controversial, representing either bone reaction to stress or a stress fracture in evolution. Chisin et al. found uncertainty of progression to stress fractures of nonfocal scintigraphic findings in suspected tibial stress fractures.[10] Disappearance of pain correlated with scintigraphic healing, and increased pain with progression to scintigraphic evidence of stress fracture; decreased or persistent pain had equivocal scintigraphic correlation. This suggests that military recruits and people training for sports who have nonfocal scintigraphic findings should be given a brief rest period before resuming training; this should be less than the usual rest period for a stress fracture in the same anatomic site. On returning to activity, the individual should be clinically monitored carefully. Early detection of tibial stress fractures prevents evolution of a micro to a macro fracture. It is therefore important to differentiate them from shin splints, a self-limiting process with no risk of frank fracture, caused by inflammation of the periosteum resulting from abnormal demands of the posterior tibialis and soleus muscles on the posteromedial border of the tibia. The scintigraphic pattern is an elongated area of moderately increased uptake along the posteromedial tibial shaft, usually without increased activity on radionuclide angiograms and blood pool images (Figure 6).[11] Exercise-induced calf pain can also be caused by compartment syndrome, due to increased pressure within the fascial boundaries of the calf. Plain radiographs and bone scintigraphy are unremarkable in this case.

Diagnosis of Pelvic Stress Fractures

The second most frequent location of stress fractures is the femur. Proximal femoral stress fractures are sometimes difficult to differentiate clinically from pelvis stress fractures. In the pelvis, stress reactions of the sacroiliac joint (Figure 7) are clinically undistinguishable from back pain due to stress reactions of the vertebral pars articularis. They commonly occur in young, healthy athletes or military recruits who begin an exercise program or who have increased their level of athletic intensity.

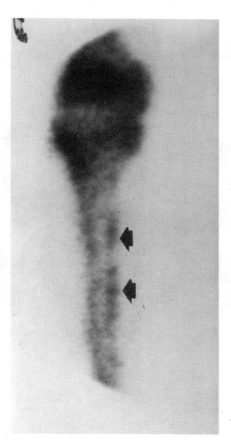

Figure 6 Arrows point to a band of increased scintigraphic activity along the posteromedial tibial cortex, representing shin splints.

Findings on plain radiographs are unremarkable, yet bone scan shows unilateral increased activity in the sacroiliac joint.[12] Sacral stress fractures among running athletes have been increasingly recognized as a potential cause of sacral and buttock pain that does not respond to treatment. Plain radiographs are typically normal.[13]

Pubic ramus stress fractures (Figure 8) often cause hip pain, and should be included in the differential diagnosis of nontraumatic thigh and groin pain in athletes and training soldiers together with femoral stress fractures of the femoral shaft, subtrochanteric region, or femoral neck.[14] Scintigraphically, it is very difficult to distinguish true biomechanical femoral stress fractures from adductor avulsion fractures.[15]

Diagnosis of Stress Fractures of Foot and Ankle

In the foot and ankle, most stress fractures occur in the metatarsals ("march fractures"), with about 90% of the cases in the second and the third metatarsi.[16] The grading system used for the long bones does not apply for the cancellous bones of

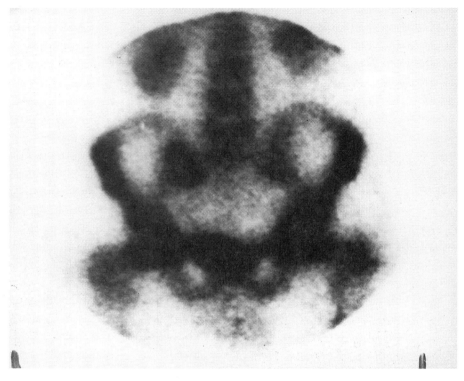

Figure 7 Anterior view bone scintigraphy showing a clear focus of increased pathological
uptake in the right sacroiliac joint.

the foot. Chisin et al. developed a separate grading system to be used for the
cancellous bones of the feet.[17] In this system, Grade 1 and 2 are not considered to
represent a stress fracture (Figure 9). Any tarsal bone can be the site of abnormal
uptake on scintigraphy, and stress fractures of the navicular, calcaneus, cuboid, and
medial and lateral malleoli have been described. Stress fractures of the central portion
of the body of the calcaneus can be encountered in activities such as parachute
jumping or prolonged standing; on scintigraphy, there is a vertical band of increased
uptake. The most difficult stress fractures to identify are those of the navicular bone.
Usually the lesion is on the middle third. A frequent cause of acute or chronic ankle
pain is the subchondral stress fracture of the talar dome.[18] This lesion is best
demonstrated by lateral and posterior views, and may benefit from the use of a
pinhole collimator. Increased ^{99m}Tc MDP uptake has also been described across the
tarsometatarsal joints after an injury to Lisfranc's joint in a 16 year-old kick boxer.[19]

The hallux sesamoids at the head of the first metatarsal may be injured acutely, or
more frequently, secondary to repetitive stress during athletic or military training. The
typical clinical presentation is one of a several-week history of pain about the meta-
tarso-phalangeal joint of the great toe. On physical examination, tenderness may be
elicited by gentle palpation of the sesamoids. Plain radiographs can identify bipartite
sesamoids and osteochondritis. Bone scintigraphy may be helpful; however, caution

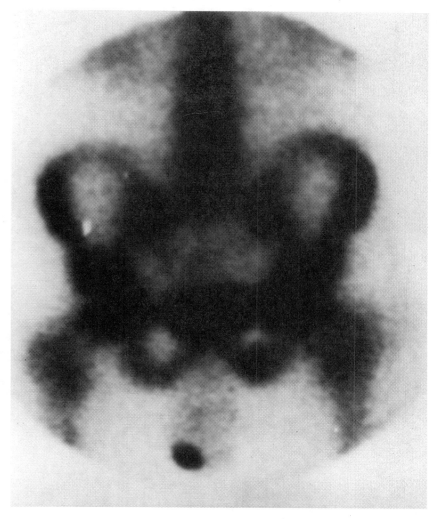

Figure 8 Anterior scintigraphy of the pelvis showing a stress fracture of the left inferior public ramus.

should be used in interpreting the meaning of mild to moderate increased scintigraphic activity. The usual tibial bone scintigraphic rating system is not valid;[5,9] for the sesamoids, only marked increased activity is likely to reflect sesamoid pathology.[20]

Asymptomatic Stress Fractures

Stress fractures can be a multifocal disease, not all foci being necessarily symptomatic. Unsuspected sites of injury may therefore be identified on whole-body bone scintigraphy since increased uptake is frequently found at asymptomatic sites of early bone stress, particularly in active patients. According to Milgrom et al., 69%

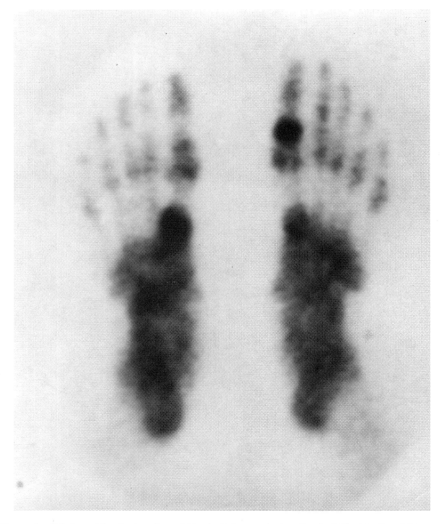

Figure 9 Scintigraphic plantar view of the feet demonstrates Grade IV foci in the right great toe and in the left first metatarsus, and a Grade I focus in the left mid tarsus (From Chisin, R., Milgrom, C., Giladi, M., Stein, M., Kashtan, J., Margulies, J., and Atlan, H., Abstracts of the 3rd Asia and Oceania Congress of Nuclear Medicine, Seoul, August 27-32, 1984.

of the femoral stress fractures, but only 8% tibial stress fractures were asymptomatic.[2] This underlines the importance of obtaining a whole body view in runners or military recruits. Limited tibial spot views are therefore to be avoided since even asymptomatic stress fractures, particularly of the femur, need to be treated. Increased scintigraphic activity of the lateral cortex of the tibia or femur is unlikely to be a stress fracture.

COMPUTED TOMOGRAPHY

Other conditions such as osteomyelitis, bony infarct, bony displasia, malignant neoplasm, osteoid osteoma, or monoarticular arthritis can also produce scintigraphic images of localized increased uptake; therefore, it is important to balance these findings with the patient's clinical picture,[4] and if necessary, with plain radiographs or CT scan.[21] Although bone scintigraphy is virtually 100% sensitive for identifying focal increases in bone turnover, it does not visualize a stress fracture. CT scans are particularly valuable when a fracture image is needed to make therapeutic decisions,[4] such as in navicular stress fractures[22] and stress fractures of the sacroiliac joint.

MAGNETIC RESONANCE IMAGING

Magnetic resonance imaging (MRI) can be used in the primary investigation of stress fractures. It is as sensitive as scintigraphy to image the medullary canal and perhaps cancellous bone, but is highly specific and can visualize soft tissue damage. However, MRI is expensive and does not image cortical bone.

A bone stress reaction on MRI shows up as bone marrow edema, and stress fractures can be typically identified as a fracture line at the level of the cortex surrounded by an intense zone of edema in the medullary cavity.[23] These signs are most evident in fat-suppressed views such as the short T1 inversion recovery sequences. Lee and Yao,[24] in five patients who had initially normal radiographs and abnormal radionuclide bone scans, described a thick intramedullary band of very low signal intensity, continuous at some point with the cortex and surrounded by an area of mildly to moderately decreased intensity in the marrow space. Sacks et al. found it difficult to distinguish stress fractures from occult intraosseous fractures or bone bruises, or even occasionally from more aggressive lesions.[25] Hodler et al., comparing the diagnostic value of MRI with two-phase bone scintigraphy in 16 patients with stress-related bone injuries and normal standard radiographs, concluded that for patients with a history compatible with stress fracture, and a low probability of other active bone diseases such as infection or neoplasm, bone scintigraphy should be the initial imaging modality.[26]

In a prospective study of 19 military subjects engaged in endurance training,[27] MRI proved to be superior to bone scintigraphy in providing an early and accurate diagnosis of the hip pain when femoral stress fracture is in the differential diagnosis: bone scintigraphy had an accuracy of 68% for femoral neck stress fractures, while MR was 100% accurate.

SUMMARY

The most valuable imaging tool to diagnose stress fracture is still bone scintigraphy. There are large databases correlating size of the scintigraphic foci with severity of the stress fracture. On this basis, early treatment of stress fractures before they are evident on plain x-rays can be given. Because of this early intervention, usually only short treatment periods are necessary. Bone scintigraphy has almost no role to play in followup of stress fracture healing. MRI is mainly useful for bone medullary imaging, and may become more utilized with the development of extremity scanners.

The Israeli Army has developed algorithms for treatment of stress fracture based on physical diagnosis and scintigraphic evaluation. Because the epidemiology of tibial, femoral, and metatarsal stress fractures is different, there are separate algorithms for each fracture. A civilian modification of these protocols has been developed for medial tibial, femoral diaphyseal, and metatarsal stress fractures. These will be discussed in Chapter 20.

REFERENCES

1. Breitheupt, M.D., Zur pathologie des menschlichen fusses, *Med. Ztg.*, 24, 169, 1855.
2. Milgrom, C., Giladi, M., Stein, M., Kashtan, H., Chisin, R., Steinberg, R., and Aharonson, Z., Stress fractures in military recruits, *J. Bone Jt. Surg., (Br)*, 67B, 732, 1985.
3. Daffner, R.H. and Pavlov, H., Stress fractures: current concepts, *Am. J. Roentgenol.*, 159, 15, 1985.
4. Brukner, P., Bradshaw, C., and Bennell, K., Managing common stress fractures: let risk level guide treatment, *Phys. Sports Med.*, 26, 39, 1998.
5. Zwas, T.S., Elkanovitch, R., and Frank, G., Interpretation and classification of bone scintigraphic findings in stress fractures, *J. Nucl. Med.*, 28, 452, 1987.
6. Silberstein, E.B., Brown, M.L., Rosenthall, L., and Wahner, H.W., *Skeletal nuclear medicine,* in Nuclear Medicine Self Study Program I, Society of Nuclear Medicine, Sigal & Kirchner, New York, 1988, 93.
7. Einhorn, T.A., Vigorita, V.J., and Aaron, A., Localization of technetium-99m methylene disphosphonate in bone using micro autoradiography, *J. Ortho. Res.*, 4, 180, 1986.
8. Matin, P., Basic principles of nuclear medicine techniques for the detection and evaluation of trauma and sports medicine injuries, *Semin. Nucl. Med.*, 18, 90, 1988.
9. Milgrom, C., Chisin, R., Giladi, M., Stein, M., Kashtan, H., Margulies, J., and Atlan, H., Multiple stress fractures. A longitudinal study of a soldier with 13 lesions, *Clin. Orthop.*, 192, 174, 1985.
10. Chisin, R., Milgrom, C., Giladi, M., Stein, M., Margulies, J., and Kashtan, H., Clinical significance of nonfocal scintigraphic findings in suspected tibial stress fractures, *Clin. Orthop.*, 220, 200, 1987.
11. Rupani, H.D., Holder, L.E., and Espinola, D.A., Three-phase radionuclide bone imaging in sports medicine, *Radiology,* 156, 187, 1985.
12. Chisin, R., et al., Unilateral sacroiliac overuse syndrome in military recruits, *Br. Med. J.,* 289, 590, 1984.
13. McFarland, E.G. and Giangarra, C., Sacral stress fractures in athletes, *Clin. Orthop.*, 329, 240, 1986.
14. Kaltas, D.S., Stress fractures of the femoral neck in young adults: a report of seven cases, *J. Bone Jt. Surg.*, 63B, 33, 1981.
15. Holder, L.E., Bone scintigraphy in skeletal trauma, *Radiol. Clin. N. Am.*, 31, 739, 1993.

16. Marymont, J.V., *Nuclear Medicine and the Sports Physician in Nuclear Medicine,* Henkin et al., Eds., Mosby-Year Book, Saint Louis, 1996, 80.

17. Chisin, R., Milgrom, C., Giladi, M., Stein, M., Kashtan, J., Margulies, J., and Atlan, H., Tc-^{99m} scintigraphic evaluation of stress fractures of the feet using a 1 to 4 grading system, *Abstracts of the 3rd Asia and Oceania Congress of Nuclear Medicine,* Seoul, August 27-32, 1984.

18. Urman, M., Ammann, W., Sisler, J., Lentle, B.C., Lloyd-Smith, R., Loomer, R., and Fisher, C., The role of bone scintigraphy in the evaluation of talar dome fractures, *J. Nucl. Med.,* 32, 2241, 1991.

19. Murray, I.P.C., *Bone Scintigraphy in Trauma in Nuclear Medicine in Clinical Diagnosis and Treatment,* Murray and Ell, Eds., Churchill Livingston, London, 1998, 92.

20. Chisin, R., Peyser, A., and Milgrom, C., Bone scintigraphy in the assessment of the hallucal sesamoids, *Foot Ankle,* 16, 291, 1995.

21. Arrowsmith, D., Radiologic appearance of stress fractures, *J. Am. Osteopath. Assoc.,* 90, 225, 1990.

22. Santi, M. and Sartoris, D.J., Diagnostic imaging approach to stress fractures of the foot, *J. Foot Surg.,* 30, 85, 1991.

23. Milgrom, C., Sigal, R., Robin, G.C., Gazit, D., Fields, S., Benmair, J., Caine, Y., and Atlan, H., Osteogenic sarcoma of the proximal tibia. A comparison of MRI and CT scan with the microscopic histopathology, *Orthop. Rev.,* 15, 91, 1986.

24. Lee, J.K. and Yao, L., Stress fractures: MR imaging, *Radiology,* 169, 217, 1988.

25. Sacks, R.H., Salomon, C.G., and Demos, T.C., Occult bone injury: diagnosis by magnetic resonance imaging, *Orthopaedics,* 13, 1408, 1990.

26. Hodler, J., et al., Radiographically negative stress bone injury. MR imaging versus two-phase bone scintigraphy, *Acta Radiol.,* 39, 416, 1998.

27. Shin, A.Y., et al., The superiority of magnetic resonance imaging in differentiating the cause of hip pain in endurance athletes, *Am. J. Sports Med.,* 24, 168, 1996.

CHAPTER 20

Early Diagnosis and Clinical Treatment of Stress Fractures

Charles Milgrom and Eitan Friedman

CONTENTS

Introduction 295
Development of the Israeli Army Stress Fracture Treatment Protocol 296
The Civilian Stress Fracture Treatment Protocol 297
Treatment of Metatarsal Stress Fractures 297
Treatment of Femoral Stress Fractures 298
Treatment of Medial Tibial Stress Fractures 300
The Stress Fracture Continuum 300
Future Directions 301
Conclusion 302
References 303

INTRODUCTION

In the century and a half since Breitheupt first described the march fracture, there is little in the literature pertaining to stress fracture treatment.[1] In a Medline search from 1986 until 1999 using the key words stress fracture and treatment, there is only one journal reference cited.[2] Brief paragraphs about stress fracture treatment can be found in some stress fracture review articles or articles focused on other aspects of stress fracture.[3]

In his classic book, *Stress Fractures*, Devas discusses specifically the treatment of each individual type of stress fracture.[4] His book was written before bone scintigraphy was used for the early detection of stress fractures. Diagnosis then was based on clinical suspicion and confirmation by radiographic evidence of stress fracture. The book's recommended treatment regimens are therefore for macro stress fractures. The clinical therapeutic goal is to detect and treat stress fractures before they are evident on radiographs, at a stage when they are still micro stress fractures. The subject of this chapter is the early diagnosis and treatment of stress fractures.

The aim of stress fracture treatment should be to heal the fracture in the shortest possible time. A major determinant of the treatment necessary is the amount of damage present. Therefore, early diagnosis will generally result in much shorter treatment regimens than when diagnosis is delayed. Ideally, any rest regimen should be tailored to limit activities that can exacerbate the stress fracture or delay its healing. Activities that do not interfere with the healing but preserve the general fitness of the patient should be allowed. Because the epidemiology of the major types of stress fractures, (tibial, femoral, and metatarsal), are very different, treatment protocols should be tailored to each.

DEVELOPMENT OF THE ISRAELI ARMY STRESS FRACTURE TREATMENT PROTOCOL

The Israeli Army has been described as a virtual laboratory for the study of stress fracture.[5] The documented high prevalence of stress fracture among Israeli infantry recruits, coupled with the unique relationship of the army medical corps and the academic community, make the Israeli infantry recruit an ideal model for studying stress fractures. Initially, stress fracture treatment in the Israeli Army was the individual prerogative of the treating physician. This, however, resulted in widely different treatments for the same injury. Recommended treatment for any given stress fracture could range from crutch ambulation to cast, to benign neglect. To unify and provide a rational basis for treatment, a stress fracture treatment protocol was developed. This protocol has been used for more than a decade to treat thousands of stress fractures. Using the protocol, no cases of stress fracture have progressed from micro to macro stress fracture while being treated. For most of the recruits, the guidelines provided by the treatment protocol were sufficient to achieve healing of the fracture in the prescribed time.

The hallmark of the Israeli Army stress fracture treatment protocol is early detection. This is accomplished first by educating trainees and their superiors about the presenting symptoms and pathophysiology of stress fractures. Second, trainees with symptoms consistent with a stress fracture have rapid access to the medical staff. Third, physicians are trained to do a comprehensive stress fracture physical examination.[6] This includes examination and palpation of the area of the chief complaint and routine palpation of the tibia, femurs, and metatarsals for tenderness. Physicians are cautioned to remember physical diagnosis alone is often not definitive for stress fractures. Fourth, trainees with a clinical suspicion of stress fracture are evaluated by radiographs, bone scintigraphy, or both. Scintigraphic areas of increased uptake are graded on the 1 to 4 rating system of Zwas et al.,[3] based on the size and intensity of the scintigraphic foci:

Grade 1: Small, ill-defined lesion with mildly increased activity in the cortical region

Grade 2: Larger than Grade 1, well defined, elongated lesion with moderately increased activity in the cortical region

Grade 3: Wide fusiform lesion with highly increased activity in the cortico-medullary region

Grade 4: Wide extensive lesion with intensely increased activity in the transcortico-medullary region.

The size of these foci are assumed to reflect the amount of microdamage. If a radiograph is positive, then obviously the stress fracture has already progressed to a macro stage. Treatment is given in proportion to the amount of damage and the specific bone involved.

When developing the stress fracture treatment protocol, one sticky issue is the so-called asymptomatic stress fracture.[7] This, by definition, is a stress fracture diagnosed by either bone scan or radiography at a site where the trainee does not have symptoms. It must be verified that the scintigraphic focus does not represent something other than stress fracture. Although some of these sites will be found to be symptomatic if the trainee is carefully re-examined, some are truly asymptomatic. The femur is typically the site of asymptomatic stress fracture. Because a high percentage of asymptomatic femoral scintigraphic foci of increased uptake will eventually show radiographic evidence of stress fracture in follow-up, the protocol treats all asymptomatic stress fractures the same as symptomatic stress fractures.

THE CIVILIAN STRESS FRACTURE TREATMENT PROTOCOL

A civilian version of the Israeli Army stress fracture treatment protocol has been developed[8] that is designed for treatment of medial tibial stress fractures, femoral stress fractures excluding those of the femoral neck, and metatarsal stress fractures. The protocol recommends the amount of rest to be given for each stress fracture. It does not state specifically, however, how absolute the rest has to be. In general, activities that produce high repetitive strains and/or strain rates in the region of the stress fracture are avoided. When a stress fracture has progressed from a microfracture to a macrofracture and a break in a cortex can be seen with little or no callus, activity must be severely restricted.

TREATMENT OF METATARSAL STRESS FRACTURES

The epidemiology of the metatarsal stress fracture is different from that of the femoral or tibial stress fracture. Metatarsal stress fracture often seems to occur secondary to cyclic overloading, without an intermediate remodeling response typical of medial tibial stress fracture. A trainee can be entirely asymptomatic at the beginning of a training session, such as a long march, and be found to have a macro stress fracture at the end. Unlike medial tibial stess fractures, radiographs may be expected to give a high diagnostic yield, either immediately after the onset of pain or within two weeks afterwards.

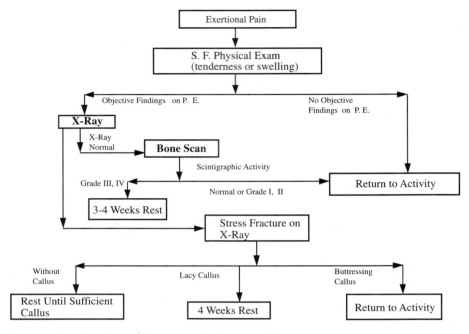

Figure 1 Treatment protocol for stress fracture of metatarsus.

Figure 1 is the treatment protocol for stress fractures of the metatarsus. It begins with physical examination. Diffuse swelling of the forefoot may be present. Standing on the toes may be painful. Typically, there is specific pain on palpation of the affected metatarsus but no pain over the intra-metatarsal spaces. Palpation of each metatarsus should be done over the dorsal surface of the foot rather than over the plantar surface where there is more soft tissue overlying the bone. When clinical suspicion is present, radiographs and bone scintigraphy are used to confirm the diagnosis. Treatment is based on the extent of damage and consists of rest according to the protocol, but some walking as tolerated can be allowed. Devas states that for some rare problem cases, a well fitting short leg walking cast may be indicated.[4] Usually, healing of metatarsal stress fractures is rapid, even if there is already a cortical break. Return to activity is gradual. A soft accommodative orthotic can help the trainee to return to activity and avoid future problems when he wears army boots or similar shoes. Likewise, when training is done in athletic shoes, a custom soft orthotic may be of value.

TREATMENT OF FEMORAL STRESS FRACTURES

Diagnosis and treatment of femoral stress fracture is more complicated than that of the metatarsus. There can be a wide discrepancy between the level of symptoms and the severity of the stress fracture. This may be explained by the relatively low sensitivity of the femoral periosteum as compared to that of the tibia and metatarsus, and the subject's difficulty in differentiating between muscle pain and bone pain in the upper femur. Devas states that the symptoms may consist of a mild ache over the thigh or a complaint of muscular stiffness in the region of the hip or knee.[4] The femoral stress fracture may even be asymptomatic until a late stage.[7] Therefore, the examiner should always have a high degree of suspicion. Deep palpation using the clenched fist and the weight of the examiner's upper torso is required to check the femoral periosteum for sensitivity.

Femoral stress fracture is most dangerous when it affects the femoral neck. Tension side (superior cortex) femoral neck stress fractures are considered to be more dangerous than compression side fractures.[9] If a femoral neck stress fracture progresses to a frank fracture, one of the complications may be avascular necrosis of the femoral head. This may lead to collapse of the femoral head, secondary osteoarthrosis of the joint, and the necessity for joint replacement surgery. This is a catastrophe for a young or active person. It should be stressed that the femoral stress fracture protocol is not for treatment of this fracture. Hospital admission is usually recommended. Treatment may consist of strict non-weight bearing ambulation, bed rest, or even prophylactic pinning of the hip. Likewise, the protocol does not treat supracondylar stress fractures of the femur, which also have a propensity to displace and require surgery.

Figure 2 is the treatment protocol for diaphyseal stress fractures of the femur. The stress fracture is graded on the basis of scintigraphic uptake and rest given according to the protocol. After the prescribed rest regimen is completed, return to

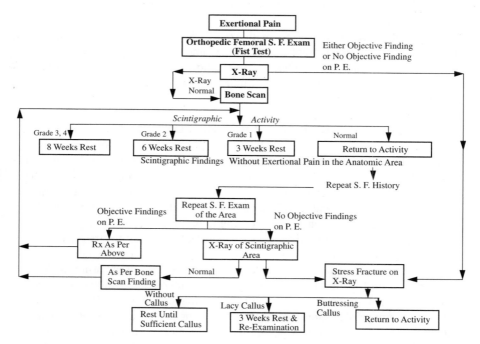

Figure 2 Treatment protocol for stress fracture of femur (not including femoral neck and supracondylar fracture).

training is gradual. Milgrom et al. noted that an Israeli infantry recruit who sustained a femoral stress fracture had 25% chance of sustaining a different stress fracture at another site in subsequent training.[10] This increased risk was not found for tibial or metatarsal stress fractures.

TREATMENT OF MEDIAL TIBIAL STRESS FRACTURES

Devas, in the era before bone scintigraphy, stated that the diagnosis of medial tibial stress fracture "must be on clinical grounds, and any patient including the athlete, must be considered to have a stress fracture without its being confirmed radiologically.[4]" This is because radiographic evidence of a tibial stress fracture may take a considerable time to appear. With bone scintigraphy, early diagnosis is possible. Milgrom et al. studied the correlation between the clinical examination suggestive of medial tibial stress fracture and bone scintigraphic results.[11] The examination was done by a single orthopedist with clinical stress fracture experience. Clinical suspicion of stress fracture was verified by scintigraphy in only 50% of the cases.

It is extremely rare for a medial tibial stress fracture to progress to a displaced fracture. Usually the high level of pain associated with this stress fracture prevents the trainee from continuing strenuous activities. The physical diagnosis of this stress fracture is relatively simple, since there are no muscle groups overlying the posteromedial border of the tibia. The posteromedial tibial border, therefore, can be easily palpated with finger pressure. Point tenderness in one or more places along the medial tibial border is consistent with stress fracture. Figure 3 is the treatment protocol for medial tibial stress fractures. The amount of rest given is according to the grade of the scintigraphic foci. Usually radiographs will be negative. Again, as for the other stress fractures, a gradual return to duty is advised.

THE STRESS FRACTURE CONTINUUM

Stress fractures are considered to arise from cylic overloading of the bone. It is this overloading, with its resultant high strains and/or strain rates that are inappropriate to the bone's geometry or quality, that produces stress fracture. Stress fracture may occur purely as a function of the number of loading cycles, before bone has a chance to remodel and strengthen, or during the remodeling response.

Roub et al. first introduced the concept of bone's response to stress as a continuum.[12] The continuum ranges from initial microcracking to reactive bone reabsorption, to coalescence of the microcracks into microfracture, to extension of microfractures to macrofracture. Repair and reaction depend on the loading circumstances and may potentially occur at any point in this damage continuum. It is thought that bone scintigraphy reflects microdamage and the bone's associated biological reaction before the stage of macrodamage occurs, after which it should be detectable by radiographs. It is assumed that the size and intensity of the scintigraphic foci increase

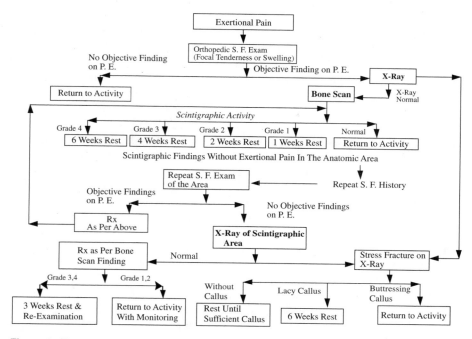

Figure 3 Treatment protocol for medial tibial stress fracture.

with increasing microdamage. This assumption is the basis for the scintigraphic grading system used to assign a severity score and the corresponding rest regimen necessary to heal the stress fracture.

To date, bone scintigraphy is our principal tool for the early diagnosis of stress fractures. It should be noted that bone scintigraphy involves significant radiation exposure to the patient. While this radiation dose is less than that of a pelvic CT scan, for example, bone scintigraphy should be ordered only when it is clinically essential to treatment. Repeated bone scintigraphy should be used sparingly.

FUTURE DIRECTIONS

Because of the radiation exposure of bone scintigraphy and its non-specificity, efforts are under way to develop alternative methods for early diagnosis of stress fractures. One promising direction is the use of metabolic markers. Little has been published about the role of bone turnover parameters as a potential diagnostic aid or an objective measure of recovery. Bennell and co-workers[13] sequentially measured serum osteocalcin and urinary pyridinium cross-links in 49 male and 46 female athletes, 20 of whom developed stress fractures, and found no differences in these parameters between athletes that developed fractures and those that did not. Similarly, Tomten et al.[14] found no differences in female athletes (n = 28) with and without stress fractures in serum IGF-1, testosterone, and cortisol, or in the biochemical markers of bone formation (osteocalcin) and bone resorption (1CTP). Both studies included a relatively small number of patients, and none of the participants was an active duty soldier. A preliminary study[15] analyzed 40 male soldiers in the Israeli Defense Forces with high grade stress fractures (Grade 3 to 4) and compared them with 40 age and ethnic matched control subjects without stress fractures (i.e., normal bone scans). The results of this study revealed that the mean bone specific alkaline phosphatase (37.6 versus 26.2 units/L; $p = 0.0001$) and osteocalcin levels (10.8 versus 8.8 ng/ml; $p = 0.00003$) were significantly higher in the high-grade stress fracture group as compared with control subjects. Moreover, bone specific alkaline phosphatase levels greater than 45 µ/l and osteocalcin greater than 12.5 ng/ml were observed only in the high-grade stress fracture group. Mean serum levels of 25–hydroxy vitamin D were significantly lower in patients with high-grade stress fractures (25.3 ng/ml) compared with controls (29.8 ng/ml; $p = 0.033$). the higher levels of osteocalcin and bone–specific alkaline phosphatase in soldiers with high grade stress fractures are not surprising, because measurements were made at a time of fracture repair. These results could potentially be used as aids in the diagnosis of stress fractures. If the exclusivity of bone–specific alkaline phosphatase levels above 45 ng/ml or osteocalcin levels above 12.5 µ/l are confirmed, then the diagnosis of stress fractures may depend on finding an abnormal biochemical profile in the appropriate clinical setting, avoiding the need for bone scan or plain radiograph.

The lower levels of 25-hydroxy vitamin D in soldiers with stress fractures as compared with control subjects are unexpected. Hypovitaminosis D is associated with low bone density and increased risk for osteoporosis and fractures.[16,17] If low 25–hydroxy vitamin D levels are found in a large proportion of patients with stress fractures in a larger series, this may provide an intervention modality to lower the rates of stress fractures. By including dietary vitamin D supplements to all training soldiers, a potential reduction in stress fracture incidence might be observed. Taken together, these realities suggest that there is more to be learned about the status of these markers in a large, unselected population of soldiers.

CONCLUSION

The stress fracture treatment protocols presented are designed to be logical guidelines for treatment of the three most common stress fractures. Like any frank fracture, the healing time of a stress fracture may be accelerated or delayed. The Israeli Army stress fracture treatment protocol, on which this civilian version is based, has been used successfully to treat thousands of cases. It is basically designed to let the bone "catch up" and sufficiently repair and strengthen the area of microdamage so training can be resumed. Physical activities that help to maintain physical fitness and produce only low strain and strain rates on the stress fracture site are allowed during the rest period. The treatment protocol should not be used as a basis for treating femoral neck or supracondylar stress fractures.

REFERENCES

1. Breitheupt, M.D., Zur pathologie des menschlicen fusses, *Med. Ztg.*, 24, 169, 1855.
2. Synder, S.J., Sherman O.K., and Hattendorf, K., Nine-year functional non-union of a femoral neck stress fracture: treatment with internal fixation and a fibular graft. A case report, *Orthopedics*, 9, 1553, 1986.
3. Zwas, T.S., Elkanowitch, R., and Frank, G., Interpretation and classification of bone scintigraphic findings in stress fractures, *J. Nucl. Med.*, 28, 452, 1987.
4. Devas, M., *Stress Fractures*, Churchill Livingston, Edinburgh, 1975.
5. Editorial, Stress fractures, *Lancet*, 2, 1326,1986.
6. Milgrom, C., Finestone, A., Shlamkovitch, N., Eldad, A., Saltzman, S., Giladi, M., Chisin, R., and Danon, Y.L., The clinical assessment of femoral stress fractures: a comparison of two methods, *Mil. Med.*, 158, 190, 1993.
7. Milgrom, C., Giladi, M., Stein, M., Kashtan, H., Margulies, Chisin, R., Steinberg, R., and Aharonson, Z., Stress fractures in military recruits. A prospective study showing an unusually high incidence, *J. Bone Jt. Surg.*, 65B, 732, 1985.
8. Milgrom, C., Finestone, A., Shlamkovitch, N., Giladi, M., Lev, B., Wiener, M., Schaffler, M., Stress fracture treatment, *Orthopedics*, 3, 363, 1995.
9. Fullerton, L.R. and Snowdy, H.A., Femoral neck stress fractures, *Am. J. Sports Med.*, 152, 45, 1987.
10. Giladi, M., Milgrom, C., Kashtan, H., Stein, M., Chisin, R., and Dizian, R., Recurrent stress fractures in military recruits. A long term follow-up of sixty-six recruits with stress fractures, *J. Bone Jt. Surg.*, 68B, 439, 1986.
11. Milgrom C., Giladi, M., Stein, M., Kashtan, H., Margulies, J., Chisin, R., Steinberg, R., Swissa, A., and Aharonson, Z., Medial tibial pain, *Clin. Orthop.*, 213, 167, 1986.
12. Roub, L.W., Gumerman, L.W., Hanley, E.N., Clark, M.W., Goodman, M., and Herbert, D.L., Bone stress: a radionuclide imaging perspective, *Radiology*, 132, 431, 1979.
13. Bennell, K.L., Malcolm, S.A., Brukner, P.D., Green, R.M., Hopper, J.L., Wark, J.D., and Ebeling P.R., A 12-month prospecive study of the relationship between stress fractures and bone turnover in athletes, *Calcif. Tissue Int.*, 63, 80, 1998.
14. Tomten, S.E., Falch, J.A., Birkeland, K.I., Hemmersbach, P., and Hostmark, A.T., Bone mineral density and menstrual irregularities. A comparative study on cortical and trabecular bone structures in runners with alleged normal eating behavior, *Int. J. Sports Med.*, 19, 92, 1998.
15. Givon, U., Friedman E., Reiner, A., Vered, I., Finestone, A., and Shemer, J., Stress fractures in the Israeli Defense Forces in 1995 to 1996, *Clin. Orthop. Rel. Res.*, (in press), 2000.
16. Baker, M.R., McDonnell, H., Peacock, M., and Nordin, B.E.C., Plasma 25 hydroxy vitamin D concentrations in patients with fractures of the femoral neck, *Br. J. Med.*, 1, 589, 1979.
17. Gloth, F.M. and Tobin J.D., III, Vitamin D deficiency in older people, *J. Am. Geriatr. Soc.*, 43, 822, 1995.

CHAPTER 21

Problematic Stress Fractures

Kenneth A. Egol and Victor H. Frankel

CONTENTS

Introduction 305
Biomechanics 306
Diagnosis 307
    History and Physical Exam 307
    Radiographic Examination 309
Treatment of Problematic Stress Fractures 310
    General Treatment Principles 310
    Tibial Stress Fractures 311
    Femoral Neck Stress Fractures 313
    Tarsal Navicular Stress Fractures 314
    Fifth Metatarsal Stress Fractures 317
Conclusion 317
References 318

INTRODUCTION

The treatment and healing of most stress fractures is straightforward and uneventful. The principles of treatment are to give the bone time to catch up to and heal the microdamage. Stress fracture healing parallels the healing of all frank fractures, where different bones and different areas within the bones generally heal at different rates. However, one can expect a small number of cases that either heal more rapidly than average or have a delayed union or nonunion. Some bones inherently have more problems than others.

Problematic stress fractures can also occur when there is difficulty in making the diagnosis and therefore a delay in treatment. A problematic stress fracture is also one which the clinical consequences of the fracture progressing to a frank fracture are significant. In this framework, a femoral neck stress fracture is a disaster and a second metatarsal stress fracture is not. For the purposes of this chapter, only the diagnosis and treatment of the problematic stress fracture will be discussed.

BIOMECHANICS

Tension stress fractures, as the name implies, occur on the tension side of the bone (i.e., superior femoral neck, anterior tibial cortex, etc.). These usually appear as transverse cracks and are sometimes identified as "the dreaded black line" (Figure 1). Tension fractures occur due to tension strains that cause debonding of osteons, eventually leading to a transverse fracture line (Figure 2). These fractures, however, often do not incite a biologic response that produces callus and healing. These cracks may persist for a long period of time before bridging callus is formed or complete displacement occurs. The presence of a tension crack acts as a stress riser. Continued exercise or loading makes it more likely that completion will occur and displacement will follow.

Compression fractures are usually oblique fractures and are due to a completely different process than tension fractures. Instead of debonding osteons, the bone fails through the formation of oblique cracks (Figure 3). These oblique cracks isolate

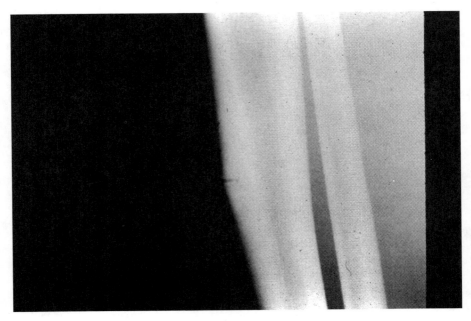

Figure 1 Lateral radiograph demonstrating "the dreaded black line" in the anterior tibial cortex.

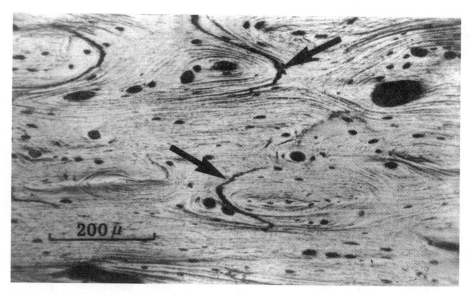

Figure 2 Electron microscopic photograph of the femur showing debonding at the osteon level.

areas of bone, which receive no nutrients and are devascularized. The result is a process of creeping substitution with an osteoclastic response. This is a slow process that usually does not result in a displaced fracture. Completion may occur if activity continues, as shear cracks coalesce, leading to an oblique fracture. Most compression type stress fractures heal with rest, external supports, or immobilization.

DIAGNOSIS

History and Physical Exam

It is critical to make the diagnosis of stress fracture early in order to institute appropriate therapy and return the patient to activities. Stress fractures can affect numerous long bones as well as the spinal column. In the lower extremities, stress fractures have been described in the femoral neck,[1-5] shaft,[6,7] and condyles,[6,8] the tibia,[8-12] medial malleolus,[13] tarsal navicular,[14-18] all the metatarsals,[19-22] and the sesamoids.[9,23] Stress fractures of the acromion and olecranon process have been described in the upper extremity.[24,25] Spondylolisthesis is the development of stress fractures in the pars interarticularis of the lumbar vertebrae.[26] The most problematic of these injuries are stress fractures of the femoral neck, anterior tibia, tarsal navicular, and fifth metatarsal.

The key to diagnosis of stress fracture lies in the patient's history. The diagnosis of stress fracture must be considered any time a patient complains of a dull, deep, aching pain. This pain may be associated with a particular activity, and worsen with

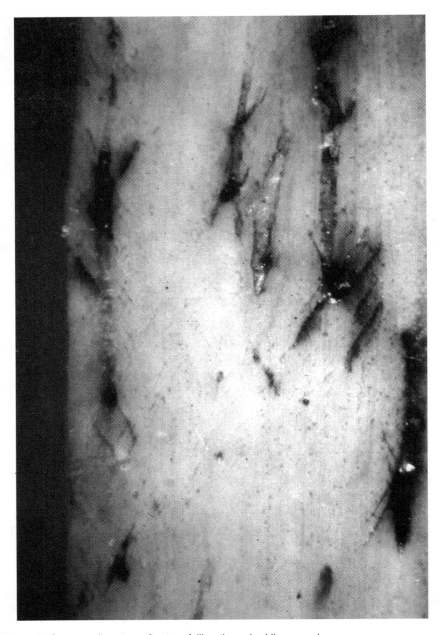

Figure 3 Compression stress fracture failing through oblique cracks.

physical activity. Patients usually deny specific trauma but often complain that pain has been present for weeks to months. The physical exam is usually positive for localized tenderness and warmth in palpable areas.

Certain patient risk factors are associated with stress fractures and should alert the treating physician to the possibility of a stress fracture. Endurance athletes, military recruits, female athletes with amenorrhea, and the presence of osteoporosis are all associated with increased risk for stress fracture.

Radiographic Examination

Standard plain radiography is often positive only late in the clinical course. It is important to remember that plain radiographs may be normal at initial presentation. When radiographic changes consistent with femoral neck stress fracture are evident on plain radiograph, they usually appear as an area of sclerosis or cortical deficiency on the superior aspect of the femoral neck as opposed to cortical irregularity of the inferior femoral neck in compression type fractures. Most anterior tibial stress fractures are transverse or oblique cracks.[27] Stress fractures of the tarsal navicular usually occur in the sagittal plane or within the dorsal margin, and may not be visualized on plain radiographs.[16,28] Stress fractures of the fifth metatarsal present as short oblique or transverse fractures of the proximal metaphyseal diaphyseal junction.[19]

Computed tomography (CT) has become an important adjunct to plain radiographs. CT has been utilized to confirm the diagnosis in selected cases and is of importance in the tarsal navicular, where the fractures occur in the sagittal plane.[28] In addition, CT scanning can be used to follow patients to union.

Until recently, bone scintigraphy with technetium[99] methylene diphosphonate has been the gold standard as an early and reliable method for the detection of occult fractures.[29] Multiple views must be attained to adequately assess affected areas. Medial and posterior views are necessary to assess the tibia; plantar views of the feet are necessary to assess tarsal and metatarsal fractures.[30] This modality is widely available, and multiple studies have attested to its sensitivity for detection of occult fractures.[30-32]

Magnetic resonance imaging (MRI) has emerged as a very sensitive technique in the diagnosis of musculoskeletal pathology. Recent studies have shown MRI to be more sensitive than radionuclide imaging for the detection of occult hip fractures (Figure 4),[33] although MRI has not yet become an established tool for diagnosing cortical stress fractures. A combination of T1 weighted images that optimize anatomic detail and depict bone marrow edema is essential. Sequences are usually performed in multiple orthogonal planes, depending on the region of interest.[30,34] Two MRI patterns of stress fracture have been described. The most common is a band–like fracture line that is low signal on all pulse sequences, surrounded by a larger, ill-defined zone of edema. The second, less common pattern on MRI is an amorphous alteration of the marrow signal without a clear fracture line. This pattern is characterized by low signal intensity on T1 images with increased signal on T2 weighted images, and is considered a stress response to injury. Advantages of MR imaging include fast results compared to radionuclide imaging, and its lack of ionizing radiation. Disadvantages include increased cost compared to radionuclide scanning. The absence of a total body image may lead the treating physician to miss asymptomatic stress fractures or multiple site stress fractures.

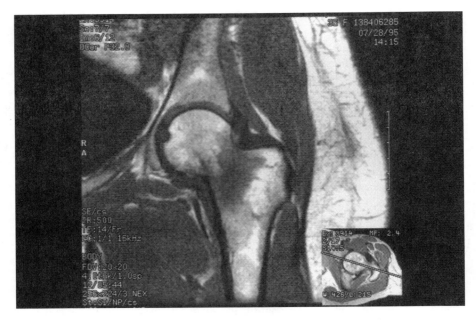

Figure 4 T1 weighted image demonstrating an occult femoral neck stress fracture.

TREATMENT OF PROBLEMATIC STRESS FRACTURES

General Treatment Principles

The common thread in the treatment algorithm for all stress fractures is a decreased level of activity. The management plan should be based on what grade stress reaction has been diagnosed[35] and the concept of imbalance between bone resorption and remodeling.[36] A grading system and a standard treatment protocol has been used at the University of Minnesota since 1990. Central to the treatment of stress fractures is keeping the patient's activity level below a painful threshold. Phase I of treatment is pain control. This is accomplished with ice, physiotherapy, anti-inflammatory drugs, protected weight bearing, and rest. Phase II begins after the patient has had five pain free days. This phase consists of light-weighted exercise and specific muscle rehabilitation, with recovery of strength lost during phase I. The average time of treatment for phases I and II is between four and eight weeks. Phase III of the treatment algorithm is gradual re-entry into sport-specific activity. This includes analysis of potential training errors with correction.

Pain–free motion is a healthy indicator that the bone is progressing towards healing.[36] Cessation of the stress will allow the repair process to dominate over bone resorption.[37] Most stress fractures heal with rest and immobilization. The morbidity associated with this successful treatment method is lack of ability to train, deconditioning, muscle atrophy, loss of cardiovascular conditioning, persistent pain, and often a long absence from competition. With this method of treatment, some fractures go on to nonunion, and at certain sites, to completely displaced fractures.

Tibial Stress Fractures

Stress fractures of the tibia account for 17 to 49% of all stress fractures,[38] and the tibia is the most common site affected. Usually seen in high performance athletes, tibial stress fractures are generally unilateral and affect the posteromedial cortex. These fractures are usually transverse or short oblique; a longitudinal stress fractures occur only rarely.[27] It should be expected that posterior medial tibial stress fractures will heal with rest. Adjunctive methods of treatment have recently been added to the orthopedic armamentarium in treating stress fractures. Ultrasound was shown to speed the healing of an elite gymnast with an Olympic deadline. (Figure 5A,B) The stress fracture showed signs of healing by 3 weeks, and the athlete returned to full workout by 4.5 weeks and won a gold medal 6 weeks post injury.[39]

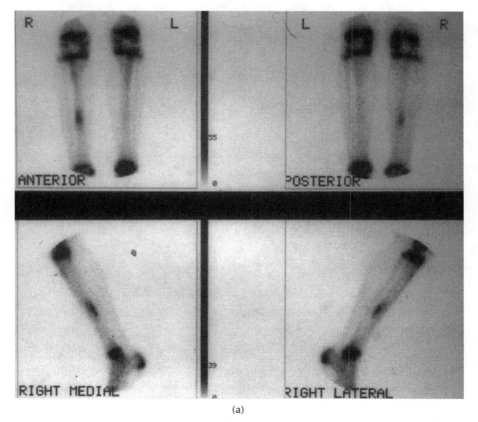

(a)

Figure 5 (a) 14 year old world-class gymnast presented in June 1996 with pain in her leg, concerned that her injury would prevent her from participating in the Olympic games. Bone scan demonstrates a tibial stress fracture. (From Jensen, J.E., *Med. Sci. Sports Exerc.*, 30, 783, 1998. With permission.) (b) MRI confirms the presence of tibial stress fracture. The patient was treated with pulsed ultrasound therapy and healed her fracture in time to win a gold medal at the 1996 Olympic games. (From Jensen, J.E., *Med. Sci. Sports Exerc.*, 30, 783, 1998. With permission.)

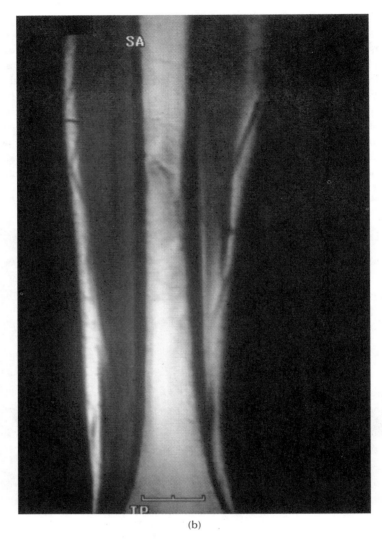

(b)

Figure 5 (continued)

Rettig et al.[10] reported on 8 patients ranging in age from 14 to 23 years who presented with anterolateral stress fractures of the tibia. Pulsed electromagnetic fields (PEMF) alone were used to treat 7 patients, and 1 required bone grafting. Complete healing with return to full activity took an average of 8.7 months. The authors recommend at least 3 to 6 months of conservative therapy prior to consideration of operative treatment. Whitelaw et al. treated 17 patients with 20 tibial stress fractures with the use of a pneumatic leg brace for 3 weeks. It is felt that the pneumatic brace unloads the tibia and fibula while allowing for full weight bearing. The authors returned the athletes to their activities 3.7 weeks sooner than other reported series, and to active competition at an average of 5.3 weeks after application of the brace.[12]

These results must be accepted with reservation, as this was an industry–supported study without an internal control group.

For patients with persistent symptoms lasting greater than 6 months, surgical treatment should be considered.[9,11] Histopathological analysis of the tibial stress fracture site has shown it to be consistent with that of atrophic pseudarthrosis.[40] Therefore, the recommendation is to excise the fissure, drill the site, and bone graft the defect.[9,11] If this fails, reamed intramedullary nailing may be utilized to heal the fracture (Figures 1 and 6).

Femoral Neck Stress Fractures

Femoral neck stress fractures are rare in young people, and more common in elderly females. Treatment depends on the type of fracture present. Tension stress fractures occur along the superior aspect of the femoral neck and are at high risk for displacement. Compression fractures occur along the inferomedial neck and are thought to be stable.[1,4,5]

Tension–sided femoral neck stress fractures can be treated nonoperatively[4] with non-weight bearing and frequent observation until pain free with radiographic signs of healing. However, the potential complications of displacement (osteonecrosis, malunion, and nonunion) outweigh the risk of surgical intervention. A tension–sided femoral neck stress fracture should be stabilized with cannulated screw fixation. The area of the stress fracture can be curetted or reamed under radiologic control to induce a biological reaction (Figure 7A, B).

Compression type stress fractures are considered stable and may be treated non-operatively. The nonoperative management must include serial radiographs to detect any changes in pattern or displacement. Treatment consists of several days of rest, followed by protected weight bearing.[41] Adjunctive modalities of PEMF or pulsed ultrasound therapy may be added to hasten the time to recovery. If serial radiographs show evidence of fracture widening or displacement, internal fixation should be performed.[4]

A displaced femoral neck stress fracture in a young person is an orthopedic emergency, and the patient should undergo open reduction and internal fixation (ORIF).[4,42] In the elderly patient, treatment options include ORIF or prosthetic replacement.

Tountas[3] reported on 13 patients with stress fractures of the femoral neck. All were elderly, average age 82 years. Nine underwent ORIF, three underwent prosthetic replacement, and one was treated nonoperatively. Most patients were able to return to full activity by 12 months.

Complications associated with femoral neck stress fractures are usually related to displacement or a delay in diagnosis.[42,43] These include delayed union, nonunion, refracture, and osteonecrosis of the femoral head.[42-44] Visuri reported a series of 12 displaced femoral neck stress fractures; five developed osteonecrosis (42%), one had a delayed union, (9%), and one had a nonunion (9%). In another series (43), 30% of patients sustained some type of healing complication. In this series five of seven patients who had a healing complication had initial displacement of their femoral neck stress fracture.[43]

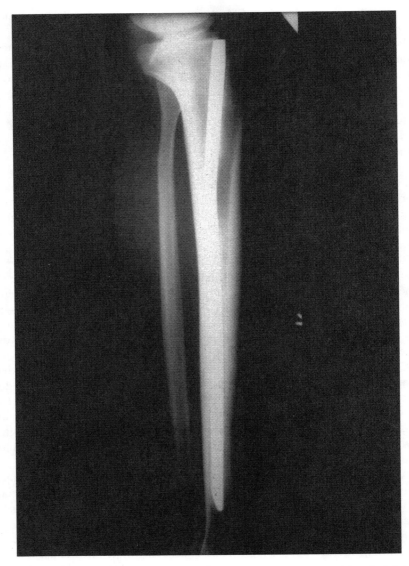

Figure 6   The tibial diaphyseal stress fracture shown in Figure 1 occurred in a ballet dancer who was followed for one year and remained symptomatic. The patient underwent drilling of the anterior cortical crack. When the fracture failed to heal, the patient underwent intramedullary nailing. By three months, the fracture healed and the patient returned to full activity.(Courtesy of Donald J. Rose, M.D.)

Tarsal Navicular Stress Fractures

After the tibia, the foot is the next most common site of stress fracture. The majority of these fractures are partial, in the sagittal plane.[16] Initial treatment consists of protected weight bearing. Delayed union or nonunion occurs in about 10% of

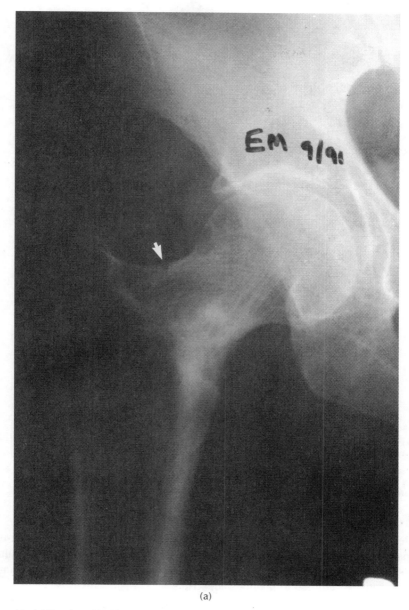

(a)

Figure 7 (a) Tension-sided femoral neck stress fracture (arrow) in a 39 year-old runner. (b) The patient underwent repair with cannulated screws. In addition, the superior cortex was curetted to induce a biologic reaction. (Courtesy of Kenneth J. Koval, M.D)

cases.[15] In a series of 82 athletes with tarsal navicular stress fracture, patients were treated with 3 different regimens: 22 patients were non–weight bearing in a cast for 6 weeks, 53 had limited activity with full weight bearing, and 6 had immediate surgery. The non-weight bearing group had significantly better results, with 86%

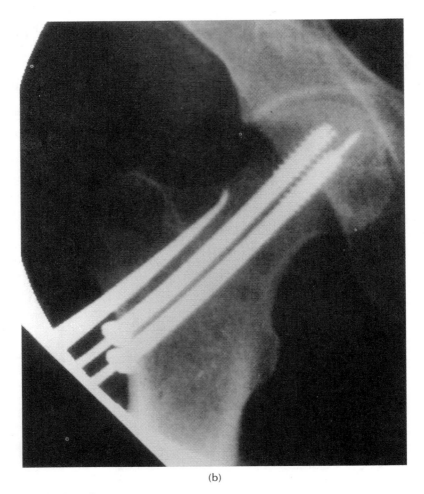

(b)

Figure 7 (continued)

healed compared to 26% in the weight bearing group. Benazzo et al.[14] treated
13 patients who had navicular stress fractures with rest and electrical stimulation
for 60 days. All patients were allowed activity at 10 weeks. There were no nonunions
and all patients returned to previous activity.

If a stress fracture of the tarsal navicular remains symptomatic with a delay in
healing, surgical treatment is indicated. Treatment at this point includes the use of
autogenous bone graft with or without internal fixation.[15,18] Fitch et al. treated
19 fatigue fractures of the tarsal navicular in 18 patients with resection of the fracture
surfaces and autogenous bone graft.[18] The authors report an 80% return to full activity
rate by one year postoperatively.

Fifth Metatarsal Stress Fractures

Fracture of the base of the fifth metatarsal at the junction of the metaphysis and diaphysis is known as the Jones fracture. It is usually a transverse or short oblique fracture secondary to repetitive overload. There are distinct differences radiographically between an acute fifth metatarsal fracture and a chronic stress fracture. In the latter there will be evidence of periosteal reaction, thickened cortical margins, and sometimes obliteration of the medullary canal. This fracture, when due to repetitive stress, is usually seen in young male athletes.[20] Intrinsic foot pathology can predispose patients to the development of fifth metatarsal stress fractures. A cavus foot is more rigid than normal, and the planovalgus foot has increased stresses along the lateral border. Both of these conditions are associated with an increase risk of developing a stress fracture.[20]

Guidelines for treatment of this fracture are controversial. Initially, nonoperative treatment can be tried.[45] Rest should be instituted, non-weight bearing with a cast. Benazzo added electrical stimulation to his nonoperative regimen for six weeks, with all patients healing and able to return to full activity.[14] The nonunion rate for stress fractures of the fifth metatarsal is approximately 50%.[19,20] For this reason, some authors recommend early operative treatment of all stress fractures of the proximal fifth metatarsal.

Surgical treatment of this injury includes open reduction, curettage, bone grafting, and internal fixation.[9,19,20,46,47] Josephson treated 22 patients with fifth metatarsal stress fracture nonunions. These patients were treated with medullary screws. All patients healed their fractures and returned to previous activity by ten weeks.[19] A diaphyseal stress fracture of the fifth metatarsal is a distraction type of injury and commonly confused with a Jones fracture. Some authors recommend surgery on this type of fracture to speed recovery and return to full activity.[48]

CONCLUSION

Stress fractures are uncommon injuries in the general population. They are commonly encountered by health care professionals who treat the elderly or high performance athletes. Fatigue fractures occur most frequently in the lower extremities in athletes who are involved in running and jumping sports. The diagnosis requires a strong clinical suspicion, as initial radiographs may be negative. Physical examination aids in determining location of the stress fracture. Radionuclide imaging or magnetic resonance imaging is usually needed to confirm the diagnosis. Treatment in most cases begins with cessation of activity and protected weight bearing. The drawback to this treatment is deconditioning of the athlete. Certain problematic stress fractures such as anterior tibial, femoral neck, tarsal navicular, and proximal fifth metatarsal fractures may require operative treatment because of a high rate of complications during healing. Of particular concern are tension–sided femoral neck fractures, which if displaced may have disastrous consequences.

REFERENCES

1. Devas, M.B., Stress fractures of the femoral neck, *J. Bone Jt. Surg.,* 47(B), 728, 1965.
2. Tountas, A.A. and Waddell, J.P., Stress fractures of the femoral neck. A report of seven cases, *Clin. Orthop.,* 210, 160, 1986.
3. Tountas, A.A., Insufficiency stress fractures of the femoral neck in elderly women, *Clin. Orthop.,* 292, 202, 1993.
4. Fullerton, L.R. and Snowdy, H.A., Femoral neck stress fracture, *Am. J. Sports Med.,* 16, 365, 1988.
5. Blickenstaff, L.D. and Morris, H.J., Fatigue fractures of the femoral neck, *J. Bone Jt. Surg.,* 48A, 103, 1996.
6. Hershman, E.B., Lombardo, J., and Bergfield, J.A., Femoral shaft stress fractures in athletes, *Clin. Sports Med.,* 9(1), 111, 1990.
7. Johnson, A.W., Weiss, C.B., and Wheeler, D.L., Stress fractures of the femoral shaft in athletes — more common than expected. A new clinical test, *Am. J. Sports Med.,* 22(2), 248, 1994.
8. Satku, K., Kumar, V.P., and Chacha, P.B., Stress fractures around the knee in elderly patients. A cause of acute pain in the knee, *J. Bone Jt. Surg.,* 76A, 918, 1990.
9. Orava, S. and Hulkko, A., Delayed unions and non-unions of stress fractures in athletes, *Am. J. Sports Med.,* 16(4), 378, 1988.
10. Rettig, A.C., et al., *Am. J. Sports Med.,* 16(3), 250, 1988.
11. Beals, R.K. and Cook, R.D., Stress fractures of the anterior tibial diaphysis, *Orthopaedics,* 14(8), 869, 1991.
12. Whitelaw, G.P., et al., A pneumatic leg brace for the treatment of tibial stress fractures, *Clin. Orthop.,* 270, 301, 1991.
13. Shelbourne, K.D., et al., Stress fractures of the medial malleolus, *Am. J. Sports Med.,* 16(1), 60, 1988.
14. Benazzo, F., Mosconi, G., and Galli, U., Treatment of stress fractures, *Clin. Orthop.,* 310, 149, 1995.
15. Orava, S., et al., Stress fracture of the tarsal navicular. An uncommon sports-related overuse injury, *Am. J. Sports Med.,* 19(4), 392, 1991.
16. Khan, K.M., et al., Outcome of conservative and surgical treatment of navicular stress fracture in athletes. Eighty-six cases proven with computerized tomography, *Am. J. Sports Med.,* 20(6), 657, 1992.
17. Khan, K.M., Tarsal navicular stress fractures in athletes, *Sports Med.,* 17(1), 65, 1994.
18. Fitch, K.D., Blackwell, J.B., and Gilmour, W.N., Operation for non-union of stress fracture of the tarsal navicular, *J. Bone Jt. Surg.,* 71(B), 105, 1989.
19. Josefson, P.O., et al., Jones fracture. Surgical versus non-surgical treatment, *Clin. Orthop.,* 299, 252, 1994.
20. Sammarco, G.J., The Jones fracture, *Instructional Course Lectures,* 42, 201, 1993.
21. O'Malley, M.J., et al., Stress fractures at the base of the second metatarsal in ballet dancers, *Foot Ankle Int.,* 17(2), 89, 1996.
22. Harrington, T., Crichton, K.J., and Anderson, I.F., Overuse ballet injury of the base of the second metatarsal. A diagnostic problem, *Am. J. Sports Med.,* 21(4), 591, 1993.
23. Dietzen, C.J., Great toe sesamoid injuries in the athlete, *Orthop. Rev.,* 19(11), 966, 1990.
24. Kuhn, J.E., Blasier, R.B., and Carpenter, J.E., Fractures of the acromion process: a proposed classification system, *J. Orthop. Trauma,* 8(1), 6, 1994.
25. Nuber, G.W., Diment, M.T., Olecrenon stress fractures in throwers. A report of two cases and a review of the literature, *Clin. Orthop.,* 278, 58, 1992.

26. Fehlandt, A.F. and Micheli, L.J., Lumbar facet stress fractures in a ballet dancer, *Spine*, 18(16), 2537, 1993.

27. Krauss, M.D. and Van Meter, C.D., A longitudinal tibial stress fracture, *Orthop. Rev.*, 23(2), 163, 1991.

28. Kizz, Z.S., Khan, K.M., and Fuller, P.J., Stress fractures of the tarsal navicular bone: CT findings in 55 cases, *Am. J Roentgenol.*, 160(1), 111, 1993.

29. Fehlandt, A.F. and Micheli, L.J., Lumbar facet stress fractures in a ballet dancer, *Spine*, 18(16), 2537, 1993.

30. Deutch, A.L., Coel, M.N., and Mink, J.H., Imaging of stress injury to bone, *Clin. Sports Med.*, 16, 275, 1997.

31. Crockett, J.P., Three phase radionuclide bone imaging in stress fractures of the iliac crest, *J. Nucl. Med.*, 31, 155, 1990.

32. Matin, P., The appearance of bone scans following fractures including immediate and long term studies, *J. Nucl. Med.*, 20, 1227, 1979.

33. Shin, A.Y., et al., The superiority of magnetic resonance imaging in differentiating the cause of hip pain in endurance athletes, *Am. J. Sports Med.*, 24, 168, 1996.

34. Lee, J.K., Yao, L., Stress fractures: MR imaging, *Radiology*, 169, 217, 1988.

35. Jones, B.H. and Kapik, J.J., Physical training and exercise related injuries. Surveillance, research and injury prevention in military populations, *Sports Med.*, 27(2), 111, 1999.

36. Arendt, E.A. and Griffiths, H.J., The use of MR imaging in the assessment and clinical management of stress reactions of bone in high performance athletes, *Clin. Sports Med.*, 16(2), 291, 1997.

37. Knapp, T.P. and Garret, W.E., Stress fractures. General concepts, *Clin. Sports Med.*, 16(2), 339, 1997.

38. Matheson, G.O., et al., Stress fractures in athletes. A study of 320 cases, *Am. J. Sports Med.*, 15(1), 46, 1987.

39. Jensen, J.E., Stress fracture in the world class athlete: a case study, *Med. Sci. Sports Excerc.*, 30(6), 783, 1998.

40. Rolf, C., Ekenman, I., and Tornqvist, A., The anterior stress fracture of the tibia: an atrophic pseudarthrosis, *Scand. J. Med. Sci. Sports,* 7(4), 249, 1997.

41. Egol, K.A., et al., Stress fractures of the femoral neck, *Clin. Orthop.*, 348, 72, 1998.

42. Visuri, T., Vara, A., Meurman, K.O.M., Displaced stress fractures of the femoral neck in young male adults: a report of twelve operative cases, *J. Trauma*, 28, 1562, 1990.

43. Johansson, C., et al., Stress fractures of the femoral neck in athletes, *Am. J. Sports Med.*, 18, 524, 1990.

44. Mendez, A. and Eyster, R.L., Displaced nonunion stress fracture of the femoral neck treated with internal fixation and bone graft, *Am. J. Sports Med.*, 20, 230, 1992.

45. Acker, J.H. and Drez, D., Non-operative treatment of stress fractures of the proximal shaft of the fifth metatarsal (Jones fracture), *Foot Ankle*, 7(3), 152, 1986.

46. Torg, J.S., et al., Fractures of the base of the fifth metatarsal distal to the tuberosity. Classification and guidelines for non-surgical and surgical management, *J. Bone Jt. Surg.*, 66A, 209, 1984.

47. Hens, J. and Martens, M., Surgical treatment of Jones fractures, *Arch. Orthop. Trauma Surg.*, 109(5), 277, 1990.

48. Lawrence, S.J. and Botte, M.J., Jones fracture and related fractures of the proximal fifth metatarsal, *Foot Ankle*, 14(6), 358, 1993.

Index

A

Accelerometry, 235
Accommodative orthotics, 239
Accumulated exposure, 4
Achievement, 28
Activation frequency, 260
  BMU, 188
  for bone remodeling, 262
Active case identification, 7
Adaptive remodeling, potential of basketball to
    influence, 251
Adolescence, stress fractures in late, 59
Adolescent(s)
  epidemiological studies of, 59
  stress fractures occurring in, 55
Adults, stress fractures occurring in, 55
Advanced infantry training, 6
Aerobic dance, 2
Aerobic fitness, 248
Age, 4, 27
  association between risk of developing injury
    and, 64
  difference, in strain, 126
  as risk factor for stress fractures, 56
Age, role of in development of stress and fatigue
    fractures, 55–71
  age as risk factor for stress fractures in sports
    and ballet, 63–65
    ballet, 65
    running, 64
    track and field, 63–64
  stress fractures in specific age categories,
    56–63
    adults, 60–63
    children age 0 to 6 years, 56
    children and early adolescents, 56–59
    late adolescence, 59–60
Alcohol, 28
Alendronate, 262, 263

Alkaline phosphatase, mean bone specific, 302
Amenorrhea, 38, 39, 40, 43
Anatomical location, distribution of stress
    fractures by, 8
Anatomical site, 3
Aneuralismal bone cyst, 272
Ankle
  dorsiflexion/plantarflexion, 25
  sprains, 235
Anorexia nervosa, 38
Anovulation, 43
Anterior mid-tibia, stress fractures of, 63
Apoptosis, 170
Arch height, foot, 238
Athletes, stress fractures in, 261
Athletic populations, see Military and athletic
    populations, incidence and prevalence
    of stress fractures in

B

Back pain, 276
Ballet, 2, 10
  adolescents engaged in, 55
  dancers, 10, 65
Ball sports, 10, 249
Basic fibroblast growth factor (b-FGF), 157
Basic fuchsin, 164
Basic multicellular unit (BMU), 185, 187, 188
Basic training
  length of, 61
  period, of military recruits, 59
Basketball, 2, 10
  playing of regularly prior to basic training, 255
  shoes, 234, 235, 236
  strain rates while playing, 250, 251
Bending
  rigidity, 266
  stress, 75

b-FGF, see Basic fibroblast growth factor
Bias, 5, 6
Bicycling, *in vivo* tibial strains during exercise,
        252
Biochemical markers, 19, 261
Biofoam®, 239
Bisphosphonates (BP), 262, 263
    gastrointestinal disturbances caused by, 264
    pharmacological activity of, 263
BMC, see Bone mineral content
BMD, see Bone mineral density
BMP2, see Bone morphogenic protein 2
BMU, see Basic multicellular unit
Body
    composition, 47
        athlete, 26
        genetically determined differences
            between genders regarding, 39
    size, 26, 27
    weight, women's preoccupation with, 36
Bone
    adaptation, 16, 45
    cell dynamics, 19, 45
    cellular dynamics, 16
    cortical, 263
    cyst, 272
    damage, 132
    densitometry, 74
    density, 16, 37, 40
        effects of oral contraceptive use on, 44
        low, 47
        lumbar spine, 43
        measurements, 65
        relationship between stress fractures and
            in females, 46
    disease, occurrence of familial, 107
    formation, 107, 264
    functional adaptation, 99
    geometry, 16, 17, 18, 36, 45, 75, 78
    grafting, 317
    hypertrophy, 98
    inertial properties of, 209
    marrow edema, 309
    mass, reduction of, 260
    microarchitecture, 16
    microcracks, 164
    mineral content (BMC), 74
    mineral density (BMD), 17, 18, 74, 80, 127
    mineralization, 263
    modeling, 98
    morphogenic protein 2 (BMP2), 157
    osteoporotic, 174
    pain, in proximal femur, 273
    pathologies, 110

remodeling, 19, 20, 87, 162, 260, see also
        Bone remodeling, role of in preventing
        or promoting stress fractures
    response, 252
    at stress fracture site, 157
    residual properties in, 167
    scan, 171, 277, 285
    scintigraphy, 272, 277, 280, 286, 288, 296
        as most valuable imaging tool in
            diagnosing stress fracture, 291
        radiation exposure of, 301
        with technetium, 309
        two-phase, 291
    sectional properties, 209
    stiffness, 93
    strain, 136, 139
    strengthening, 247, 248
    strength index, 76
    trabecular, 175, 263
    tumor, 277
    turnover, 19, 20, 40, 263
        in athletes, 261
        intracortical, 265
        parameters, 301
    width, 75
    work to failure of, 265
Bone fatigue, stress fractures and, 85–103
    creep and damage, 90–97
    factors affecting fatigue strength, 86–90
    fatigue damage and skeletal adaptation, 98–99
    mathematical modeling, 99–100
    trabecular bone, 97–98
Bone fatigue and remodeling, in development of
        stress fractures, 161–182
    bone behavior when fatigue-loaded at lower,
        more physiological strains, 162–164
    fatigue microdamage in compact bone,
        164–167
    microdamage accumulation in bone, 174–177
    range of physiological strains and cycles, 162
    remodeling and repair of microdamage in
        bone, 167–170
    stress fracture occurrence, 170–174
Bone remodeling, role of in preventing or
        promoting stress fractures, 183–201
    discussion, 198–200
        failure of homeostatic damage control,
            199–200
        remodeling and homeostatic damage
            control, 198–199
    theory, 185–198
        mathematical model, 186–192
        model results, 192–198
Boots

comparison of types of, 236
military, 234, 236
BP, see Bisphosphonates
Bulk stain technique, 153

C

CA, see Calcaneal angle
Caffeine, 28
Calcaneal angle (CA), 237
Calcaneal stress fracture, 276
Calcitonin receptor (CTR), 110, 111
Calcium, 28, 37
intake, 36, 42
metabolism, 27
Calf girth, as predictor of stress fracture in
women, 64
Caloric intake, low, 38
Candidate genes, 107, 110, 111
Cantilever bending
fatigue experiments, 86
loads, 85
Career soldiers, 59, 62
Cartilage growth, mechanical regulation of, 99
Case
ascertainment, 4, 6
definition, 2, 3
identification, 7
series, 6, 56
Cellular dynamics, 21
Children, stress fractures in, 56
Clinical setting, 6
Cohort
denominator, 4
studies, 56, 60
COLIA1 gene, 110, 111, 112
COLIA2 gene, 110, 111, 112
Collagen
N-telopeptides of type 1, 20
turnover, 261
Comparing rates, 4
Competitive runners, 2
Composite materials, 164
Compression, 93, 99
fractures, 306
fully-reversed, 93
Compressive strains, 88
Compressive stress, 99
Computed tomography (CT), 80, 276, 291, 309
Computerized medical records, 6
Confocal microscopy, 167
Cortical bone, 120, 263
Cortical specimens, 85

Cortical thickness
manual measurements of, 17
mean, 76
COX-2, see Cyclooxygenase-2
Crack density, 260
Creep
behavior, 90
mechanism, 141
Crew, 2, 10
Cross-sectional geometry, 80
Cross-sectional moment of inertia, 17, 75, 266
Crucible, The, 7
CT, see Computed tomography
CTR, see Calcitonin receptor
Curettage, 317
Cyanoacrylate glue, 121
Cycles to failure, 88, 89, 98
Cyclic bending, 90
Cyclic damage, 96
Cyclic loading, effect of on ultimate strength of
compact bone, 87
Cyclic training, 254
Cyclooxygenase
inhibition of by indomethacin, 265
synthesis, 264
Cyclooxygenase-2 (COX-2), 157, 265
Cytokines, 157

D

Damage
accumulation, 177, 261
biological response to, 264
due to cyclic compression, 93
formation rate, 187
Dancing, adolescents engaged in, 55
Database, of outpatient encounters, 8
Data collection, 5
Delayed union
femoral head, 313
foot, 314
Denominators, 2
Density, 4
Diagnostic criteria, 3
Diagnostic methods, 61
Diaphyseal femoral stress fractures, 272
Diet, 259
Dietary deficiencies, 28
Dietary intake, restricted, 36
Differential diagnosis, of stress fracture, 272
Disordered eating patterns, 38
Dissipation energies, 96
Distance running, 10

Dreaded black line, 306
Drop jumping, 124
Drop landing, 121
Drug treatments, 266
Dual energy x-ray absorptiometry (DXA), 17, 74, 80
Durometry tests, 234
DXA, see Dual energy x-ray absorptiometry

E

Early bone strengthening exercises, 248
Early diagnosis and clinical treatment, of stress
        fractures, 295–303
    civilian stress fracture treatment protocol, 297
    development of Israeli Army stress fracture
        treatment protocol, 296–297
    stress fracture continuum, 300–301
    treatment of femoral stress fractures, 298–300
    treatment of medial tibial stress fractures, 300
    treatment of metatarsal stress fractures,
        297–298
Eating disorders, 36, 38
Elastic modulus, 89, 187, 191, 265
Endocrine disorders, 17
Endogenous hormones, 27
Endurance, 26
    athletes, risk of for stress fracture, 309
    stress limit, 97
Energy
    absorbing device, foot as, 238
    absorption, 134, 135, 263
    dissipation, 93
Environmental influences, bone health and, 16
Epiphyseal stress fractures, 59
Equilibrium
    state, 192
    time to reach new, 194, 198
ER, see Estrogen receptor
Estrogen, 36, 37
    deficiency, 45
    exogenous source of, 44
    low-circulating, 40
    receptor (ER), 110, 111
Etidronate, 263
Excessive jumping model, rabbit, 229
Exercise-induced pain, 10
Exercise programs, prevention or delay of onset
        of stress fractures by, 247–257
    bone strengthening in American military,
        253–254
    bone strengthening exercises in Israeli
        infantry recruit model, 248–250

home exercises that strengthen bone and limit
        stress fractures, 255
measurement of *in vivo* tibial strains during
        exercises, 250–252
prior training activities associated with stress
        fracture risk, 248
Exertional anterior compartment syndrome,
        physical examination of, 273
Exposure-time, measures of, 7
Extensometer, 124
External loading kinetics, 22
External validity, 6
Ex vivo testing, 120

F

Familial stress fractures, 106
Family history, as risk factor for stress fracture,
        106
Fatigue, 20, 151
    behavior, 163
    damage, 93, 99, 162, 163, 184, 260
    failure
        of skeleton, 170
        strain rate in, 119
    fracture, 2
        distinguishing between insufficiency
            fractures and, 65
        of pars interarticularis, 57
    in vitro, 207
    life, 86, 90
    muscular, 26
    resistance, 91
    strength, decrease in, 87
    uniaxial, 90
Fat intake, 38
Feedback loop, 185, 186
Female athlete(s)
    with amenorrhea, risk of for stress fracture, 309
    triad, 38, 43
Female chromosomes, 36
Femoral neck stress fractures, 63, 275, 299, 306,
        313
Femoral scintigraphic foci, asymptomatic, 297
Femoral stress fractures, 273, 274, 275, 286, 290,
        292
    in older athletes, 63
    treatment of, 298
Femur, 10
    bone pain in proximal, 273
    paradigm, 140
    supracondylar stress fractures of, 299
    trabecular bone from, 263

Fibula
    paradigm, 140
    stress fracture of, 56
        in children, 56
        in younger athletes, 63
Field training, 8
Figure skating, 2, 10
Fist test, 274, 275
Flurbiprofen, 265
Foot
    alignment, 22
    as common site of stress fracture, 314
    as energy absorbing device, 238
    high arched, 22
    low arched, 25
    planovalgus, 317
    type, 23, 25
Football, 10
Footwear, 22
FOR, see Forefoot angle
Forefoot angle (FOR), 237
Forefoot varus, 24
Fracture(s)
    compression, 306
    Jones, 317
    march, 275
    rapid healing of, 259
    site of, 10
    stress, see Stress fracture
    tension, 306
    treatment protocol, 296
Fully reversed bending, 86
Functional stimuli, 16, 20, 45

G

Gaenslen's sign, 276
Gait, alteration in muscle force during, 251
Gastric ulceration, 265
Gaucher's disease, 111
Gender differences, in bone geometry, 78
Generalizing, 6
Genetic basis for stress fracture, 105–117
    candidate genes, 110–111
    evidence of existence of genetic basis,
        106–109
    relationship between candidate genes and
        stress fractures, 111–112
    risk factors for stress fractures, 105–106
Genetic disorders, 110
Genetics, 27, 36
Genu recurvatum, 23
Genu valgum/varum, 23

Genu varum, 25
Greyhound models, stress fractures in, 221
Ground reaction forces, 22, 26
Gymnastics, 2, 10
Gymnasts, incidence of fatigue fracture in female,
    57

H

Healing, primary, 207
Heel spur syndrome, 276
High arched foot, 22
High arch subjects, 237
Hind foot, semi-rigid varus, 238
Hip rotation/extension, 25
Histological appearance of stress fractures,
        151–159
    evidence for microdamage accumulation
        association with stress fracture,
        154–158
        biopsy of stress fracture, 154–157
        cytokines and bone remodeling at stress
            fracture site, 157
    staining microdamage, 153–154
        bulk stain technique, 153
        types of microdamage, 153–154
Histologic structure, of specimens, 86
Histopathological analysis, of tibial stress fracture
        site, 313
Homeostatic damage control
    failure of, 199
    remodeling and, 198
Home program, of hopping and zigzag hopping,
    255
Hormonal disturbances, 62
Hormonal status, 59
Horse models, stress fractures in, 221
Horses, bucked shins in, 203–219
    classical etiology/pathogenesis, 204–207
    experimental studies to determine
        etiology/pathogenesis, 207–213
    natural history, 203–204
    prevention, 213–216
    synthesis, 216–218
Human stress fracture tissues, 171
Humerus paradigm, 140, 141
Hurdlers, percentage of stress fractures among,
    62
Hydrostatic compression, 99
Hydrostatic tensile stress, 99
Hydroxyapatite crystal, 167
Hydroxyproline, 262
Hysteresis, 87

I

IDF, see Israeli Defense Forces
IGF1, see Insulin-like growth factor 1
Imaging modalities, role of in diagnosing stress
        fractures, 279–293
    bone scintigraphy, 280–290
        appearance of developing and healing
            stress fractures, 286
        asymptomatic stress fractures, 289–290
        classification by image characteristics,
            283–284
        diagnosis of pelvic stress fractures,
            286–287
        diagnosis of stress fractures of foot and
            ankle, 287–289
        soft tissue versus bony lesions, 285–286
    computed tomography, 291
    magnetic resonance imaging, 291
    plain radiographs, 280
Impact attenuation, 20, 25
Impulsive loading, 171, 222
Incidence rates, 6
Independent predictors, 64
Indomethacin, 264, 265
Infantry unit, Israeli, 249
Inflammation, treatment of, 259
Injury(ies)
    association between age and risk of
        developing, 64
    duration of, 3, 5
    ligament, 262
    tendon, 262
Insidious onset, 5
Insoles
    material appropriate for making, 239
    neoprene, 234
    sorbothane polymer, 234
Insufficiency fractures, distinguishing between
        stress or fatigue fractures and, 65
Insulin-like growth factor 1 (IGF1), 110, 111
Interleukin 6 (IL-6), 157
Internal fixation, 313, 317
Intracortical porosity, 172
Intracortical remodeling, 171
In vitro fatigue, 207
In vivo strain data, 210
Ischemia, 273
Israeli Defense Forces (IDF), 107, 111
Israeli infantry
    model, 253
    unit, 249
Israeli recruit populations, 7
Isthmic spondylolysis, 57

J

Joint range of motion, 25
Jones fracture, 317
Jumpers, percentage of stress fractures among, 62

K

Knee flexion/extension, 25

L

Lacrosse, 2, 10
Leg length
    difference, 23, 24
    discrepancy, 25
Leg presses, in vivo tibial strains while
        performing, 252
Ligament injuries, 262
Linear microcracks, 165, 169
Load cycles, 120
Loading
    frequency, 87, 88, 91, 93
    regimen, 22
    repetitive, 260
Load magnitude, 22
Long bones, structural properties of, 59
Long distance runners, 249
    adolescent, 59
    mean age of, 64
Low arched foot, 25
Low arch subjects, 237
Lower extremity alignment, 22
Lumbar vertebrae, fatigue fracture of pars
        interarticularis of, 57
Lumbosacral spine, stress fractures of, 57
Luteal phase cycles, 43

M

Macrofracture, 297
Magnetic resonance imaging (MRI), 280, 291,
        292, 309
Magnitudes, 123
Marathon runners, mean age of, 64
March fractures, 275
Mathematical model, 99, 186
Matrix
    cracking, at sub-lamellar level, 167
    damage, diffuse, 165, 169
MDP, see Methylene disphosphonate

Mean age, as distribution between competitive and recreational athletes, 62
Mean strain, 88
Mechanical environment, 19
Mechanical loading, 20, 21, 22, 45
Mechanical microdamage, 99
Mechanical stimuli, 16, 20
Mechanosensory systems, 19, 45
Mechanostat, 16, 79
Medial tibial stress fractures, 280
Men, risk of stress fracture for, 126
Menarche, 43, 44
    age of, 64
    delayed, 39
Menstrual disturbances, 36, 38, 39
    deleterious effects of, 40
    risk of stress fracture in athletes with, 45
    stress fractures in athletes with, 41
Menstrual status, 47
Metastatic lesion, of bone, 272
Metatarsal(s)
    paradigm, 137
    risk of ballet dancers for stress fracture of, 65
    stress fractures, 56, 138, 275, 287, 292
        in children, 56
        related to vertical forces, 235
        treatment of, 297
Methylene diphosphonate (MDP), 280, 282
Microcracks, 164, 169
Microdamage, 99, 163, 164
    accumulation of, 152
    biological repair of, 152
    repair of bone, 19
    staining, 153
Microfracture, 204, 297
Middle-aged people, participation of in sports, 65
Middle distance runners, adolescent, 59
Military and athletic populations, incidence and prevalence of stress fractures in, 1–14
    incidence, 6–10
        athletic populations, 9–10
        military populations, 6–9
    problems in estimating incidence and prevalence, 2–6
        active versus passive surveillance, 4–5
        case definition, 3
        duration of injury, 5
        estimating population base, 3–4
        individual risk variation, 5
        study design, 5–6
Military boots, 234, 236
Military populations, motivated, 4
Military recruits, 2, 6, 59

basic training period of, 59
body size as risk factor in, 27
risk of for stress fracture, 309
Military training, adolescents engaged in basic, 55
Miner's rule, 99
Misclassification bias, 4
Modulus reduction, 93, 163
Motivation, 28
MRI, see Magnetic resonance imaging
Multiple sites, 3
Multivariate analysis, 56, 62
Muscle
    conditioning, 135, 136
    contraction, 132, 133
    cross-sectional area, 79
    fatigue, 26, 79, 124, 133, 136, 138, 140
    flexibility, 25
    force(s)
        alteration in during gait, 251
        repetitive, 142
    size, 26
    strength, 26
Muscular force and fatigue, role of in stress fractures, 131–149
    mechanics of muscular contraction, 132–133
    molecular mechanisms of muscular contraction and fatigue, 133
    muscular fatigue and stress fractures, 134–140
        muscular force in musculoskeletal energy absorption, 134–135
        relationship between muscular conditioning and stress fractures, 135–136
        relationship between muscular fatigue, bone strain, and stress fractures, 136–140
    muscular force and stress fractures, 140–144
        femur paradigm, 140–141
        fibular paradigm, 140
        humerus paradigm, 141
        patella paradigm, 141
        rib paradigm, 142–144
        tibia paradigm, 141
        ulna paradigm, 142
Musculotendinous injury, 273
Mutation, within gene involved in bone formation, 107

N

Neoprene insoles, 234
Neutral subtalar position, 239
Non-military athletic populations, 2

Nonsteroidal anti-inflammatory drugs (NSAIDS),
    264, 265
Nonunion
    in foot, 314
    of femoral head, 313
    rate, for fifth metatarsal stress fractures, 317
NSAIDS, see Nonsteroidal anti-inflammatory
    drugs
N-telopeptides of type 1 collagen, 20
Nutrition, 27, 28, 62, 259

O

OC, see Osteocalcin
OCP, see Oral contraceptive pill
Officer
    cadets, U.S. Army officer, 8
    candidate program, 8
    training, 6
25 OH-vitamin D, 27
Older people, participation of in sports, 65
Older runners, stress fractures of femoral neck in,
    63
Oligomenorrhea, 39, 40
Open reduction and internal fixation (ORIF), 313
Operational populations, 6, 8
Oral contraceptive pill (OCP), 36, 44, 45
ORIF, see Open reduction and internal fixation
Orthotics, 22, 239
Ossification, cartilage, 99
Osteoblasts, 168
Osteocalcin (OC), 20, 157, 302
Osteoclasts, 168, 169, 264
Osteocytes, 168, 170
Osteogenic sarcoma, 272
Osteogenic stimulus, 98
Osteon, 168
Osteonecrosis, of femoral head, 313
Osteopenia, 38, 162
Osteoporosis, 17, 174, 263, 309
Osteotomy, 264
Outpatient
    encounters, database of, 8
    problems, 4
    records, 6
Overuse injuries, of adolescent athletes, 59

P

Pain
    exercise-induced, 10
    treatment of, 259
Pamidronate, 263

Parathyroid hormone (PTH), 27, 265, 266
Pars interarticularis
    of lumbar vertebrae, fatigue fracture of, 57
    stress fractures of in children, 56
Passive methods, 5
Passive surveillance, 2, 4, 7
Patella paradigm, 141
Pathologic fracture, 2, 8
Pathologic sites, 3
Peak incidence, definition of, 120
Pelvic stress fractures, 56, 276
PEMF, see Pulsed electromagnetic fields
Periosteal expansion, 200
Periosteal inflammation, 265
Periosteal modeling, 195
Periosteal response, 195, 199
Periosteal woven bone, 260
Periostitis, 2, 272, 273
Peripheral quantitative (pQCT) scanners, 80
Person-time, 4, 7
Pharmaceutical treatments, prevention or delay of
        onset of stress fractures by, 259–270
    potential pharmaceutical therapies to enhance
        healing of stress fractures, 265–266
    potential pharmaceutical treatments to prevent
        stress fracture, 262–265
        bisphosphonates, 262–264
        indomethacin and NSAIDS, 264–265
Pharmacological stimuli, 16, 20
Phosphorus, 28
Physical activity, high risk recruits with low levels
        of prior, 21
Physical diagnosis of stress fractures, 271–278
    awareness, 277
    calcaneal stress fractures, 276
    femoral stress fractures, 273–275
    metatarsal stress fractures, 275–276
    navicular stress fractures, 276
    pelvic stress fractures, 276–277
    stress fracture history, 272–273
    tibial stress fractures, 273
Physical examination, stress fracture, 275, 296
Physical fitness, 21
    poor, 253
    scores, 254
Physical intensity, 8
Physical rigor, 6
Physical stressor,
Physiological stimuli, 16, 20
Piezo-electric properties, 98
Pin firing, 204
Plain radiographs, 279, 286, 287
    bipartite sesamoids identified by, 288
    sensitivity of, 280
Planovalgus foot, 317

Plantar fascitis, 276
Plantar foot pressures, 238
Plastazote®, 239
Plaster of Paris, 239
Pneumatic brace, 312
Polymethylmethacrylate, 121
Population(s)
    at risk, 4
    base, 2, 4, 6
    impact of stress fracture on, 5
    Israeli recruit, 7
Porosity, 162, 191
Positive feedback, 162
    loop, 174
    mechanism, stress fracture occurring as, 177
Post-yield deformation, 167
pQCT scanners, see Peripheral quantitative
        scanners
Predicted fatigue life to failure, of compact bone,
        162
Prediction of stress fractures, 73–83
    bone mineral density and stress fracture,
        74–75
    future of, 81–82
    reason some bones weaker than others, 75–79
        bone geometry, 75–79
        measuring muscle, 79
    stress fracture prediction, 80–81
        technical difficulties in measurement of
            bone and muscle properties, 80–81
        where to measure, 81
Predisposing factors, for stress fracture, 106
Prevention techniques, use of in military
        populations, 65
Primary bone, 87
Primary healing, 207
Principal strains, 123
Problematic stress fractures, 305–319
    biomechanics, 306–307
    diagnosis, 307–309
        history and physical exam, 307–309
        radiographic examination, 309
    treatment, 310–317
        femoral neck stress fractures, 313
        fifth metatarsal stress fractures, 317
        general treatment principles, 310
        tarsal navicular stress fractures, 314–316
        tibial stress fractures, 311–313
Procollagen type 1, 110
Progesterone, 43
Pronation, 25
Prospective cohort designs, 6, 7
Prospective studies, 10
Prostaglandin synthesis, 264
Prosthetic replacement, 313

Protein, 28
Psychological traits, 27, 28, 36
PTH, see Parathyroid hormone
Pulsed electromagnetic fields (PEMF), 312, 313
Putative genes, 107
Pyridinium cross-links, 20

Q

Q angle, 23, 25, 39

R

Rabbit impulsive loading model, 260
Rabbits, as animal model for stress fractures,
        221–232
    excessive jumping model, 229–230
        advantages of excessive jumping model,
            229–230
        limitations of excessive jumping model, 230
    impulsive loading model, 222–229
        advantages of impulsive loading model,
            226–228
        limitations of impulsive loading model,
            228–229
Racehorse(s), 126, 127
    with stress fracture, 171
    Thoroughbred, 203
Racket sports, 10
Radiation exposure, of bone scintigraphy, 301
Radiograph(s), 3, 276, 277, see also Plain
        radiographs
    false-negative, 280
    limitation of, 280
Radionuclide, 3
Range of motion, joint, 25
RAP, see Regional acceleratory phenomenon
Reamed intramedullary nailing, 313
Rearfoot inversion/eversion, 25
Rearfoot valgus, 24
Recreational runners, 9, 64
Recruits, high risk, 254
Recurvatum, 25
Refracture, of femoral head, 313
Regional acceleratory phenomenon (RAP), 264
Rehabilitation, 5
Remodeling, 177
    activity, 154, 157
    homeostatic damage control and, 198
    response, 261
    space, 185, 266
    specificity factor, 189
    suppression, 263, 264

Repetitive loading, 260
Resorption, 169, 261
    depth, 262
    space, 162, 168
Rib paradigm, 142
Risk factors, for developing stress fractures,
        15–33
    constraints, 27–28
        nutrition, 28
        psychological traits, 28
    controller, 19–20
    functional stimuli, 20–27
        mechanical, 20–27
        physiological, 27
    measurable bone components, 17–19
        bone density, 17
        bone geometry, 17–19
Rotating bending, 87
Rotating cantilevers, 86
Runners, 9
    adolescent, 59
    collegiate female, 9
    percentage of stress fractures among, 62
    prospective studies of, 9
    recreational, 64
    ultramarathon, 261
Running, 10, 124
    health benefits of, 9
    injuries, 9
    long distance, 249
    strain rates during, 251

                    S

Sacroiliac joint, 276, 277
Salt, 28
Sampling, 6
Scanning acoustic microscope, 265
Scintigraphy, 4
    abnormalities, 272
    foci, 248
    grading system, 301
SEALS, U.S. Navy, 8
Secant modulus, 93
Secondary bone, 87
Section modulus, 75
Self-report, 6
Set points, genetically defined, 45
Sex hormones, 20, 27, 39
Shear
    loading, 99
    strains, 123, 251
    stress, 99

Shin splints, 273, 286
Shock
    attenuation, of basketball shoes, 234
    wave, heel strike, 234
Shoe(s)
    effects related to, 233
    last, 233, 236
    shock absorbing properties of, 234
Shoe wear, prevention of stress fractures by
        modifying, 233–245
    arch height and stress fractures, 237–239
    custom-made orthotics, 239–243
    heel strike shock wave and stress fractures,
        234–236
    shoe fit and shoe last effects, 236
Sine's method, 99
Skeletal adaptation, 98
Skeletal alignment, 23, 24, 39
Skeletal loading, 75
S-N curve, 86
Soccer, 2, 10
Somatotype, athlete, 26
Sorbothane polymer insoles, 234
Sports
    adolescents engaged in, 55
    associated with pars interarticularis stress
        fracture, 59
    ball, 249
    participation of children and adolescents in
        organized, 65
Statistical methods, 61
Stepmaster, *in vivo* tibial strains while using,
        252
Stiffness, 87
Strain(s), 119, 132, 134, 162, 163
    age difference in, 126
    data, *in vivo*, 210
    error distribution hypothesis, 251
    gage, 121
    histories, 99
    in vivo, 250
    magnitudes, high, 123
    maximum, 121
    principal, 121
    range, 88, 89, 96
    rates, occurring during basketball, 250
Strain and strain rates, role of in stress fractures,
        119–129
    ex vivo studies, 120
    in vivo studies, 120–126
        role of muscle fatigue on strain and strain
            rates, 124–126
        strains and strain rate in human metatarsal,
            124